Robotics in Physical Medicine and Rehabilitation

AF754169

Robotics in Physical Medicine and Rehabilitation

DOUGLAS P. MURPHY, MD
RAC Medical Director
Central Virginia Veterans Health Center
Richmond, VA

ELSEVIER

Elsevier
1600 John F. Kennedy Blvd.
Ste 1800
Philadelphia, PA 19103-2899

ROBOTICS IN PHYSICAL MEDICINE AND REHABILITATION

ISBN: 978-0-323-87865-4

Copyright © 2025 by Elsevier Inc. All rights reserved.

No part of this publication may be reproduced or transmitted in any form or by any means, electronic or mechanical, including photocopying, recording, or any information storage and retrieval system, without permission in writing from the publisher. Details on how to seek permission, further information about the publisher's permissions policies and our arrangements with organizations such as the Copyright Clearance Center and the Copyright Licensing Agency, can be found at our website: www.elsevier.com/permissions.

This book and the individual contributions contained in it are protected under copyright by the publisher (other than as may be noted herein).

Notice

Practitioners and researchers must always rely on their own experience and knowledge in evaluating and using any information, methods, compounds, or experiments described herein. Because of rapid advances in the medical sciences, in particular, independent verification of diagnoses and drug dosages should be made. To the fullest extent of the law, no responsibility is assumed by Elsevier, authors, editors, or contributors for any injury and/or damage to persons or property as a matter of products liability, negligence or otherwise, or from any use or operation of any methods, products, instructions, or ideas contained in the material herein.

Content Strategist: Humayra R. Khan
Senior Content Development Specialist: Akanksha Marwah
Publishing Services Manager: Shereen Jameel
Project Manager: Nandhini Thanga Alagu
Design Direction: Margaret M. Reid

Printed in India
Last digit is the print number: 9 8 7 6 5 4 3 2 1

Working together to grow libraries in developing countries
www.elsevier.com • www.bookaid.org

To The Lawrenceville School- in gratitude for excellence in teaching.

LIST OF CONTRIBUTORS

Blessen C. Eapen, MD
Chief
Physical Medicine and Rehabilitation Service
VA Greater Los Angeles Healthcare System
Associate Professor
Department of Medicine
Division of Physical Medicine and Rehabilitation
University of California, Los Angeles (UCLA)
Los Angeles, California
United States

Sara Flores, MD
Associate Professor
Department of Medicine
University of California, Los Angeles (UCLA)
Los Angeles, California
United States

Riya Fukui, MD
Resident Physician
Physical Medicine and Rehabilitation
The University of Texas Health Science Center at Houston
Houston, Texas
United States

Ashraf S. Gorgey, MPT, PhD, FACSM, FACRM
Director of SCI Research
Spinal Cord Injury Service and Disorders
Richmond VA Medical Center
Professor
Physical Medicine and Rehabilitation
Virginia Commonwealth University
Richmond, Virginia
United States

Andrew Hanna, DO
Medical Director and CEO–Axios Medical Group
Interventional Pain Medicine Physician
Physical Medicine and Rehabilitation
Manhattan Beach, California
United States

John Hermansen, MD
Medical Director
Polytrauma Rehabilitation Center
Central Virginia Veterans Healthcare System
Richmond, Virginia
United States

Hope Jervis-Rademeyer, MPT, PhD
Postdoctoral Fellow
Medicine
University of Alberta
Edmonton, Alberta
Canada

M. Rehan Khan, MD
Staff Radiologist
Radiology
VAMC Richmond
Professor of Radiology
Radiology
Virginia Commonwealth University
Richmond, Virginia
United States

Dean J. Krusienski, PhD
Professor
Biomedical Engineering
Virginia Commonwealth University
Richmond, Virginia
United States

Denise D. Lester, MD
Director, Peripheral Nerve Stimulation Implant Program
Interventional Pain Clinic
Central Virginia Veterans Healthcare System
Richmond, Virginia
United States

William Lovegreen, MS, CPO
Prosthetist-Orthotist Regional Clinical Director
Physical Medicine and Rehabilitation
Veterans Administration
Richmond, Virginia
United States

Douglas P. Murphy, MD
Associate Professor of PM&R
PM&R
VCU College of Medicine
Regional Amputation Center Medical Director
PM&R
Central Virginia Veterans Health Care Center
Richmond, Virginia
United States

Kenichiro Ono, DO
Neurologist
Neurology
VA Central Virginia Healthcare System
VCU Health
Richmond, Virginia
United States

Kavya Pramod Puthuveetil, BS
PhD Student
Robotics Institute
Carnegie Mellon University
Pittsburgh, Pennsylvania
United States

Robert Trainer, DO, MBA, FASAM
Staff Interventional Pain Physician
Central Virginia VA Healthcare System
Richmond, Virginia
United States

Grace Zhang, MD
Doctor of Medicine
Physical Medicine and Rehabilitation
VA Greater Los Angeles
Los Angeles, California
United States

FOREWORD

Robots, real and imagined, have been a part of human civilization for millennia and have had roles ranging from workers to protectors to companions. Although the 500-year-old sketches of humanoid robots by Leonardo da Vinci are best known to Americans and contributed to the naming of the popular DaVinci surgical robot, designs for these automata have pervaded the work of early Egyptian, Muslim, Japanese, Greek, Chinese, and many other cultures. The use in health care of machines that can be programmed to perform a specified set of simple or complex tasks, with or without human assistance, formally began in the 1980s and has increased dramatically. Although many of these devices perform mundane, repetitive tasks such as sterilizing operating rooms or securely delivering medications in a hospital, others are straining the boundaries of belief by fostering safe gait and providing environmental control. This groundbreaking textbook by Dr. Douglas P. Murphy and his team of innovative clinicians and researchers brings together cutting-edge information on a dazzling array of common and novel robots and robotic applications across health care. While never losing sight of the practical application of automated machines and programs and the importance of preserving the very human side of medicine, this book can also serve as a resource for their roles and potential uses in the health care of tomorrow. In this 21st-century guide, you can learn about some of the everyday uses of robots across many areas of health care, from operating rooms to radiology suites to rehabilitation gyms. As you turn the pages, you will also be able to read about some of the 22nd-century applications that are being tested across the human-machine interface, from brain-controlled prosthetics to computer-guided artificial intelligence data processing to autonomous battlefield medical drones. Truly, this is a work that will function as a manual for many of the everyday uses of robots in health care today, while serving to lay the foundations that allow you to imagine and visualize the potential for the automation of tomorrow. I encourage you to use this guide to allow you to explore the past, get to know the present, and dream of the future of robots in medicine.

David X. Cifu, MD
Associate Dean of Innovation and System Integration
Herman J. Flax, MD Professor and Chair, Department of Physical Medicine and Rehabilitation
Virginia Commonwealth University School of Medicine
Rehabilitation Consultant, the Sheltering Arms Institute
Senior TBI Specialist, US Department of Veterans Affairs
Richmond, Virginia

PREFACE

The world of robotics and artificial intelligence (AI) inspires a range of emotions in most people that extends from fascination and great hopes to fear and uncertainty. Currently the field is undergoing such rapid development and progress that it is emerging into virtually all sectors of our culture. Perhaps medicine is one of the sectors that is gathering the most benefit and thus undergoing the most changes. Are robots relegated to relieving humans of the most repetitive and tedious of chores in the medical setting? Hardly. Robots and AI are addressing the most challenging and demanding areas such as diagnosis, surgery, and research.

If you were to break down the entire infrastructure of this service industry from administration to billing to hospital supplies to pharmacy to the actual care of patients, robots can be seen assisting human workers to make processes faster, more efficient, more cost-effective, more accurate, and safer. Are robots outperforming their human counterparts? In some ways perhaps they are. An alternative way of viewing their role is that they allow human workers to perform those interventions and tasks that require skills that are irreplaceable, that robots cannot perform, and for which robots and AI will have no counterpart within their programs and intelligence systems.

However, that is not to say that robots will not try and perhaps come close. There are emotional support robots that can ease the anxiety of patients underdoing tests and treatments. There are robots than can add to the hospitable, friendly, and helpful approach of a hospital.

Robots can perform surgeries and can perform certain surgeries independently. They cannot do this without a human programing human knowledge and skill into the apparatus of a surgical robot. Additionally, surgical robots perhaps perform optimally as facilitators of human surgeons, adding elements of precision and control that were previously unattainable.

So where is all of this leading us?

In a way we do not really know. This book will illuminate the current panorama of robotic options and attempt to project this into the future. However, since the ability to self-develop is being built into robotic programs and AI and since this is a brand-new vista, the distant destinations of this technology cannot be completely anticipated. Such a future brings great hope but also great responsibility. Humans must guide and control this process so that this technology provides the optimum service to humanity.

Open the door and take a look. These mechanical friends await you to bring a new vision of medicine previously unanticipated but stunning in its scope and capacity.

ACKNOWLEDGMENT

Chris Kapogiannis

CONTENTS

1

Introduction—The Growing Role of Robotics in Health Care

Sara Flores ■ Andrew Hanna ■ Grace Zhang ■ Blessen C. Eapen

KEY POINTS

- Robotics is taking an increasingly larger role in the delivery of health care.
- The field supports all phases of medicine from acute care to rehabilitation.
- This technology is making battlefield medicine safer and more efficient.
- This industry is growing and changing the economics of health care.
- With the advent of artificial intelligence and other advancements, robots can offer increasingly more sophisticated capabilities for direct patient care and for health systems infrastructure.

The advancement of technology has grown exponentially in the commercial and public sectors over the last several decades, with health care being no exception. Robotics, in particular, serves as a pivotal tool in improving the delivery of high-quality, personalized health care in the realm of battlefield medicine, rehabilitation therapy, and functional assistance using exoskeletons and orthoses.

Robot-assisted rehabilitation can complement conventional therapy methods by increasing the amount of time patients can participate in therapeutic exercises, reducing burden on therapists, improving secondary health conditions, and personalizing the recovery process.[1] The MIT Manu, one of the first robotic devices designed for neurorehabilitation, was shown to improve overall function in the upper extremity following stroke by guiding patients to trace patterns on a screen with an end-effector device.[2] Since then, several functional robotic devices for upper and lower extremity training have been introduced to the market, which similarly work through guided facilitation of movement and sensorimotor functional training. These include, but are not limited to, wearable exoskeletons, grounded exoskeletons, and end-effector devices.[3] Robotics supports repetitive exercises for motor relearning, which encourages plasticity while also reducing therapist burden, and these machines may be a useful tool in telerehabilitation for patients who cannot access traditional rehabilitation facilities. In a study following patients with spinal cord injury of C5 or lower, the use of a lower extremity exoskeleton was shown to reduce spasticity, as measured by patients' own subjective reports as well as the Modified Ashworth Scale.[4] Furthermore, use of the Indego exoskeleton, which was comprised of hip, knee, and bilateral ankle-foot orthoses units, decreased patients' Borg Scale of Perceived Exertion while walking indoors.[4]

In this chapter, we will explore how the growing field of robotics in rehabilitation has affected both practitioners and patients, examine its role in acute and battlefield medicine, as well as take a look at the major leaders in the industry and future developments in the area, including artificial intelligence.

How Robotics Will Affect the Practice of Medicine for Practitioners

The use of robotics serves as a complementary tool to traditional therapy methods, the delivery of which is often limited by time, cost, and availability of staff. For example, early mobilization has been widely accepted as a method for improving outcomes and functional mobility for critically ill patients in the intensive care unit.[5] In a study examining mild patients with to moderate intracranial hemorrhage, early out-of-bed mobilization was seen to be beneficial in improving functional independence measure motor scores and reducing length of stay in the stroke center compared with those patients who received only in-bed rehabilitation.[6] Unfortunately, mobilizing every patient may not be possible due to lack of trained personnel. Robotics such as exoskeleton-assisted walking devices can help assist with this often-difficult task. Studies have shown that exoskeletons can contribute to significant health benefits, such as cardiovascular health, bowel function, bone health, and quality of life, by aiding patients with spinal cord injury with early mobilization.[1]

Although acute rehabilitation can offer patients in-person therapy 3 hours a day, patients often spend the rest of the day inactive, despite being encouraged to continue self-directed exercises taught by their therapists. Robotics may serve as a useful adjuvant to in-person therapy by encouraging additional mobility and may even be utilized to increase therapy time in group settings through robotic-assisted group training.[7] In doing so, robotics can improve provider productivity and decrease delays to initiation of rehabilitation. Studies have shown in poststroke populations, robotic-assisted therapy is comparable in improving upper limb functional outcomes to conventional therapy.[8] In a study of patients after stroke, robotic therapy reduced upper limb impairment in patients with both chronic and subacute stroke, with evidence of improvement in several kinematic parameters, including speed.[9] Additionally, robotics can help practitioners monitor improvement during therapy by collecting data throughout recovery. Information such as progress with range of motion, precision, accuracy, and kinematic data across multiple joints can be useful with adjusting the intensity and focus of therapy.[10]

Telerehabilitation is a growing field, especially in the era of the SARS-CoV-2 pandemic, where compliance with in-person therapy may not be feasible or safe. Faced with the challenge of providing accessible care, practitioners are looking for ways to augment traditional routes for delivery of care. Robotics can increase access to therapy for patients in remote areas with limited resources, while also increasing overall therapy time. Specifically, home-based rehabilitation with the use of end effectors, and exoskeletons can be utilized for highly repetitive exercises while also giving the patient a sense of control over their rehabilitation progress in a remotely supervised setting.[11] Robotic upper limb rehabilitation devices designed for in-home use have been shown to be similar in usability and performance compared with their commercial counterparts.[12] In a study of rural veterans following unilateral or ischemic stroke, the use of in-home robotic rehabilitation devices, in conjunction with remote monitoring by a therapist, resulted in an overall increase in upper and lower extremity mobility, as well as perceived independence.[13] In the maintenance step of therapy, commercial gaming systems such as Nintendo and PlayStation have been utilized to encourage continued activity and self-directed therapy.[10]

Overall, robotics can complement conventional therapy by standardizing training environments, increasing access to care, and reducing burden on therapists.

How Robotics Will Affect the Experience of Health Care for Patients

In the field of rehabilitation, robotics plays a significant role in neurorehabilitation, functional training, and assistive technology. For patients undergoing rehabilitation, these technological advancements have the potential to not only improve functional outcomes but also provide social and psychological benefits as well.

The incorporation of biorobotics in the field of prosthetics assists patients in experiencing a more natural setting with the use of sensory integration and feedback. Incorporating visual, auditory, and tactile feedback improves user experience through an engaging and stimulating process. The use of biofeedback provides a method through which patients can decrease compensatory movements and work on spatial, cognitive, and visual integrative skills training. Furthermore, the utilization of sensors to monitor position and movement, and respond in real time, aims to mimic a realistic environment. Robotic training can enhance kinematics and improve function through the use of exoskeletons and robotic end effectors. Several studies have shown that utilization of robotic rehabilitation devices can enhance motor outcome after stroke through biofeedback and repetitive task training.[14]

The incorporation of virtual reality and augmented reality in rehabilitation training can also complement traditional therapy. In fact, utilizing a gaming interface may be highly motivational and encourage patients to participate in therapy to improve fine movements to aid in activities of daily living. Robotics are ideal for consistent, repetitive motion training and functional exercises during intensive therapy following central nervous system (CNS) damage, while also being engaging for the patient. Studies have shown that augmentation of therapy with robotics may give patients a sense of control over their progress, thereby improving their sense of independence and mood.[13] Neuromodulation, vibration, and continuous passive motion may be passive modalities that can address spasticity and improve range of motion.

Brain-computer interfaces are an emerging technology with the capability of amplifying and translating brain signals to produce a desired outcome on an external device.[15] Several studies have shown the effectiveness of brain-computer interfaces in motor retraining for CNS injuries, by aiding neuroplasticity and bypassing damaged tissue. With this technology, electrodes can be placed over the cortex to record neural signals, which are then converted to a prosthetic output. In other cases, intracranial implants transmit electroencephalographic signals to external devices.[16] Neurostimulation and cortical activation in both sensory and motor pathways using neuroprosthetics provide a promising future for modulating neuroplasticity. The continuing development of neuroprosthetics will hopefully serve as a tool for patients with neurologic disorders to regain previously lost function.

The Growing Industry of Robotics—Taking a Look at Some of the Major Companies

THERAPY ROBOTS

Bionik, the developer of InMotion Arm therapy, has been used in the inpatient setting for several years to improve range of motion, strength, speed, and coordination in the upper arm following stroke and other CNS injuries. Furthermore, this tool can be used to decrease spasticity by activating muscles that otherwise would not be used. According to the developer, patients can achieve a minimum of 600 movements per hour with the assistance of the InMotion arm device. With the success of the inpatient model, Bionik is in the process of developing an in-home device.[17]

Ekso Bionics, pioneers in wearable exoskeletons, has been creating robotics to help with gait training in patients with limited lower extremity mobility or paralysis. EksoGT and EksoNR exoskeletons can allow previously nonambulatory patients to stand and walk and are approved by the Food and Drug Administration for gait training in patients with strokes, traumatic brain injuries, and spinal cord injuries. The company has several products, ranging from load carriers to SmartAssist software for pregait training.[18] A unique feature of this device is its ability to adjust power to either side of the body, thereby making it easier or more difficult for the patient to move the limb.

Hocoma, a rehabilitation technology company out of Switzerland, has added several wearable exoskeletons to the market as well, including its products Erigo, Lokomat, and Andago. These devices aid with early mobilization by improving muscle strength and joint range of motion. Erigo allows for bedbound patients to be slowly verticalized, while simultaneously performing cyclical leg movements with functional electrical stimulation at the lower limb. Small studies have shown this device to be a safe, useful tool for early sensorimotor rehabilitation and vestibular rehabilitation in patients after stroke.[19]

AUGMENTED FEEDBACK

Hocoma also has delved into the realm of augmented feedback therapy with its product Valedo, a wearable sensor. Placed on various points on the low back, the device claims to reduce low back pain by encouraging range of motion, lumbar stabilization, and general movement therapy. The device provides real-time feedback in an encouraging and motivating setting, which has been shown in small studies to be similar to conventional exercise led by physical therapists in terms of adherence, improvement in disability, and movement control.[20]

PROSTHETICS

Össur Touch Solutions, formerly known as Touch Bionics, is a world leader in prosthetic technologies, manufacturing prosthetics for upper and lower limb amputees. Its products range widely from multiaxial, myoelectric, microprocessor, and high-performance carbon prostheses for amputees of all activity levels. The company manufactures knees, feet, legs, and hands, as well as liners, sockets, and bracing.[21]

Robots in Acute Medicine

Robots in medicine can fulfill a wide range of functions to assist doctors, nurses, and other medical staff and to enhance the delivery of care. Hospital robots can distribute medications and laboratory specimens around the hospital. Pharmacy robots can process, return, and restock medications, helping to reduce costs and errors in hospitals. Robotic systems are also being designed to disinfect devices and equipment in health-care settings.[22]

Aethon has developed a robot, TUG, made specifically for hospitals. It uses a built-in map and sensors to navigate hospital halls and communicates with elevators, fire alarms, and automatic doors via Wi-Fi. TUG can deliver medicine, meals, and supplies through the hospital and to hospital units.[23] It also uses biometric security and pin codes to transport lab specimens safely.[24]

There are three main types of robots currently in use in the surgical field—active, semi-active, and master-slave systems. Active systems work autonomously, while remaining under the control of the surgeon, and undertake preprogrammed tasks. Semi-active systems allow for a surgeon-driven element to complement the preprogrammed element of these robot systems. Master-slave systems (of which the da Vinci and ZEUS platforms were forerunners) lack any of the preprogrammed or autonomous elements of the other systems. They are entirely dependent on surgeon activity. Surgeon hand movements are transmitted to laparoscopic surgical instruments, which reproduce surgeon hand activity inside the patient's body.[25]

Some of the most used medical robots are artificial intelligence–assisted surgical robots, which can analyze data from preoperative medical records to physically guide a surgeon's instrument in real time during a procedure. Such surgical robots are used in neurologic, orthopedic, and laparoscopic procedures, being operated both locally and remotely.[26] Robot-assisted operations are often minimally invasive, offering an alternative to open surgeries, which have more associated risks and require a longer period of recovery.[27]

HOW ROBOTS CAN SERVE IN BATTLEFIELD MEDICINE

Approximately 86% of all battlefield deaths occur within the first 30 minutes after injury. Therefore, the ability to rapidly locate, diagnose, and provide appropriate initial treatments are vital to improving the historical outcomes of battlefield injuries. Before attending to the injured, frontline medics must quickly locate the soldier and extract him or her from the battlefield, often under fire. This can take up costly minutes, as well as expose medics as targets.[28]

Military robotic combat casualty care has three main goals: safely extracting the injured soldier from harm's way, rapidly diagnosing life-threatening injuries, and delivering lifesaving interventions. In the short term, extraction robots will decrease the risk to the soldier and combat medic by safely moving wounded war fighters out of the line of fire. In the longer term, teleoperated and autonomous surgical robots will deliver surgical care on the battlefield as well as during transport to military treatment facilities.[29]

The US military recognized the potential of stationing trauma surgeons remotely, allowing them to tend to the wounded via a robotic platform. This would allow for a timely response while reducing mortality and morbidity of service personnel on the battlefield.[25]

Therefore, the US Department of Defense funded the development of unmanned medical treatment systems for the battlefield.[30] The goal of these "Trauma Pods" was to stabilize injured soldiers within minutes after a battlefield trauma. The trauma pod could assist a surgeon in administering lifesaving medical and surgical care prior to evacuation, as well as during transport. With the help of the trauma pod, a surgeon could conduct all the required surgical procedures from a remote location using a system of surgical manipulators. The system's actions could then be communicated wirelessly to the surgery site. Automated robotic systems would provide necessary support to the surgeon to conduct all phases of the operation. The Trauma Pod system also included x-ray capabilities for fluoroscopic guidance, if needed, for interventions.[30] The trauma pod system was successfully teleoperated by a surgeon to perform a bowel anastomosis and an iliac artery shunt placement on a phantom patient with no human assistance.[30] However, Trauma Pod never moved into final animal trials, which would have included control of hemorrhage as well as airway and intravenous line insertion, due to a command transition and funding issues from federal budgeting processes.[31]

Telecommunication and robotic limitations that restrict robust intervention at a distance are areas of continued military research and development. As these limitations are overcome, medical robots will provide robust casualty extraction and battlefield care that will save the lives and limbs of our soldiers.[29]

The Defense Advanced Research Projects Agency, or DARPA, founded a prosthetics program in 2006 for Wounded Warrior amputees and military personnel with spinal cord injury. These programs have funded the ongoing research and development of neuroprosthetic technology, such as the LUKE arm, a highly advanced bionic arm with the capability of mimicking dexterous upper limb movements. The LUKE arm is a multi-articulated prosthesis controlled by multiple input devices, including surface electromyography electrodes and wireless foot controls. Furthermore, it is the only commercially available prosthesis with a powered shoulder in addition to 10 other powered joints, with the capability of refining highly specific movements and regulating pressure and sensation.[4,16]

ARTIFICIAL INTELLIGENCE AND ROBOTICS (AND BRAIN-COMPUTER INTERFACE)

Many patients who are seen for rehabilitation have undergone functional changes that require adaptation. The most common example of functional change is seen with patients after stroke who suffer from hemiparesis, dysphagia, and/or aphasia. In addition to medication management, therapy is used to treat and assist patients in adapting to their new physiologic changes.

Artificial intelligence is used to collect and interpret data, then subsequently deliver a unique and tailored response through a robot. An example of this is Google's Street View, which took billions of pictures of cars, and based on the types of cars within communities, were able to determine the community's income, race, education, and political affiliations.[32,33]

In rehabilitation, artificial intelligence and robotics are used in the form of exoskeletons, prosthetics, social robotics, and smart environments.[33,34] An applicable example of artificial intelligence and robotics with use of a brain computer interface is the National Aeronautics and Space Administration's X1 powered lower limb exoskeleton. The X1 was introduced as a potential therapeutic tool for the leading cause of neurologic disability, stroke.[34] The X1 uses electroencephalogram (EEG), electromyogram, and goniometers to establish a brain computer interface.[34] Decoding of the goniometers, electromyograms, and EEGs allowed the exoskeleton to reconstruct gait kinematics of the hip and knee joints in the hemiparetic patient.[34]

Brain-computer interfaces have also been used to control robotic and prosthetic arms.[35] The brain-computer interface records neural activity through an EEG or electrocorticography, decodes the neural activity through a computer, and finally sends these decoded commands to a robot to perform an action.[35] Of note, EEGs are placed on the external surface of the cranium leading to limited topographical resolution and frequency range, whereas electrocorticographs are placed on the cortical surfaces of the brain allowing for better topographical resolution and improved accuracy.[36]

THE ECONOMICS OF THE ROBOTIC INDUSTRY

The robotic industry continues to grow and integrate within our health-care system. Robotics can assist with diagnosis, prognosis, and treatment in rehabilitation by analyzing and interpreting live data to assist with rehabilitative therapy. [37] In rehabilitation, we see the use of robotics to address therapy for postneurologic deficits such as hemiparesis, amputees with prostheses, and gait dysfunction. These advancements come at a premium cost. Examples of rehabilitation robots are therapeutic robots, assistive robots, exoskeleton robots, and prosthetic robots. A study performed by McCabe et al., which focused on comparing robotics and functional electrical stimulation and motor learning in patients with upper extremity dysfunction poststroke, noted that the cost of using robotics with motor learning was significantly more expensive when compared with functional electrical stimulation plus motor learning or motor learning alone. There was also no difference in treatment response across the different interventions.[38]

In contrast, the US Department of Veterans Affairs' Robotics Study analyzed the economics of robot-assisted therapy for long-term upper limb impairment after stroke and found at 36 weeks there was no significant differences between the intensive therapy group, robot-assisted therapy group, and usual care group.[39] Thirty-six-week averages were $12,364 for the intensive therapy group, which included 50 individuals; $12,679 for the robot-assisted group, which included 49 individuals; and $19,098 for the usual care group, which included 19 individuals.[39] Due to the number of individuals in the usual care group, the 36-week average was skewed.[39] The study ultimately concluded that the robot-assisted therapy group used less Veterans Affairs care and had a lower average cost when compared with the intensive therapy group.[39]

The global medical robots market is projected to reach $25.4 billion by 2028 from $ 9.2 billion in 2022.[40] This market includes therapeutic, surgical, rehabilitation, and hospital automated robots.[40] It is expected to grow at a compound annual growth rate of 18.5% from 2022 to 2028.[40]

ROBOTS OF THE FUTURE

Many ideas regarding the future of robotics are currently in development. One idea theorizes that surgically placed electrodes within the brain could allow for neural spikes to be interpreted almost immediately. This would allow for accurate recording of neural activity, which could result in improved decoding and robotic output. There is also plenty of room for growth within the realm of brain-computer interfaces.[36] The future of brain-computer interfaces will focus on improving function, reliability, safety, and convenience.[36] Those who have lost the ability to control their neuromusculoskeletal system, such as patients with spinal cord injuries, amyotrophic lateral sclerosis, or locked-in syndrome, will be able to control a neuro-prosthesis with their brain waves.[41] Instead of only decoding brain signals, future brain-machine interfaces will also be able to induce a signal back to the brain, allowing for CNS neuroplasticity to restore motor function.[36,41]

References

1. Mekki M, Delgado AD, Fry A, Putrino D, Huang V. Robotic rehabilitation and spinal cord injury: a narrative review. *Neurotherapeutics*. 2018;15(3):604–617.
2. Hogan N, Krebs HI, Charnnarong J, Srikrishna P, Sharon A. MIT-MANUS: a workstation for manual therapy and training. I. *Proceedings IEEE International Workshop on Robot and Human Communication*. IEEE; 1992:161–165.
3. Gassert R, Dietz V. Rehabilitation robots for the treatment of sensorimotor deficits: a neurophysiological perspective. *J Neuroeng Rehabil*. 2018;15(1):1–15.
4. Juszczak M, Gallo E, Bushnik T. Examining the effects of a powered exoskeleton on quality of life and secondary impairments in people living with spinal cord injury. *Top Spinal Cord Inj Rehabil*. 2018;24(4):336–342.
5. Zang K, Chen B, Wang M, et al. The effect of early mobilization in critically ill patients: a meta-analysis. *Nurs Crit Care*. 2020;25(6):360–367.
6. Yen HC, Jeng JS, Chen WS, et al. Early mobilization of mild-moderate intracerebral hemorrhage patients in a stroke center: a randomized controlled trial. *Neurorehabil Neural Repair*. 2020;34(1):72–81.
7. Holanda LJ, Silva PM, Amorim TC, Lacerda MO, Simão CR, Morya E. Robotic assisted gait as a tool for rehabilitation of individuals with spinal cord injury: a systematic review. *J Neuroeng Rehabil*. 2017;14(1):126.
8. Norouzi-Gheidari N, Archambault PS, Fung J. Effects of robot-assisted therapy on stroke rehabilitation in upper limbs: systematic review and meta-analysis of the literature. *J Rehabil Res Dev*. 2012;49(4):479–496.
9. Mazzoleni S, Sale P, Tiboni M, Franceschini M, Posteraro F, Carrozza MC. Upper limb robot-assisted therapy in chronic and subacute stroke patients: a kinematic analysis. *Am J Phys Med Rehabil*. 2013;92(10 Suppl 2):e26–e37.
10. Laut J, Porfiri M, Raghavan P. The present and future of robotic technology in rehabilitation. *Curr Phys Med Rehabil Rep*. 2016;4(4):312–319.
11. Akbari A, Haghverd F, Behbahani S. Robotic home-based rehabilitation systems design: from a literature review to a conceptual framework for community-based remote therapy during COVID-19 pandemic. *Front Robot AI*. 2021;8:612331. https://doi.org/10.3389/frobt.2021.612331
12. Catalan JM, Garcia JV, Lopez D, et al. (2018, August). Patient evaluation of an upper-limb rehabilitation robotic device for home use. In: *2018 7th IEEE International Conference on Biomedical Robotics and Biomechatronics (Biorob)*. IEEE; 2018:450–455.
13. Cherry COB, Chumbler NR, Richards K, et al. Expanding stroke telerehabilitation services to rural veterans: a qualitative study on patient experiences using the robotic stroke therapy delivery and monitoring system program. *Disabil Rehabil Assist Technol*. 2017;12(1):21–27.
14. Langhorne P, Coupar F, Pollock A. Motor recovery after stroke: a systematic review. *Lancet Neurol*. 2009;8(8):741–754.
15. Shih JJ, Krusienski DJ, Wolpaw JR. Brain-computer interfaces in medicine. *Mayo Clin Proc*. 2012; 87(3):268–279.
16. Eapen BC, Murphy DP, Cifu DX. Neuroprosthetics in amputee and brain injury rehabilitation. *Exp Neurol*. 2017;287:479–485.
17. BIONIK. (n.d.). Overview: Bionik Laboratories Corp. (BNKL). https://www.bioniklabs.com/about/overview
18. Ekso Bionics. Published August 19, 2021. https://eksobionics.com/

19. Calabrò RS, Naro A, Russo M, et al. Do post-stroke patients benefit from robotic verticalization? A pilot-study focusing on a novel neurophysiological approach. *Restor Neurol Neurosci*. 2015;33(5):671–681.
20. Hügli AS, Ernst MJ, Kool J, et al. Adherence to home exercises in non-specific low back pain. A randomised controlled pilot trial. *J Bodyw Mov Ther*. 2015;19(1):177–185.
21. Össur Prosthetics. http://www.ossur.com/en-us/prosthetics/
22. Bell J. Four types of medical robot leading the way in healthcare… they are taking over, but they're here to help. Published January 3, 2020. Accessed August 17, 2021. https://www.ns-healthcare.com/analysis/medical-robots/
23. High-tech "TUG" robots will do heavy lifting at Mission Bay. UCSF Benioff Children's Hospital. Accessed August 17, 2021. http://www.ucsfmissionbayhospitals.org/articles/high-tech-tug-robots-do-heavy-lifting-at-mission-bay.html
24. Mobile robots for healthcare—pharmacy, laboratory, nutrition And evs. (n.d.). TUG. Change Healthcare: Mobile robots improve patient care, employee satisfaction, safety, productivity and more. Accessed August 20, 2021. https://aethon.com/mobile-robots-for-healthcare/
25. Lane T. A short history of robotic surgery. *Ann R Coll Surg Engl*. 2018;100(6 suppl):5–7. https://doi.org/10.1308/rcsann.supp1.5
26. Chen M, Decary M. Artificial intelligence in healthcare: an essential guide for health leaders. *Healthc Manage Forum*. 2020;33(1):10–18. https://doi.org/10.1177/0840470419873123
27. Lanfranco AR, Castellanos AE, Desai JP, Meyers WC. Robotic surgery: a current perspective. *Ann Surg*. 2004;239(1):14–21. https://doi.org/10.1097/01.sla.0000103020.19595.7d
28. Combat Casualty Care Research Program (CCCRP). US Army MEDICAL RESEARCH AND DEVELOPMENT COMMAND. Published 2019. Accessed August 20, 2021. https://Mrdc.Amedd.Army.Mil/Index.Cfm/Program_areas/Medical_research_and_development/Ccc_overview
29. Gilbert GR, Beebe MK. *United States Department of Defense Research in Robotic Unmanned Systems for Combat Casualty Care*. NATO: 2010.
30. Garcia P, Rosen J, Kapoor C, et al. Trauma Pod: a semi-automated telerobotic surgical system. *Int J Med Robotics Comput Assist Surg*. 2009;5:136–146. https://doi.org/10.1002/rcs.238
31. George EI, Brand TC, LaPorta A, Marescaux J, Satava RM. Origins of robotic surgery: from skepticism to standard of care. *J Soc Laparoendosc Surg*. 2018;22(4):e2018.00039. https://doi.org/10.4293/JSLS.2018.00039
32. Gebru T, Krause J, Wang Y, et al. Using deep learning and google street view to estimate the demographic makeup of the US. *arXiv preprint arXiv:1702.06683* (2017).
33. Barry DT. Adaptation, artificial intelligence, and physical medicine and rehabilitation. *PM&R*. 2018;10(9S2):S131–S143. https://doi.org/10.1016/j.pmrj.2018.04.013
34. Venkatakrishnan A, He Y, Nathan K, et al. An integrated neuro-robotic interface for stroke rehabilitation using the NASA X1 powered lower limb exoskeleton. *Conference proceedings: Annual International Conference of the IEEE Engineering in Medicine and Biology Society*. IEEE Engineering in Medicine and Biology Society; 2014:3985–3988. https://doi.org/10.1109/EMBC.2014.6944497
35. Vilela M, Hochberg LR. Applications of brain-computer interfaces to the control of robotic and prosthetic arms. *Handb Clin Neurol*. 2020;168:87–99. https://doi.org/10.1016/B978-0-444-63934-9.00008-1
36. Daly JJ, Wolpaw JR. Brain-computer interfaces in neurological rehabilitation. *Lancet Neurol*. 2008;7(11):1032–1043. https://doi.org/10.1016/S1474-4422(08)70223-0
37. Krebs HI, Caurin G, Battistella L Rehabilitation robotics, orthotics, and prosthetics for the upper extremity. In: *Textbook of neural repair and rehabilitation*. 2016;177–189. https://doi.org/10.1017/CBO9780511995590.019
38. McCabe J, Monkiewicz M, Holcomb J, Pundik S, Daly JJ. Comparison of robotics, functional electrical stimulation, and motor learning methods for treatment of persistent upper extremity dysfunction after stroke: a randomized controlled trial. *Arch Phys Med Rehabil*. 2015;96(6):981–990.
39. Wagner TH, Lo AC, Peduzzi P, et al. An economic analysis of robot-assisted therapy for long-term upper-limb impairment after stroke. *Stroke*. 2011;42(9):2630–2632. https://doi.org/10.1161/STROKEAHA.110.606442
40. Research and Markets. Medical robots market forecast to 2028 - COVID-19 impact and global analysis by product, application, and end user, and geography. Report 4617877. Published May 2022. https://www.researchandmarkets.com/reports/4617877/medical-robots-market-to-2025-global-analysis
41. Bullard AJ, Nason SR, Irwin ZT, et al. Design and testing of a 96-channel neural interface module for the Networked Neuroprosthesis system. *Bioelectron Med*. 2019;5:3. https://doi.org/10.1186/s42234-019-0019-x

2

How Robotics Will Affect the Practice of Medicine for Practitioners

John Hermansen

KEY POINTS

- Through the performance of repetitive and time-consuming tasks, robots can help prevent practitioner burnout.
- Robots can add greater safety and efficiency such as in pharmacy systems.
- Tremendous flexibility exists to automate functions such transport systems, hospital admissions, and infusion devices.
- Devices can extend and enhance practitioner skills such as through gait trainers and robotic surgical systems.

Historically the practice of medicine has been consumed by repetitive, albeit important, tasks. In today's world, the number of independent tasks a practitioner may need to accomplish per patient has increased dramatically. Especially with the emergence of electronic medical records, or electronic health records, and value-oriented healthcare management, the additive burden of small tasks and redundant charting has become an inordinate obstacle directly associated with increasing burnout across all fields in health care.[1] It has been reported that primary care providers may spend as much as 2 hours on electronic medical record–related tasks for every hour of direct patient care.[2] Robots are well suited for repetitive, technically defined tasks and are being increasingly adopted in the health-care field. The global medical robotic systems market is expected to surge to $10.7 billion by 2026.[3] Although we are still far from the Star Trek/Star Wars vision of a robotic future, many advances have been made and robots are currently widely used throughout the globe in the multifaceted world of health care.

In this chapter we will look at the current applications of robotics, artificial intelligence (AI), and technologic advances improve the efficiency of various practitioners, attempt to reduce burnout, and most importantly improve patient outcomes. As the field of health care is incredibly broad, multidisciplinary, and traditionally grounded in physical and face-to-face interactions, we will also discuss the role these technologies play in the entire realm of health care delivery, including environmental services, dining and nutrition, and hospital logistics. Due to the breadth of the health-care field, and the myriad of robots available, it is beyond the scope of this chapter to discuss every currently available option. Instead, we will focus on one or two exemplars of robotic applications in each setting. Lastly, as the COVID-19 pandemic has changed the way people interact with health-care systems across the globe, we will even touch on applications in telemedicine, telehealth, remote health management, and new modalities of infection control.

"Keeping It Safe"

A pharmacy, both inpatient or outpatient varieties, is a prime example of where small mistakes can have big consequences. Pharmacists and their team (including pharmacy technicians, or techs) may be expected to serve many patients on a daily basis, attempting to both provide timely and useful service as well as mitigating or eliminating potentially dangerous situations. For reference, there are approximately 115,000 actively practicing full-time pharmacists in the United States.[4] Pharmacists manage teams of technicians to help receive and process dozens to hundreds of prescriptions daily, whether brought in by hand by the customer or sent by electronic means, telephone calls from the health provider, or even mail order. The average volume of medications provided in the United States is 259 prescriptions per day based on a 2013 Pharmacy Survey.[4]

Additionally the pharmacy may, and in many cases must, perform cross-checking of prescriptions against already prescribed medications, narcotics monitoring boards, and a myriad of potential side effects.[5] Mistakes can be annoying at best and deadly at worst. More than 100,000 Americans die each year of adverse drug reactions. Adverse drug reactions have become one of the six leading causes of death in the United States.[6] This is not unique to the United States: a 2018 report from the University of York estimates that as many as 237 million medication errors occur in England every year.[7]

Teams must also maintain, catalog, and stock hundreds of varieties of medicine and supplies, some with incredibly similar shape and design. Similar medications can look alike or their names can sound alike, commonly referred to as LASA medications.[8] There are currently more than 20,000 prescription medications approved by the Food and Drug Administration in the United States.[9] These prescriptions change in quantity, packaging, generic versus brand name and can even be occasionally counterfeit. Pharmacies often change suppliers of a particular generic drug, or a pharmacy wholesaler may continually rotate supply companies, contributing to innocuous shifts in pill descriptions that may lead to further confusion.[10] The US-based Drug Enforcement Administration reported in 2021 that there has been a sharp increase in fake prescription pills containing fentanyl and meth.[11]

There have been many strategies aimed to prevent pharmacy errors and adverse drug events as well as increase overall efficiency. Robotics is playing a significant role in accomplishing these goals. One approach is the use of AI-powered pharmacy dispensing platforms. The Fred Dispense Plus platform, recently deployed in Australia, is a computer-based tool that "uses AI and big data to support clinical and business decision making. As it predicts medication directions, the AI tool allows pharmacists to quickly and safely enter directions for dispensing labels through shortcuts instead of manual typing. Another smart tool on the same software platform can perform pricing comparison."[12] This platform also integrates with other third-party software to help provide comprehensive medication management.[12]

Automated pharmacy dispensing and robotic filling devices are becoming more ubiquitous in developed countries, and as the capabilities and storage potential of these robots grow so will their role in health care.[8,13] A relatively small, nonmobile robot such as the Kirby Lester KL60 Dispensing Robot (from Capsa Healthcare) (Fig. 2.1) fully automates 60 high-moving oral solids; that is 35% to 40% (or more) of a pharmacy's total daily prescriptions in a device that is less than 4′ deep. With the KL60 automatically handling more than one-third of orders, pharmacy staff are freed up to concentrate on important priorities like immunizations and customer service.[12,14] Larger robotic prescription robots are also available that can handle up to 108 high-moving tablets or capsules stored in locked cassettes, which can constitute automation of 50% or more of average daily prescriptions.

Even larger systems, such as the PillPick by Swisslog Healthcare, can automate unit-dose packaging, storage, and dispensing, while also providing additional safety measures like a vision-based sorting and verification system (Fig. 2.2A and B). Their solution is termed PickView and can

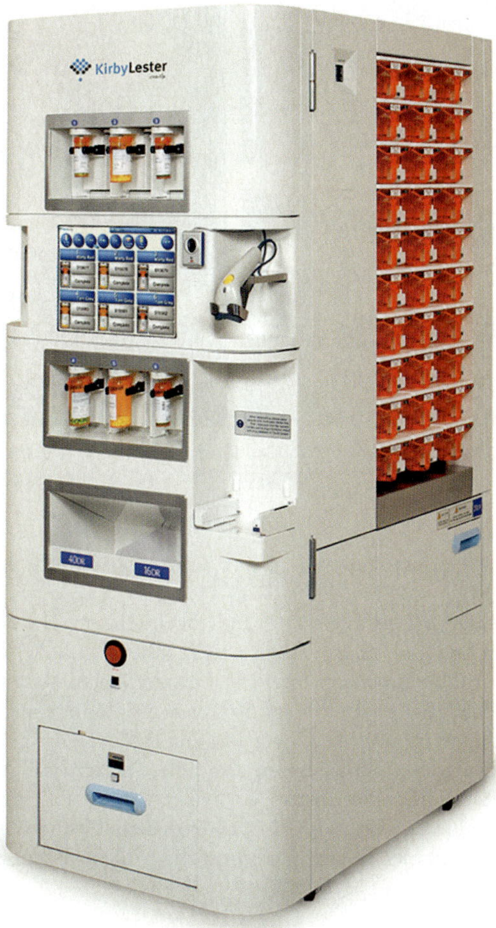

Fig. 2.1 The Kirby Lester (from Capsa Healthcare) KL60 Dispensing Robot. Capable of automating 30% or more of a pharmacy's daily prescription volume. (Courtesy Capsa Healthcare.)

help reduce or eliminate dispensing of look-alike or soundalike medications, as well as enabling hospitals to provide documentation that the right drug was in the right package.[15]

Smart infusion pumps have become more common in health-care systems[16] and are a popular method of delivering medication during inpatient hospital or outpatient clinic visits. These pumps may be combined with bar code–based scanning of medications and patients to develop "closed-loop" systems. Closed-loop systems help automatically regulate a process, in this case drug delivery, without human intervention. As human error is a significant factor in 70% to 80% of industrial adverse events,[17] the more routine human interference can be automated, the greater the opportunity for improved efficiency and decreased mistakes.

There are multiple groups working on bringing AI-enabled infusion pumps to market. One such effort began in an attempt to coordinate complex and real-time changes in patients' blood pressures during labor and delivery and notably during Cesarean sections. "We're doing all of these things simultaneously while taking care of an anxious, awake patient and preparing for major abdominal surgery. In a couple of minutes, the math becomes too complex for any human

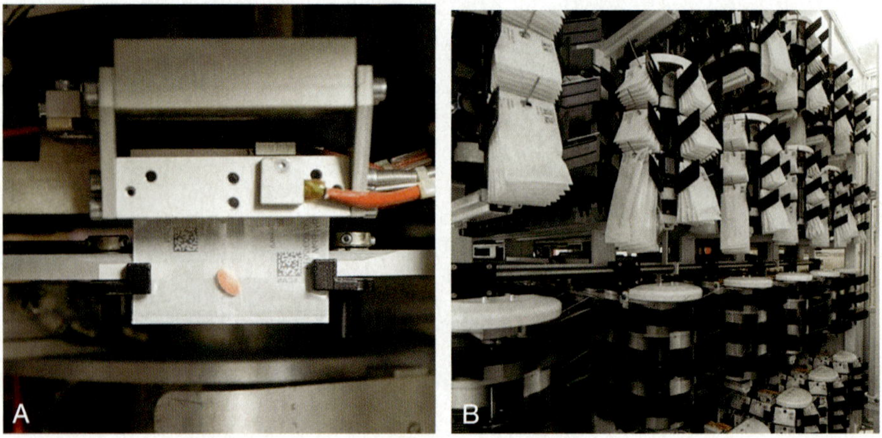

Fig. 2.2 Pictured are parts of the PillPick machine. (A) An example of the processing, identification, and verification capabilities. (B) The myriad of packaging materials the machine can use to appropriately dispense the medications.

to do, and we may under- or over treat the patient" as described by Dr. Kovacheva with Brigham and Women's Hospital.[18]

The current health-care and business landscapes dictate the priority of dispensing medications accurately, precisely, and on an ever increasingly tight schedule. A 2016 look at time utilization of pharmacists at a typical US pharmacy found that dispensing still consumes more of a pharmacist's time than any other activity—an average 39%, versus 22% for consultation, 15% for medical record interaction, and 19% for drug therapy management.[19]

Interacting with insurance companies can also take an immense amount of time to check approvals, arrange preauthorizations, assess copayments, and collect payments. Additionally, patient interaction and education by a pharmacy employee can be up to 2 hours per day.[4] Reducing a pharmacy worker's labor burden in any way possible is critically to ensuring comprehensive and robust health care.

"Keeping It Effortless"

Health care providers in hospital-based or outpatient clinic–based settings encounter significant barriers to consistent and efficient patient care. For many patients the first step toward care is either establishing care with a provider or undergoing admittance to a hospital system. Admission to a hospital is no simple or small feat, whether by way of the emergency department or direct admission from another health-care provider or facility. An analysis led by Thibodaux Regional Medical Center, located near New Orleans, Louisiana, looked at the hospital's inpatient admission process.[11] Although every medical center has its own unique population, needs, and challenges, many of the issues the analysis found can be generalized to many hospitals in the United States. According to their report: "While Thibodaux had invested millions in its EHR [electronic health record] and other information technologies designed to improve patient care, the hospital's inpatient admission process was still entirely manual, involving documentation on paper and faxing. This led to errors such as lost faxes, and to cumbersome processes such as multiple phone calls to track down information while patients waited. The manual process also led to inefficient handoffs, redundant data collection, as well as delays in getting necessary information, doctor's orders, and bed assignments so care could be initiated."

Processes to help automate admissions are being implemented in hospitals around the world. These automations tend to focus on improvements in data acquisition (for example, from surrounding third-party health provider records), patient reporting of medical histories, present illness, and reviews of systems, as well as integration of health-care reporting measures. Although fascinating and incredibly potent catalysts within the health-care field, most are software-driven or data science–driven processes and beyond the scope of this chapter. However, there are also many attempts to integrate robotics in health care in a customer service–based perspective.

In a 2016 study published in the *Journal of Medical Practice Management*, customer service in health-care settings was by far the most frequent complaint by patients.[20] While having a (knowledgeable and friendly) human as a point of contact with in a health-care setting is currently indispensable, several companies are developing potential solutions to the "always available" customer service need. First created in 2014, Pepper is an interactive robot designed to identify, process, and empathize with human emotions. With the inclusion of multiple cameras, 19 different languages, and 20 degrees of freedom, Pepper is able to meaningfully interact with people in many settings. The robot is being trialed in several environments but with its emotion-processing capacity and ability to speak and direct people in multiple languages, a hospital or health-care setting is a great fit. Several hospitals in Belgium and Canada are using Pepper robots to meet, greet, and direct incoming visitors.[21] As previously mentioned, creating a consistent and helpful welcome to a hospital is paramount to establishing an overall positive experience.

Among the many changes instilled by the COVID-19 global pandemic, and secondary to the critical need to minimize human exposure to pathogens, institutions initiated new methods of collecting vitals and screening hospital employees and visitors. One hospital system, Brigham and Women's Hospital in Boston, Massachusetts, collaborated with researchers to place contactless vital sign monitors on autonomous quadruped robots.[22] These technologic chimeras, referred to as Dr. Spot by the development teams, have proven viable, and there are plans to for them to deploy the robots in the emergency department and potentially on inpatient floors as well. The machines that collect vital signs without direct touch are not novel, but integrating them onto a robotics platform that allows safer and more effective deployment of resources exemplifies several of the advantages of robotics in the health-care system.[23]

Health care is much more than direct interactions with a patient; on a daily basis a typical health-care provider may be expected to check a plethora of laboratory values, obtain and evaluate imaging, access and navigate medical records (both physical and electronic in nature), communicate various test results to patients, document physical examination findings, write prescriptions, and cross-check against other current prescriptions including from outside providers, among other responsibilities. These tasks are in addition to the face-to-face time spent with the patient, whether in person or virtually, and can add up to immense amounts of time. One study cited by the American Medical Association reports that up to a third of physicians spend 20 or more hours a week performing tasks outside of direct patient contact.[24]

Companies are both currently deploying and developing robots in an effort to offload provider burdens, especially those involving repetitive motions or labor-intense but cognitively light tasks. One common theme is transportation of materials within a large hospital. For example: Relay, built by Savioke, provides trackable and secure chain of custody for biospecimens such as collected blood samples, especially for ones that cannot be transported via pneumatic tube systems existing in many hospitals. Deployed examples have reported an average of 400 deliveries per month with quicker and more cost-effective results than human full-time equivalents.[25] Notably, this example comes from before the COVID-19 SARS-CoV-2 pandemic with the concurrent increased need for aseptic techniques and a global shortage in health-care workers. Savioke estimates that one Relay machine can save close to $500,000 in costs over 3 years compared with a full-time labor equivalent.

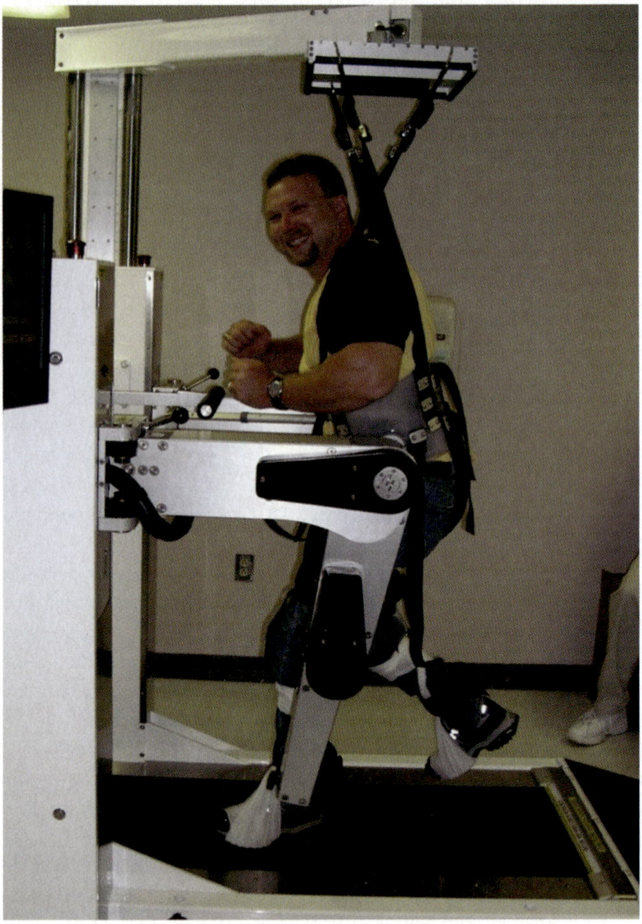

Fig. 2.3 AutoAmbulator by Encompass Health.

Patients presenting for outpatient clinic appointments with physical, occupational, or other therapists often find themselves interacting with robots. Advanced treadmill platforms with weight support and robotic functions are growing in popularity, with some version present at many rehabilitation centers. Sensors and motors help provide a safe and variable gait pattern to help reproduce and reinforce normal ambulation. A popular treadmill in the United States is the AutoAmbulator by Encompass Health (Fig. 2.3). It can provide robotic therapy assistance for patients of various conditions at levels that would normally take three or more human therapists. Additionally, the precise and consistent feedback provided by the treadmill on patient contribution to the task has proven incredible helpful to health-care providers in prescribing exercise or monitoring results of interventions. Potential patient conditions include spinal cord injuries and disorders, brain injury, multiple sclerosis, stroke, Parkinson disease, and other orthopedic or neurologic conditions resulting in mobility changes.[26]

No discussion of robotics in health care would be complete without mention of da Vinci, a robot-assisted minimally invasive surgery system (Fig. 2.4). Approved by the Food and Drug Administration in 2000, the systwem has gained in popularity due to ease of use and faster

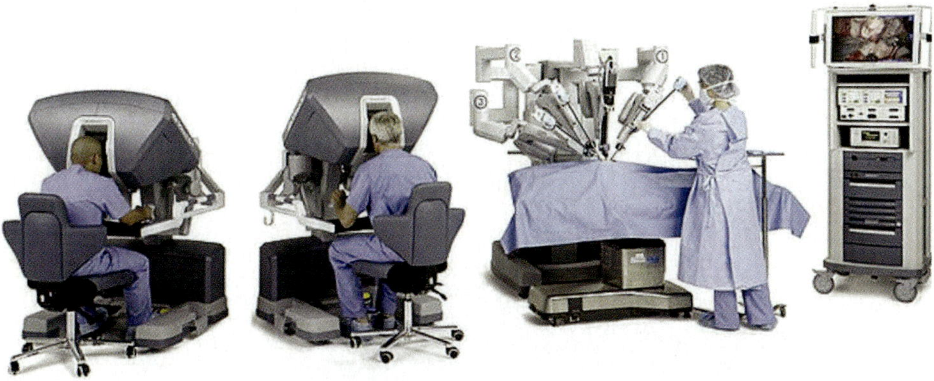

Fig. 2.4 Da Vinci image. (From Pietrabissa A, Vinci A, Pugliese L, Peri A. Robotic surgery: current controversies and future expectations. *Cir Esp*. 2013;91(2):67–71.)

operative times.[27] Overall cost-effectiveness in many surgical fields is still equivocal.[28,29] This system will be discussed more in depth in a separate chapter.

"Keeping It Clean"

Keeping environments free of infectious, dangerous, or just inconvenient material has been a significant challenge for health-care systems. Modern germ theory, as first introduced by Robert Koch in the late 19th century, still exists as the framework for overall cleanliness and infection control.[30] The COVID-19 pandemic, emerging at a time where technology and robotics are enabling revolutionary changes in environmental controls, has helped to accelerate the adoption by health-care systems.

Room turnover, or preparing a room for the next occupant, is a significant logistics obstacle in many realms of health care. In a hospital, long or inefficient turnovers can hamper patient transfers and increase anxiety on the behalf of the patient and staff responsible for care. Inefficiencies here can compound to the point where people requiring more intense care may be unable to be admitted from an emergency room or lower-complexity health care setting in a safe time frame. This can affect everything from the quality of patient care to the overall operating costs of the system. One of the larger components of room turnover is human labor involved with cleaning, disinfection, and restocking of supplies.

Cleaning a room involves physical removal of waste, whether debris from patients, procedures, or tests or organic matter such dust, fluids, or hair. Robots that assist in these processes are quickly becoming popular. The robots help increase efficiency of cleaning services as well as reduce contact between humans and potentially dangerous materials. Whiz is an autonomous vacuum sweeper, made by SoftBank Robotics, for industrial environments that its creators have termed a cobot. "Cobot," a portmanteau of collaborative and robot, is a term coined in 1996 by J. Edward Colgate and Michael Peshkin, professors at Northwestern University, to refer to robots intended for direct human interaction.[31] The term is relatively uncommon; however, there is a recent global increase in usage as a search term. Much like the gallant, but much smaller, variants of household robotic vacuums that have surged in popularity, industrial-sized models are helping to efficiently keep large areas of floor clean. Currently used in hotels, airports, and hospitals, autonomous vacuums help reduce the labor hours of environmental service teams and allow them to focus on more critical tasks such as deep cleaning and disinfection of surfaces.

Disinfection is a distinct process from cleaning. As opposed to cleaning, which involves physical removal of material, disinfection kills germs present on surfaces to reduce or prevent the risk of spreading infection. There are many ways to disinfect a surface, including chemical and physical methods like heat and pressure, but ultraviolet light–based systems are growing in favor. Using ultraviolet light allows contactless interaction with irregular surfaces as well as better penetration into difficult to reach areas such as seams and holes. One such robot is the LightStrike, created by Xenex, that uses full-spectrum ultraviolet light to disinfect a hospital room in 5 minutes (Fig. 2.5).

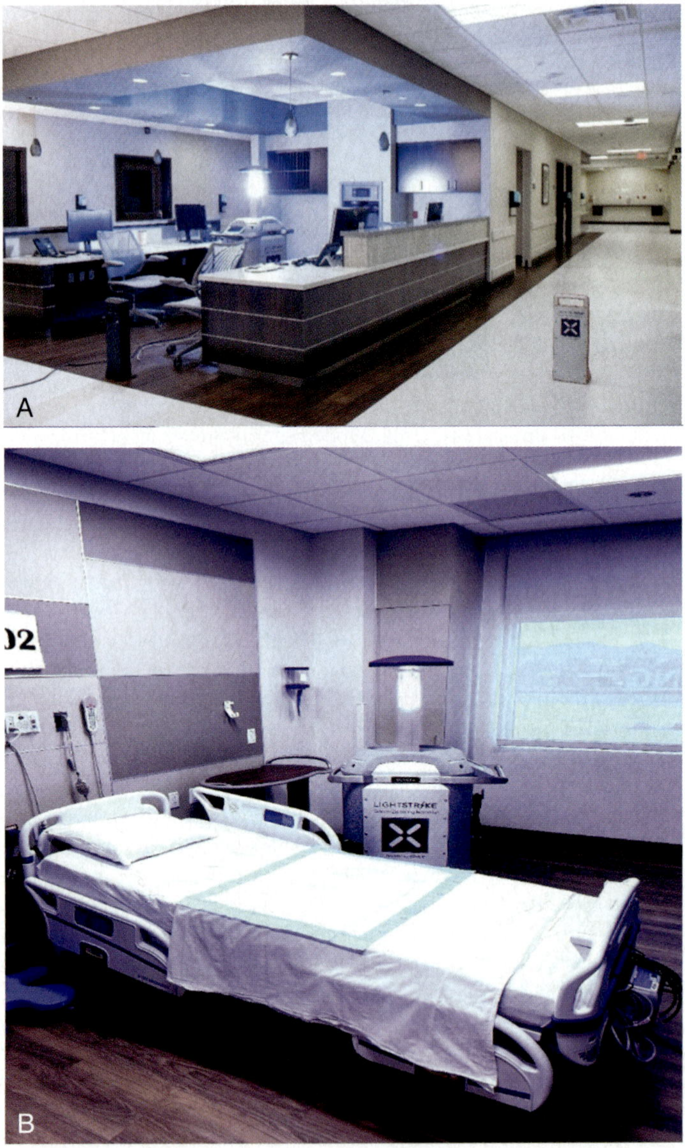

Fig. 2.5 LightStrike LS6 disinfection robot at work in a nursing station (A) and patient room (B).

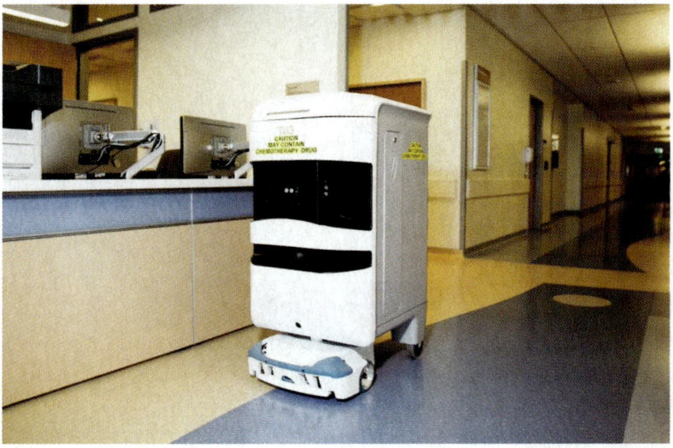

Fig. 2.6 TUG, robotic delivery system by Aethon. Traversing the halls of a hospital.

This technology is especially compelling as we enter (and may already be in by some measures) a postantibiotic era where germs are resistant to current medications—with deadly outcomes. A study by the United Nations predicts drug-resistant infections will kill more than 10 million people globally by 2050.[32] Xenex reports that a basic quick clean of a room plus treatment by the LightStrike can save 20 to 30 minutes per room for full *methicillin-resistant Staphylococcus aureus* disinfection. Methicillin-resistant S. aureus infections acquired during a hospital stay can add 14 days to the admission, which may also be the financial responsibility of the hospital.[33] Disinfecting robots are also frequently used outside of health care in schools, airports, and hotels.

Distribution of supplies and delivery logistics within health-care settings are areas ripe for the application of robotics. Robotic delivery systems are gaining traction throughout the world. One example is TUG, developed by Aethon (Fig. 2.6).[34] TUGs have been adopted by many hospitals to ease in-hospital delivery burdens and streamline and automate logistics. These robots can carry from 500 to 1400 pounds of secured and tracked payload, autonomously navigate through environments including use of elevators, and in several variations are able to automate both pickup and drop-off of loads. Payloads can include medications, clinical supplies, biospecimens, secure documents, meals and dietary items, linens, and more. TUGs can operate continuously for 14 out of 24 hours a day, 7 days a week. Including the possibility of charging between deliveries, the functional duty cycle can be even greater. Additionally, preplanned movement of supplies can be biased toward nighttime, or predictably less busy time frames, to free up hallways for patients, families, and clinicians. A large hospital system has reported each TUG has accumulated approximately 500 miles and over 4000 stops over the last year of use.[25] These are miles, hours, and interactions that a human no longer has to complete, and instead people may focus on patient-centric situations such as decision-making, caring, and supporting.

"Keeping It Friendly"

Telemedicine and telehealth have recently found a place at the front line of medicine. This shift in services was already gradually gaining in popularity, but the rise of the COVID-19 pandemic thrust virtual health care into the spotlight. It is important to differentiate between the two terms: "telemedicine" is the practice of medicine using technology to deliver care at a distance, and "telehealth" refers broadly to electronic and telecommunications technologies and services used to provide care and services at a distance. Even more broadly, telepresence refers to the use of virtual

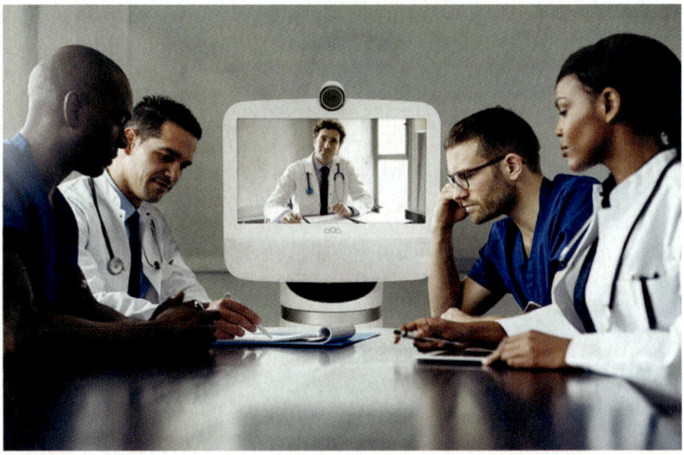

Fig. 2.7 Ava 500 by Ava Robotics.

reality technology, especially for remote control of machinery or for apparent participation in distant events. The use of modern technology, including high-speed telecommunications and the ubiquitous high-fidelity audio and video capabilities found in computers and cellular phones, have allowed health-care providers to provide critical patient care. This care can now be provided in settings of infectious concerns and where providers are not able to meet patients due to mobility, financial, or geographical restrictions. Telehealth and telemedicine have previously been performed primarily through video streams or audio communication; however, the use of telepresence robots is becoming more popular. One of the first complete systems was initially developed in the 1990s by the US Air Force's Armstrong Labs. Telepresence robots are most commonly used as night watchmen, tour guides, and factory inspectors and in settings dangerous to human health. One prominent player in the health-care telepresence sector is iRobot. The company was first founded in 2002 with the release of the Roomba autonomous vacuum but in 2009 announced a Healthcare Robotics division that would go on to become Ava Robotics (Fig. 2.7). Their current flagship telepresence robot is the Ava 500. Multiple video screens and cameras allow the participants to have real-time and meaningful interactions. The robot itself can be piloted by the user from anywhere in the world and is also capable of full autonomy using depth cameras and lidar. This autonomy can be paired with user control to create a moveable robot that simultaneously avoids static and dynamic obstacles without input from the primary user, creating a safer environment for all. All communications are Health Insurance Portability and Accountability Act compliant and the entire robot is easy to clean and disinfect.[35] Not limited to just primary care providers, any health-care worker can leverage telepresence robots to engage in more intimate and interactive patient care. Additionally, the mobile form factor allows the user to navigate the environment and interact with other providers or people in the same building. Multiple telepresence robots can even interact with each other, allowing further flexibility for the user.

Social interaction, or lack thereof, is well known to affect mental health, behavior, physical health, and mortality risk.[36] Traditional social interactions in the health-care setting require significant amounts of time, time that is increasingly being diverted to other requirements such as medical record charting. A 2017 study, published in the *Journal of Alzheimer's Disease*, demonstrated that patient interactions with robotic pets decreased stress and anxiety and resulted in reductions in the use of psychoactive medications and pain medications in elderly clients with dementia.[37] It follows that simulated interactions may confer some of the benefits of "flesh-and-blood" interactions

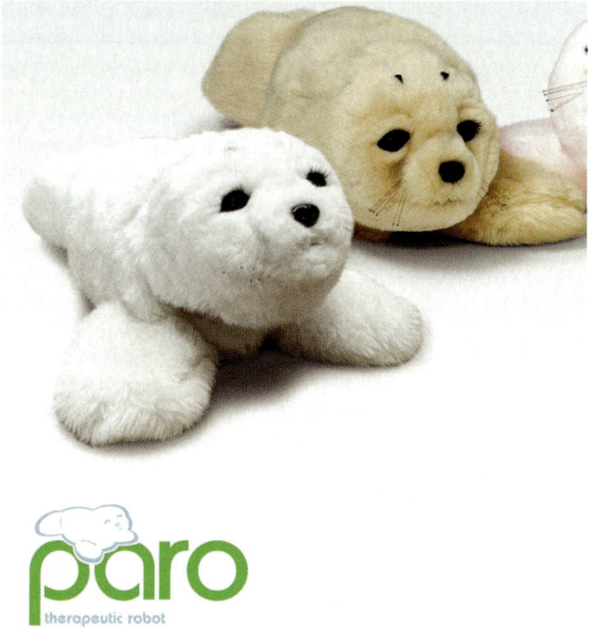

Fig. 2.8 PARO Therapeutic Robot.

without the significant use of human resources. PARO is a therapeutic robot, classified as a Food and Drug Administration Class 2 medical device since 2009, that assists with biofeedback therapy (Fig. 2.8). It is covered by Medicare in the United States for patients with dementia, brain injury, posttraumatic stress disorder, cancer, or other conditions associated with anxiety, depression, pain, or agitation. Many of these symptoms have been found to be exacerbated by the isolation due to COVID-19 restrictions.[37] Interestingly, this isolation is similar to that found during space travel. Isolation in space is being studied as astronauts can spend months in space at a time. A proposed trip to Mars could take as long as 9 months each way and would impose the additional constraint of a time delay in Earth communication as high as 20 minutes.[38] Interestingly, a space version of PARO has been proposed to help mitigate the effects of isolation. It is likely simulated social interaction, especially combined with physical touch and feedback, will play a significant role in not just astronaut health but in those of patients here on Earth in the future. Therapeutic robots could be very beneficial in the health-care setting where there are simply not enough providers and care givers to go around.

Despite many current applications in the health-care field, robotics is still in its infancy in scope, capabilities, and future potential. There are many promising concepts being developed and tested, which will be discussed in a later chapter. The question is not if, but when, robotics and AI will play a prominent role in medicine and health. It is clear that there are not enough human resources currently available in health care to provide the needed care, and this problem will only grow with increasing population levels and longer life spans. The human species will have to do what it does best: reach into our bag of tools and leverage technology to craft the solutions.

References

1. Robertson SL, Robinson MD, Reid A. Electronic health record effects on work-life balance and burnout within the I3 population collaborative. *J Grad Med Educ*. 2017;9(4):479–484.

2. Arndt BG, Beasley JW, Watkinson MD, et al. Tethered to the EHR: primary care physician workload assessment using EHR event log data and time-motion observations. *Ann Fam Med.* 2017;15(5):419–426.
3. Medical robotic systems market size, share and industry analysis by product (surgical robots, telepresence robots, rehabilitations robots), by end user (hospitals, ambulatory surgery centers, rehabilitation centers) and regional forecast 2019-2026. *Fortune Business* Insights. Accessed September 19, 2022. https://www.fortunebusinessinsights.com/industry-reports/medical-robotic-systems-market-100957
4. Kantar media readership study ranks Pharmacy Times #1 among pharmacists for two years in a row. *Businesswire.* Published May 6, 2015. Accessed September 19, 2022.
5. Agency for Healthcare Research and Quality. Medication errors and adverse drug events. Published September 7, 2019. Accessed September 19, 2022. https://psnet.ahrq.gov/primer/medication-errors-and-adverse-drug-events
6. Lazarou J, Pomeranz BH, Corey PN. Incidence of adverse drug reactions in hospitalized patients: a meta-analysis of prospective studies. *JAMA.* 1998;279(15):1200–1205.
7. Elliott R, Camacho EM, Campbell F, et al. Prevalence and economic burden of medication errors in the NHS in England. Rapid evidence synthesis and economic analysis of the prevalence and burden of medication error in the UK. EEPRU Medication Errors. Published 2018. https://www.researchgate.net/publication/323457145_Prevalence_and_Economic_Burden_of_Medication_Errors_in_The_NHS_in_England_Rapid_evidence_synthesis_and_economic_analysis_of_the_prevalence_and_burden_of_medication_error_in_the_UK
8. Kerslake R. How look-alike, sound-alike drugs are commonly confused. Singlecare. Published March 17, 2021. Accessed September 19, 2022. https://www.singlecare.com/blog/look-alike-sound-alike-drug/
9. US Food and Drug Administration. Fact sheet: FDA at a glance. Published November 2021. Accessed September 19, 2022. https://www.fda.gov/about-fda/fda-basics/fact-sheet-fda-glance
10. Why do my pills look different each time I fill the same prescription? Consumer Reports News. Published May 25, 2012. Accessed September 19, 2022. https://www.consumerreports.org/cro/news/2012/05/why-do-my-pills-look-different-each-time-i-fill-the-same-prescription/index.htm
11. How to significantly reduce inpatient admission times and improve patient satisfaction. Health Catalyst. Published 2016. https://www.healthcatalyst.com/success_stories/inpatient-admission-process-thibodaux/
12. Ang A. Latest AI-powered pharmacy dispensing platform launched in Australia. Mobihealthnews. Accessed September 19, 2022. https://www.mobihealthnews.com/news/anz/latest-ai-powered-pharmacy-dispensing-platform-launched-australia
13. Drake E, Srinivas P, Trujillo T. Using computerized prescriber order entry to limit overrides from automated dispensing cabinets. *Am J Health Syst Pharm.* 2016;73(14):1033–1035.
14. Kirby Lester KL60 dispensing robot. Capsa Healthcare. Accessed September 19, 2022. https://www.capsahealthcare.com/product/kl60-dispensing-robot/
15. PillPick® automated packaging and dispensing system. Swisslog Healthcare. https://www.swisslog-healthcare.com/en-us/products/pharmacy-automation/pillpick-automated-packaging-and-dispensing-system.
16. Trbovich PL, Pinkney S, Cafazzo JA, Easty AC. The impact of traditional and smart pump infusion technology on nurse medication administration performance in a simulated inpatient unit. *Qual Saf Health Care.* 2010;19(5):430–434.
17. Preventing human errors in healthcare. Managed Healthcare Executive. Published March 25, 2016. Last accessed September 19, 2022. https://www.managedhealthcareexecutive.com/view/preventing-human-errors-healthcare
18. Artificial intelligence to automate drug infusions for safer C-sections. Brigham and Women's Hospital. Last accessed September 19, 2022. https://www.brighamhealthonamission.org/2019/11/27/artificial-intelligence-to-automate-drug-infusions-for-safer-c-sections/
19. Fisher AM, Ding MQ, Hochheiser H, Douglas GP. Measuring time utilization of pharmacists in the Birmingham Free Clinic dispensary. *BMC Health Serv Res.* 2016;16(1):529.
20. Gooch K. Patients' no. 1 complaint? Front desk staff. Published April 26, 2016. Accessed September 19, 2022. https://www.beckershospitalreview.com/hospital-management-administration/patients-no-1-complaint-front-desk-staff.html
21. Aldebaran United Robotics Group. *Pepper the humanoid and programmable robot.* Last accessed January 26, 2023. https://www.aldebaran.com/en/pepper.

22. Trafton A. Robot takes contact-free measurements of patients' vital signs. Mobile system could reduce health care workers' exposure to Covid-19 virus. MIT News. Published August 31, 2020. Accessed September 19, 2022. https://news.mit.edu/2020/spot-robot-vital-signs-0831
23. Huang HW, Chai PR, Ehmke C, et al. Agile mobile robotic platform for contactless vital sign monitoring. TechRxiv. https://www.techrxiv.org/articles/preprint/Agile_mobile_robotic_platform_for_contactless_vital_signs_monitoring/12811982
24. Kane, L. *Medscape Physician Compensation Report 2018*. Last accessed January 26, 2023. https://www.medscape.com/slideshow/2018-compensation-overview-6009667
25. Horowitz BT. Nonsurgical robots keep hospitals clean and capable: from sanitizing rooms to delivering supplies, the machines offer relief and boost morale in busy environments. HealthTech. Published May 29, 2020. Last accessed September 19, 2022. https://healthtechmagazine.net/article/2020/05/nonsurgical-robots-keep-hospitals-clean-and-capable
26. AutoAmbulator at Encompass Health. Last accessed January 26, 2023. https://healthscopemag.com/health-scope/autoambulator
27. Patel MN, Hemal AK. Does advancing technology improve outcomes? Comparison of the Da Vinci Standard/S/Si to the Xi Robotic platforms during robotic nephroureterectomy. *J Endourol.* 2018;32(2):133–138.
28. Crew B. Worth the cost? A closer look at the da Vinci robot's impact on prostate cancer surgery. *Nature.* 2020;580(7804):S5–S7.
29. Pietrabissa A, Vinci A, Pugliese L, Peri A. Robotic surgery: current controversies and future expectations. *Cir Esp*. 2013;91(2):67–71.
30. National Research Council (US) Committee to Update Science, Medicine, and Animals. Science, Medicine, and Animals. A theory of germs. Published 2004. https://www.ncbi.nlm.nih.gov/books/NBK24649/
31. Van J. Mechanical advantage. *Chicago Tribune*. Published December 11, 1996. Last accessed January 26, 2023. https://www.chicagotribune.com/news/ct-xpm-1996-12-11-9612110101-story.html
32. Minor L. Welcome to the post-antibiotic era. Will we save ourselves in time? Stanford Medicine. Published December 6, 2019. Accessed September 19, 2022. https://scopeblog.stanford.edu/2019/12/06/welcome-to-the-post-antibiotic-era-will-we-save-ourselves-in-time/
33. Li X, Chen Y, Gao W, Ouyang W, Wei J, Wen Z. Epidemiology and outcomes of complicated skin and soft tissue infections among inpatients in Southern China from 2008 to 2013. PLoS One. 2016;11(2):e0149960.
34. TUG Autonomous Mobile Robots for Healthcare and Hospitality. Last accessed January 26, 2023. https://www.aethon.com/products/
35. Gardner M. Ava telepresence: hospital emergency department transformation. Ava Robotics. Published ay 23, 2020. Accessed September 19, 2022. https://www.avarobotics.com/post/ava-telepresence-hospital-emergency-department-transformation
36. Umberson D, Montez JK. Social relationships and health: a flashpoint for health policy. *J Health Soc Behav*. 2010;51(Suppl):S54–S66.
37. Petersen S, Houston S, Qin H, Tague C, Studley J. The utilization of robotic pets in dementia care. *J Alzheimers Dis*. 2017;55(2):569–574.
38. https://www.nasa.gov/hrp/social-isolation

3

How Robotics Will Affect the Experience of Health Care for Patients

Kenichiro Ono

KEY POINTS

- Patients will increasingly encounter robotic service delivery as they access health care.
- This technology can fill in gaps of care and improve access to care such as with telemedicine.
- Patients will encounter a responsiveness to their needs that is faster, more accurate, and more complete through enhanced data collection.
- Home robotic systems will provide companionship and the delivery of services.
- The "human touch" will not be lost as emotional support and responsiveness will be part of robotic behavior.

Health-care delivery is constantly evolving for the patient, resulting in increased demand from providers and technology developers. Health-care delivery and the technology used to perform these services have grown and been refined at an exponential pace. One only needs to casually peruse through technology journals or websites of various vendors to realize there is an electronic tool that can aid in various tasks, ranging from using utensils with artificial limbs, communicating over vast distances, or performing the most intricate of surgeries with minimal recovery time. Software improvements have enhanced our phones and tablets to deliver, collect, and monitor a wealth of medical information. The possibilities of utilizing robotics and technology for health care seem limitless at first glance. However, the practice of medicine is still rooted in a traditional, unidirectional transaction from a content expert (provider) to a recipient (patient). With more ubiquitous adoption of technology in daily life, patients have an ever-increasing stake in not only managing but delivering their own care. This begs the question: Should health care be delivered the same way it has been done for centuries?

Most of the robotic product development currently appears strongest in the physical rehabilitation industry, which encompasses clinical practice, product development, and the technology market. The industry as whole has a wide scope, for example, of improving mobility, function, and independence for patients with various physical and/or neurologic disabilities. Yet many products have a narrow focus on manual tasks or augmentation in gait. This is not to criticize the industry on prioritizing resources on fundamental tasks such as regaining hand function or transferring one's weight from seated to standing. It does, however, illustrate a disconnect from what patients seek from their health-care providers and what we actually deliver. There is a need for a call to arms involving patients, their caretakers, medical teams, and robotics developers to better understand and deliver products that address what patients want the most.

To better understand how robotics *could* affect the experience of health care for patients, one should understand what patients and their caregivers truly want from health care. This is an incredibly complex and often misunderstood concept. Traditional Western medical training emphasizes predefined (prescribed) "models" of care, where a patient-provider relationship dyad (patient centric vs. paternalistic) trades information and creates a management plan. But what if robotics could step in and transform this for both parties? The dyad model could still exist but with replacement of a human clinician with a robotic medical provider, or a triad model with a patient–robotic assistant–clinician arrangement. The robotic assistant could serve to monitor a patient's health, provide daily home health needs, and perhaps inform the clinician of health data elements or history that a patient could not provide in sufficient detail or in a competent way. The robotic assistant could also provide these updates in a more frequent fashion in between formal clinic visits. On the other hand, the clinician could instruct the robotic assistant to automatically intervene for certain health care needs such as wound care, medication administration, or more complex actions such as cardiopulmonary resuscitation when family or other health-care workers are not available.

Robotics goes beyond the past movie interpretations of a stiff, cold machine with slow-moving arms and a comical stammering digital voice that serves you a beverage. Transparent use of robotic technology today such as vacuums, food delivery, and various toys may indicate growing acceptance with consumers. Availability, affordability, and ease of use are only the most basic of requirements for technology to be integrated in everyday life, not just for health care. Much like a household appliance, the functions and more importantly the consumer (patient) experience and acceptance of robotics into one's life would strongly influence a product's market success in health-care delivery. Caution should be exercised, as market success may not necessarily translate to good clinical outcomes or high-quality care. In addition, cultural differences in the expectations and family involvement of a patient's care should be considered. Most importantly, the large socio-economic gap separating patients who not only get access to but are literate of health care and its capabilities is paramount. To assume that each patient gets the same kind of care even within one's own facility would be as careless as assuming all types of water taste the same. In an ideal world, all health care is truly individualized, However, the so-called personalized care should be scrutinized for bias between the haves and have-nots.

Though health-care administrators use patient surveys to gain feedback following a hospital stay, Nepal et al.[1] dove much deeper to engage patients in conversation during an acute hospitalization. This effort found that the patient experience is rooted in empowerment and independence, in understanding the medical problem at hand across the clinician-patient continuum, and in having a clear line of communication across stakeholders. Some of the issues raised in this study may not be an area easily filled by robotics, such as room design or the taste of hospital food; however, much of the patient experience involves engagement, compassion, as well as efficiency and overall sense of comprehensive care.[1] This puts a large burden on clinical as well as ancillary health-care workers. Employees of health-care organizations thus need to deliver not only medical care, but also an experience much akin to what is provided in the hospitality industry.

An unfortunate reality of health-care delivery is that staffing has been, and continues to be, insufficient. This does not excuse a poor experience when in the clinic or hospital. A robotic or digital guide could to some extent supplement where the human touch is lacking. Routine cleaning could be automated much like appliances used in people's homes. Medications could be routed quickly and efficiently within the medical center using high-capacity robotic carts that could deliver at least some of their cargo directly to patients (consumers) via self-navigating delivery vehicles and drones. Navigation within a large medical center could be assisted in an app-based or motorized companion that may guide or physically accompany or shuttle patients who have difficulty walking or decipher signs and directions to get to a clinic. Ma et al.[2] studied how a real example of a companion robot could work in a large hospital or clinic setting. This intelligent guidance robot addressed various questions in a natural language environment. Though its initial intent was to serve almost as a tour guide, the majority of the inquiries involved requests for medical information. This is an intriguing concept and may be alarming to some. This clearly demonstrates that some populations have far more comfort engaging in a conversation to discuss and learn about their medical problems with a robot. It also demonstrates the thoroughness of the patient-clinician interaction may be incomplete and patients are left to fill those needs with a robot. There are various explanations, such as insufficient time, use of overly complex language by the clinician, or simply having many sometimes unrelated medical problems that may not have been asked by the patient or adequately answered by the clinician. This boils down to one thing, that the communication between clinician and patient was insufficient to comprehensively meet the patient's needs.

Despite the innovation in physical robotics design, none of these devices would be of benefit or have as much adoption as we are seeing today without cutting-edge software. We live in an era where cell phone and wearable technology use is exponentially higher than just a few years ago. Though there is debate on whether this amount of screen time is appropriate, the reality is that digital devices are here to stay. Rather than fixating on the negatives of screen time, health-care workers and robotics developers could leverage our reliance on technology to bridge the patient experience. This adaptation would start even before a patient logs into a telehealth visit or leaves their home to come to the clinic or hospital and may continue after the visit is finished. Patient acceptance of robots or electronic interfaces with health-care providers is profiled by Chai et al.[3] In that study, patients answered a survey regarding their general opinions on the utility of a robot for certain tasks such as taking vital signs or simple clinical tasks that a human nurse or assistant would routinely perform. This information may then be entered in the medical record and prepared for use by the provider prior to engaging with the patient. It was generally perceived useful, particularly in the advent of the COVID-19 pandemic, to use a robot to perform these tasks. Furthermore, human attention can be better dedicated to more critical needs, medical decision-making, and patient education and may promote social distancing and time-efficient evaluation (limiting exposure) between patient and provider. These perceptions were further assessed by deploying a quadruped robot with a tablet that would round on different patients and facilitate a screening evaluation by a human clinician. This allowed the delivery of care from human to human via a mobile communication platform. Overall acceptance and willingness of patients to use this system was high, ranging from mid-80% to 90% of survey respondents.[3]

Although it is not clear whether this mode of video clinical communication and evaluation would have garnered such acceptance prior to the COVID-19 pandemic, it appears now patients are far more willing to receive their medical care through a digital interface. From a bird's-eye view, the use of a motorized robot to transport an audiovisual communication device around an emergency room or clinic would solve some of the problems of a strained health-care infrastructure and may allow direct and efficient care delivery. Depending on your point of view, the existence of a motorized, robotic communication device may exemplify that on-demand patient care delivery equipment is in high demand. Patients can already contact and participate in a video evaluation with providers through their cell phones. Thus, it would not be unreasonable for video evaluations to replace or supplement parts of the patient evaluation and reallocate direct human interaction to when physical examination or contact is absolutely needed. These technologies can potentially allow patients to seek and obtain emergent and/or specialist care within a safe space and over long distances. It is unclear whether the robot transporting the telecommunications device or just the option to telecommunicate itself was perceived positively by the patients in the study by Chai et al.[3] A motorized patient interview platform deployed within a clinic or from one home to another would have a place in health care when telecommunication is not readily available or is too costly. A few dedicated platforms could move from site to site to fulfill the needs of patient evaluation and management. Such a technology may even fill health-care gaps in rural or low-income areas of the world, where a dedicated clinic may not exist.

The acceptance of human interactions through medical telecommunications devices and the actual autonomous use, assessment, and intervention by a medical robot could radically transform health-care delivery. The current simplicity, portability, and accessibility of video telecommunication with a health-care provider today may indicate that future evaluations with a medical robot, perhaps with humanlike appearance could be done the same way. But is it enough that the robot *looks* human? Cresswell et al.[4] interviewed select volunteers of various ethnic and professional backgrounds on their general views of robotics in health care. The respondents were mostly highly educated individuals from Europe, the United States, and Australia who either had some understanding or experience discussing and thinking about how robots play a significant role. Though this population of respondents may not represent the world's view, one thing is clear—there is a general lack of experience and a fear of the unknown when it comes to an integrated human-robot interaction. In this study, references were made to a reportedly negative perception of robots, based on their appearance, mistrust of its reliability, potential threat to replacing or significant change to established human tasks, ethical concerns revolving supervision, and liability toward the robot and/or its operator.[4]

The demand and use case for telemedicine was witnessed in full swing during the COVID-19 pandemic; however, its existence and benefit have been established long before the pandemic. One key benefit is the delivery of specialized care across long distances and into the safety and comfort of patients' homes. The need for lengthy and potentially expensive transportation costs to the patient would also be reduced. Patients could potentially attend clinic visits with minimal interruption to their workday or other responsibilities. The social distancing requirements put forth by COVID-19 were also mitigated safely by telemedicine. Depending on the type of care needed, telemedicine has some distinct advantages and disadvantages. Clinicians need to rapidly pivot their style of patient examination, relying more on the interview and elaborately described symptoms and physical details when direct contact is not possible. Visual inspection of various parts of the body rather than tactile examination has become the mainstay. On the other hand, video evaluations may not lend well to visits needing detailed examination of tissue texture, shape, or consistency; joint manipulation; or close inspection of the body such as the skin or genital regions.

Though the current delivery of video telemedicine may not seem pertinent to the robotics industry, the overall simplification of the patient visit, its repetitive nature, and delivery of care on demand and in the patients' desired location may lend well to robotic integration. Clinicians have a typical limited set of interview questions to determine what course of action would need to be taken. If the questions are broken down into their components—what, where, when, exacerbating or alleviating factors, and so on—an artificial intelligence programmed to analyze language could potentially determine a most likely diagnosis and initiate a testing or treatment recommendation. With the current state of mobile phone and Internet-based apps possessing seemingly unlimited data resources, now more than ever, there is a possibility that simple medical visits could be fulfilled by a robot. With the appropriate set of detailed and adaptive questions; attached tools such as a thermometer, blood pressure cuff, pulse oximeter; advanced microphones to auscultate the body; and cameras and software to detect superficial lesions or abnormal movements, a physical examination could be performed on demand for patients without ever making contact with the human clinician.

Before one starts to fear that robots will replace the medical provider workforce, consider this—many medical visits could be evaluated in a primary care or urgent care setting with quick and limited interview and examination. The use of a health screening or triage robot could potentially deliver simple, preventive primary care functions regardless of whether a patient has access to a human clinician or even a physical clinic. By offsetting simple medical visits to robots, this could potentially allow human clinicians to focus their time and effort on more complex cases. The notion of "simple visit" is obviously up for interpretation and subject to debate. On one hand, a complex case could genuinely involve the presence of too many or too difficult a problem for the robots' programming to solve. It could alternatively involve care for a patient who simply cannot operate or interact with a robot appropriately to benefit from its care algorithms. Finally, the level or detail or truthfulness of information provided by patients would influence the nature of the visit. Note that this is not simply a limitation in the robots' functions, but also of human willingness, acceptance, and access to a robot.

If the simplest of primary care visits involve a series of health screening questions, vital signs, and point-of-care blood tests (biometrics), it is plausible that visits may be fully automated. Medication and vaccine administration could be performed on demand. Prescription generation and monitoring could be automated as well. Supplies could be delivered by mail in bulk, reordered and replenished automatically, and medication adherence could be monitored with accessory devices at home. Adherence monitoring would require additional ingenuity and forethought. We currently employ simple methods to approximate treatment adherence based on the interview, use of a pill box, physical examination findings, or blood work. Through the clinician-patient relationship, we could then counsel a patient based on the history or test data whether there is evidence to confirm or doubt a patient's adherence to a treatment plan. How would a medical robot reconcile this? The accuracy of interpreting a patient's responses could lead a robot to correctly or incorrectly determine that a patient has been compliant with health recommendations and medications. Take, for example, the act of taking an anticoagulant medication for atrial fibrillation. Optimal dosing of the anticoagulant is paramount to ensure the patient is sufficiently protected from a devastating stroke but also from catastrophic bleeding. If a medical robot is tasked with monitoring the administration of anticoagulants, how would it verify this? Monitoring the pill count may not be enough. Would a camera monitoring the ingestion of the medication be needed? Results of point-of-care testing to confirm a drug is therapeutic may determine whether the robot releases the next dose. What would the robot do if the patient did not take his or her medication? Would the robot be allowed to enforce medication compliance against the will of a patient? The ethics of how a medical robot could monitor and enforce patient compliance needs to be well thought out.

The clinician-patient relationship is delicate and based on trust. The patient must not only be provided with but must also follow a clinician's recommendations. With a detailed history, certain physical examination findings, or laboratory tests, the physician could monitor patient adherence to medication guidelines. This information could be used to counsel patients on their performance. In certain clinical scenarios, accurate information from the patient is paramount for safety. For example, if anticoagulant pill count or video monitoring of pill ingestion happens to be circumvented, without verification via blood test a robot could potentially administer an inappropriate dose and risk injury to the patient. To what end will the robot be allowed to intervene, adjust the medication dose, or counsel (encourage) the patient to adhere to the treatment plan? Would this be the decision point where the robot requires contact by a human clinician? Perhaps this could be done without human verification? Would the robot reprimand the patient for not strictly adhering to the treatment plan? What if the therapeutic relationship (transaction) were to not be conducive? A highly trained robot could thus play a pivotal role in on-demand clinical decision-making.

Interventions may become automated, ranging from simple checking of vital signs to more skilled tasks such as interpreting laboratory or imaging data, mental health counseling and crisis intervention, and emergent procedures such as endotracheal intubation or minor surgery. This question can be made further complex if the industry allows robots to perform these tasks independently with artificial intelligence. Perhaps future clinical robots can synthesize and act on care plans generated on their own rather than being supervised by attending clinicians. Would robots have a role to play in the actual early diagnosis and management of a patient or would it simply augment the decisions made by a human clinician? The process to verify whether a medical robot can independently solve medical problems is discussed by Ashrafian et al.[5] The age-old Turing test is discussed, which challenges whether a human can distinguish between human (control) or computer-generated responses. Though no actual decision-making comparison is performed, they propose a relatively simple and powerful modification. Rather than having a blinded examiner determine whether two interpretations of a medical problem was either computer or human generated, a third response that is human generated is randomly and blindly mixed with the computer-generated response. As a result, the blinded examiner could be tasked to distinguish between responses from a human and a computer (replicating the classic Turing test) or two different humans. This delivers a more stringent examination generating true-or-false, positive-or-negative detection of a computer response, as the response combination would not be consistently and predictably originating from either a computer or a *single* human. The authors challenge the industry by proposing this methodology be used to distinguish responses during a hypothetical medical interview of a patient to a clinician, where the clinician responses could be computer generated.

An oversimplified but current example can be seen in various "chat bots" that offer customer service on websites. Here, customers are engaged via text messaging where a keyword-based program interprets customers' queries to navigate questions regarding a product or service. Take this example and develop it with robust natural verbal conversations with a lifelike display of a human clinician. If designed to exhibit emotion and body language, coupled with the ability to interpret spoken language to perform a medical interview, this could simulate a video telemedicine visit that has become so omnipresent today. Though there are some limitations to examinations over video, history taking remains key, and the automated medical interview may potentially transform the way patients receive and manage their own medical care. What is unclear is whether it is enough for an intelligent robot to simply display a photorealistic image of a clinician, with background office decor to replicate the experience of a human-to-human video visit. If it were enough to simulate human appearance and behavior on video, with enough medical proficiency built in, a true virtual medical visit could be conducted without ever needing human-to-human contact.

One needs to periodically look at his or her own profession or daily routine and ask, "Is there a way I can do this better with a robot?" This is not to say that human actions will *all* be replaced or improved with robots. The dichotomy of human- and robot-specific functions has become blurred over time, where actions we take for granted could either not be performed at all or not be performed as proficiently without the assistance of robots. Performance of repetitive health-care tasks by robots are just the tip of iceberg. The real benefit is the endurance and reproducible precision of performing said repetitive task. At the time of this writing, robots do not complain of excessive work hours or poor working conditions. Robots do not fatigue and decline in task performance as readily as humans unless there is equipment failure. The expectation of robot endurance is far higher with less empathy compared with human performance. There is no influence on robotic performance as a result of criticism or praise. Many may view technology and robots as tireless workhorses that are replaceable when it no longer serves its purpose. To treat a human in such a fashion could be viewed as discrimination.

Robotic assistance in health care is now readily seen in the operating room. Surgical robots have allowed the delivery of extremely precise, minimally invasive operations where a surgeon may not even need to make prolonged physical contact with the patient. Very small incisions are all that may remain to indicate a patient had radical surgery that previously may have resulted in large unsightly scarring. In my own profession of epilepsy neurology, our practice has advanced to collaborate with neurologic surgeons to plan very complex implantations of electrodes in the brain to target precisely, on the order of millimeters, the areas of seizure onset. Though these and other surgeries may be performed manually by a well-trained surgeon, the use of robots to assist in a reproducible and tireless manner has markedly improved not only the accuracy but the aggressiveness, confidence, and complexity of these procedures. However, how can we ensure medical centers or surgeons are competent with robot-assisted surgery? Many may be unaware that these options even exist, so how can the medical community expect patients are given all of these options? Say a patient needs surgery to remove a tumor or other potentially life-threatening lesion located in a delicate area where the margin for error is very small. Say this procedure's risk can be lowered or recovery time can be decreased in half with a robot-assisted surgery. Will patients be influenced to seek this care at the most advanced centers, potentially traveling great distances and at cost to obtain this procedure? We live in a time where online reviews, elaborate infographics, and incredibly high, sometimes unrealistic, expectations are put upon clinicians to deliver the most complex, comprehensive care. Will patients instead drive the advancement for surgeons' use of robotics, or will they trust tried-and-true manual techniques that may have been performed for decades?

Lam et al.[6] writes that with "digital surgery" comes massive amounts of data, not only regarding the surgeon's performance but also for patient information as well. They emphasize that scrutiny of technique, data security, and the ability for surgeons to adapt to new techniques are core pillars to develop and protect. Yet what entity should champion this? Is this push for innovation in the best interest of the patient and driven by patient demand? If robot-assisted surgeries have better outcomes and shorter recovery times, then shorter hospital stays and increased profitability may result. Yet at what other costs? With the drive to shorten hospital length of stay from a payment, quality, and complication perspective, clinicians and administrators also need to strongly consider the risks and overall health-care experience for the patient undergoing technically complicated surgeries. The cost of robotic surgical assistants is currently incredibly high. Though the prospect of minimal invasiveness and shorter recovery time may be attractive to the patient, the robotic operation itself, given its complexity, will likely cost much more in terms of upfront equipment, training, and maintenance compared with a traditional manual operation.

In the home setting, robots may be categorized into (1) service type or assistants for daily activity or (2) companions that are designed with the intent to engage humans socially and emotionally when a human or animal equivalent may not be capable or available. At its face value, this is an admirable goal: to allow patients to live independently with minimal hardship in the comfort of their own home. Chiu et al.[7] profiled a Taiwanese population's opinions following video observation of robots of various physical forms, human, animal, or nonbiological. They showed that acceptance of companion robots into one's life was high regardless of one's previous experience or lack thereof. Superficially, patients appeared to gravitate to certain physical forms that may be visually appealing, such as a friendly face or a cute animal. This would be important for product design to understand what drives the market to a certain type of robot. But should service or companion robots exist purely for the patient's pleasure, or should they have a specific purpose such as performing physical tasks that a disabled or socially isolated human cannot reliably perform? Ideally both purposes would be satisfied.

In a 2017 interview of Maja Matarić, PhD,[8] socially assistive robots and the intended gaps in health care they are intended to fill are profiled. One important point she makes is that a robot's discrete functions or features are less important than how it motivates and encourages patients to facilitate their own recovery. This is a more holistic approach to robotics development than a simple appliance that has unique attributes to improve sales figures. It bridges the human touch, that warm feeling someone gets when given the right words of encouragement to take control of one's health and to actually get better. Traditionally this may be achieved by separate visits with a provider, a therapist, or a social worker. With the right programming, this therapeutic relationship could be combined and achievable at the home regardless of the presence or absence of advanced technical features. We should all be realistic about the physical, mental, and emotional effort involved as well as the limitations to motivate a patient to be adherent to a treatment regimen. Sometimes the right human or right type of motivation may not be available. Dr. Matarić realizes very well that there is a disconnect when care is simply delivered via a large video display. Having a robot small enough for a patient to hold, with different textures or colored "skin," possibly temperature changes, all add to the experience of interacting with a living being. Consider how emotional support animals have different appearances, hair color, breathing patterns, mannerisms in response to a patient's state of well-being. Robots that detect these physiologic changes in humans and adapt their responses and tangible characteristics accordingly could provide very therapeutic effects. She recognizes that to pioneer robots to help people, the robots in essence may need to become more "human."

This also illustrates a complex social problem impacting patients and the role of robots at home. Human interactions, not just between clinician and patient but on a larger societal scale, could be supplemented, if not replaced, by robots. Depending on your point of view, this may or may not be desirable. One needs to exercise caution and determine whether living with a robot is not only appropriate but truly desirable by the patient. The obvious altruistic explanation would be that the patient has a genuine physical or psychologic benefit from a robot or companion. Alternatively, this may be the result of insufficient human effort or financial resources to provide this type of care direct at the bedside or in the home environment. This is not to say that human-to-human care is not possible—some patients may prefer the interaction with a support animal or robot for a number of reasons. However, health-care workers, administrators, robot developers, and most importantly patients' family members should consider whether the use of a robot is truly of direct benefit to the patient and not preferential to other stakeholders seeking respite from the caretaker role.

Care of patients with cognitive impairment can be very demanding, and caregivers deserve respite from these duties, which many times can be an all-day affair. This is a very popular area of research focusing on neuropsychiatric disorders such as autism spectrum disorder, attention deficit hyperactivity disorder, and various forms of cognitive impairment and dementia.[9] Having a robot engage and occupy a patient would allow the caretaker to satisfy other needs of the household, perhaps go to work or engage in his or her own social needs while the loved one is kept occupied. There would be a delicate balance between augmenting the daily activities/interactions of a patient with impaired cognition and simply offloading the effort involved to monitor this patient. This challenge is not unlike parenting in general. Young children have individual likes/dislikes and needs. Not all of these may be met to their satisfaction by the parent or caretaker. The complexity of these interactions may not need to be very sophisticated. Like toys that are designed to entertain and occupy a child, robots may provide simple activities to patients with neurocognitive impairment. The caretaker as well as the clinician would need to decide whether this is appropriate, as it may not be socially acceptable for an adult to behave and interact with objects like a child. There is negative social stigma toward patients with disabilities in the general public, particularly cognitive impairment. The root of this is most commonly insufficient knowledge, experience, and understanding by the lay public on the challenges patients and their caretakers face. The crude example of a "large baby" who can only communicate in simple grunts or vocalizations and only interacts with playthings does not do this justice. Older children or adults with neuropsychiatric dysfunction may exhibit disinhibited behavior, require very constant or repetitive stimulation, and may act out or behave negatively when their needs are not met. This is typically due to insufficient understanding of a disabled patient's needs and assumptions made by caretakers and clinicians alike—such as hunger, pain, television, and so on.

Robots can also provide more reliable and trackable data on a patient's behavioral patterns. This can range from tacking daily habits such as feeding, toileting, and medication administration but can also be very individualized such as patterns of interest toward certain activities, other people, or interactions with the environment. It may be possible that robots and artificial intelligence can continuously monitor these and detect and predict trends in a patient's behavior better than a human caretaker. These human-robot interactions are not without merit and go beyond simple entertainment or consumption of time. Some case reports have shown improvement in independence, initiation of social interaction, and improved (more detailed) expression of wants and needs in patients with autism.[10] Other studies reported improvement in following or reproducing movements and following musical cues. Objective findings of reduced cortical thinning involving the anterior cingulate have been reported in the elderly.[9] Though some of these achievements may seem simple, given the severity of cognitive dysfunction within this population, any improvement in social interaction would be deemed significant given the time and effort necessary to appreciate even the smallest of gains.

Perhaps some patients have personalities or mannerisms that are not conducive to companionship with another human. This would then question whether a patient's actions resulting in incompatibility with a human are appropriate to subject to an animal or robot companion. Where do robots stand in this spectrum of patient-companion relationship? Say the barrier to a patient-human caregiver relationship was due to negative, possibly abusive, mannerisms by the patient. Would it be appropriate to then subject an animal or a robot to this kind of behavior? One can assume that "robots don't have feelings, therefore patients can treat them however they please," yet this may miss the point of what a companion robot was initially designed for. We assume that companions help and enhance a human's behavior such that future interactions—be they with other humans, animals, or objects—regardless of whether real or virtual, occur in a societally accepted manner. However, if a patient with abusive or negatively interpreted mannerisms is allowed to continue this behavior onto a robot that may not act in defense, what rehabilitative benefit is provided to the patient? In this hypothetical situation, negatively interpreted behavior may be perpetuated, potentially at the detriment of the patient's contribution to or reintegration with society.

Doring et al.[11] provide a very detailed review of the current literature of sex dolls and sex robots and their impact on human sexuality. Where this article truly exemplifies itself is how it challenges the reader and the medical/science community as a whole to consider how advances in robotics can impact not just how we interact with one another, but how human-robot interaction can mold the way humans seek relationships. On one hand, the unidirectional relationship of user and robot (product) can be seen as a predictable transaction of commands resulting in set responses. The sexual health and desires of the user are either satisfied or unsatisfied by the constraints of what the robot is designed to perform. The human-robot relationship could be taken a step further if the supportive or companion functions of the robot surpass those that a human partner or caretaker is capable or *willing* to provide. This again partly returns to the notion that robots in this day and age are primarily compliant objects. This can have significant benefits as well as consequences. Whereas the tireless nature of robots would be of benefit for repetitive tasks, if the relationship is more involved, say with sexual health, the user or patient in this case could become accustomed to not only the functions (service) but the compliance (willingness) of the robot. Doring et al. discuss existing literature raising concerns that this could perpetuate dysfunctional sexual behavior. Say a patient uses a sex doll and explores his or her desires fully and without judgment. This may involve intercourse as well as nurturing functions such as supportive conversations, which is assumed to be therapeutic. Should the patient instead exhibit verbally or physically abusive tendencies onto an otherwise compliant robot, this would potentially perpetuate deviant behavior, which may possibly be inflicted on future human partners. Robot developers, clinicians, patients, and caretakers alike would need to acknowledge and agree that robots with advanced companion functions may not only supplement relationships but can facilitate pathologic behavior as well.

In conclusion, the use of a medical robot would not just revolve around patient monitoring, trust or mistrust, but most importantly independent self-care. Medical robot use has the potential to accelerate the delivery of care simply by increasing access. The analysis and guidance a medical robot provides could facilitate earlier intervention to common medical comorbidities such as obesity, hypertension, and diabetes and its sequelae on a daily basis rather than from one clinic visit to another. Robotics developers and clinicians would need to determine how much of simpler, primary care should be automated. Medical errors and accuracy would need to be scrutinized. Should there be future determination that the robot misdiagnosed or incorrectly administered a medication, what entity would be responsible? Would the robot undergo human supervision of some or all recommendations? If an error was made, would the robot developer or its human supervisor (if one exists) reconcile this? How much would user (patient) error be a factor? We would need to imagine that given the technology gap that already exists in the general population, there will be at least an initial limitation to the comfort and engagement by patients in their own care delivered by a robot. Socioeconomic differences are likely to impact the availability and acceptance of medical robots. The research and development of an artificial intelligence that is capable of accurately diagnosing basic conditions or is compact enough to readily deploy in the homes of patients will likely come at great cost. It is thus assumed that early adoption of this technology would be limited to patients who not only are accepting and competent with technology but who have the purchasing power to obtain these devices and services.

Services, both medical and technical, will likely require upkeep and may necessitate (or monetize) a subscription akin to Internet, phone, or television services. This is bound to impact how health insurance companies in the United States or government health services regulate the reimbursement of medical robotics. If a robot with the promise of personalized care can provide lower-cost preventive care in an automated fashion, it would be advantageous for developers to leverage this not only for profit but also for a reasonable cost to patients. The potential for lower cost per patient care via a medical robot may influence insurance companies to reward patients with the use of a robot over a human clinician. Clinicians who are early to adopt these technologies for supervision could potentially monitor the health of a greater number of patients remotely. Remote monitoring with a theoretically higher volume may result in higher productivity and reimbursement. If used effectively, this may fill the primary care gap. If not implemented appropriately, these systems may instead add to the workload burden and burnout of clinicians practicing today. The prospect of medical robotics is boundless and no longer just a dream or a science fiction fantasy; however, strong collaboration among patients, clinicians, and developers is more important than ever to ensure its implementation is successful and beneficial.

References

1. Nepal S, Keniston A, Indovina KA, et al. What do patients want? A qualitative analysis of patient, provider, and administrative perceptions and expectations about patients' hospital stays. *J Patient Exp.* 2020;7(6):1760–1770. https://doi.org/10.1177/2374373520942403. In press.
2. Ma AC, Meng Z, Ding X. Performance review of intelligent guidance robot at the outpatient clinic setting. *Cureus.* 2021;13(8):1–4. e16840. https://doi.org/10.7759/cureus.16840. In press.
3. Chai PR, Dadabhoy FZ, Huang H-W, et al. Assessment of the acceptability and feasibility of using mobile robotic systems for patient evaluation. *JAMA Network Open.* 2021;4(3):1–13. e210667. https://doi.org/10.1001/jamanetworkopen.2021.0667. In press.
4. Cresswell K, Cunningham-Burley S, Sheikh A. Health care robotics: qualitative exploration of key challenges and future directions. *J Med Internet Res.* 2018;20(7):1–11. e10410. https://doi.org/10.2196/10410. In press.
5. Ashrafian H, Darzi A, Athanasiou T. A novel modification of the Turing test for artificial intelligence and robotics in healthcare. *Int J Med Robotics Comput Assist Surg.* 2015;11:38–43. https://doi.org/10.1002/rcs.1570. In press.
6. Lam K, Purkayastha S, Kinross JM. The ethical digital surgeon. *J Med Internet Res.* 2021;23(7):1–3. e25849. https://doi.org/10.2196/25849. In press.
7. Chiu C-J, Hsieh S, Li C-W. Needs and preferences of middle-aged and older adults in Taiwan for companion robots and pets: survey study. *J Med Internet Res.* 2021;23(6):1–15. e23471. https://doi.org/10.2196/23471. In press.
8. Abbasi J. Socially assistive robots help patients make behavioral changes. *JAMA.* 2017:317(24):2472-2474. In press.
9. Yuan F, Klavon E, Liu Z, et al. A systematic review of robotic rehabilitation for cognitive training. *Front Robot AI.* 2021;8:605715. https://doi.org/10.3389/frobt.2021.605715. In press.
10. Scassellati B, Boccanfuso L, Huang C-M, et al. Improving social skills in children with ASD using a long-term, in-home social robot. *Sci Robot.* 2018;3:eaat7544. https://doi.org/10.1126/scirobotics.aat7544. In press.
11. Doring N, Mohseni MR, Walter R. Design, use, and effects of sex dolls and sex robots: scoping review. *J Med Internet Res.* 2020;22(7):1–28. e18551. https://doi.org/10.2196/18551. In press.

4

Robot and Artificial Intelligence Companies Around the Globe

Douglas P. Murphy

KEY POINTS

- Health-care robotic companies are thriving on every continent.
- Every sector of the health-care industry is being targeted for robotic support.
- Most of these companies are thriving economically.
- Artificial intelligence is driving the robotic industry to vast new capabilities.

The undeniable presence of robotics in the health field can easily be seen in the emergence of numerous robotic companies that are well funded and often thriving through sales and service to the health sector. Many hospitals now have at least some version of robotic offerings to enhance the health-care environment and improve service to patients. In the following chapter some of the leading robotic companies around the world will be profiled for what they have achieved and for how they plan to improve and expand their robots through research and development. Each of these companies play an international role and seek to change in dramatic and positive ways the nature of health-care delivery.

The number of categories for robotic applications continues to increase. Nearly every facet of medicine has seen some developments from this type of technology. Types of robotic applications include (1) training robots; (2) emotional support robots; (3) rehabilitation robots; (4) surgical robots; (5) rescue robots; (6) robots for pharmaceutical applications; (7) robots for transport within hospitals; (8) nursing robots; (9) avatar robots; (10) robots for blood draws; (11) disinfection robots; (12) robotic process automation; and (13) patient simulation robots. There are even robots that attempt the physician functions of diagnosis and treatment. The fields of artificial intelligence (AI) and the brain-computer interface are closely linked to these fields if not actually integral to them. For each of these areas, there are companies working vigorously to create products that propel the practice of medicine forward. Although some companies strive for robotic and AI products that are specifically geared to certain roles, others offer more generic types of solutions that can be adapted to any given facility's individual needs.

The drive to integrate robots into our culture and health-care delivery systems thrives in countries throughout the world. Some of the leaders in these efforts include the United States, China, Japan, South Korea, and Germany.

Not all developments come through private industry. Academic centers throughout the world compete to bring forward newer and more spectacular technological achievements. In the United States many colleges and universities and colleges feature departments devoted to this field. Certain universities such as Massachusetts Institute of Technology (MIT) and Stanford are well known for their work in this field. The interchange between academic programs, robotic companies, and governments is often significant.

The third leg of the system for development in the United States involves the Department of Defense, which funds projects among its own ranks, in industry and in academics. Some of those areas relate to the medical management of soldiers on the battlefield. Nevertheless, the Department of Defense plays a role in the activities of industry and academics, a role with substantial importance in terms of funding and influence for future directions. A separate chapter will be devoted to these efforts.

The following is a tour around the world of some companies that are playing crucial roles. There are many more but unfortunately only a sample can be feasibly highlighted.

United States

DILIGENT ROBOTICS

Diligent Robotics[1] has two cofounders who have created the engaging but equally as useful Moxi, the robot who functions as a frontline aid to health-care workers in a hospital. Andreas Thomaz is chief executive officer and has worked hand in hand with Vivian Chu, the chief technology officer. Dr. Chus's bio includes an undergraduate degree in electrical engineering and computer science at the University of California at Berkeley and a master's degree at the University of Pennsylvania, where she worked at the GRASP lab in the Haptics Research Group. Her doctorate in robotics came at Georgia Tech. Here she met and received training from Andrea Thomaz, her future partner. In addition to her role as an adjunct professor and senior research scientist in the Department of Electrical and Computer Engineering at the University of Texas at Austin, Dr. Thomaz received her bachelor's of science degree in electrical and computer engineering at the University of Texas at Austin and then both her master's of science and doctor of philosophy degrees from MIT.

Robots can take different tracks in health care, and the Diligent Robotics model includes support of clinical staff through fielding tasks such as the delivery and transport of patient care items that can include medicines and laboratory samples. The service includes automation so that the robot can independently access medical records and receive instructions from an electronic system. After internalizing a map, the robot can navigate throughout the hospital and interface with different wards and clinics. An increase in need in any given area can be addressed.

Moxi has multiple features that provide significant advantages to a hospital system (Fig. 4.1). Its robotic arm can manipulate items in the environment and can be used to access elevators and

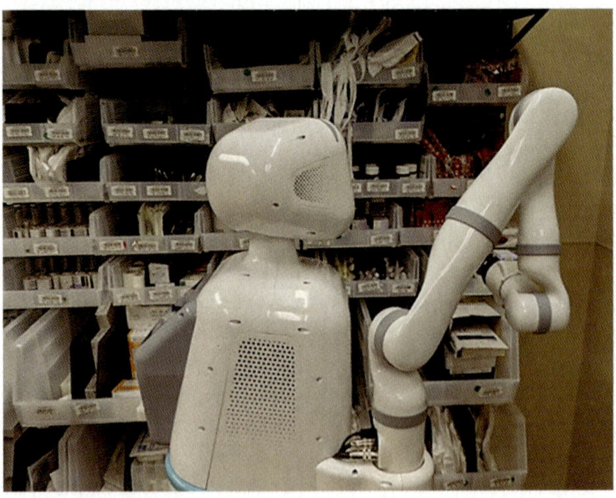

Fig. 4.1 Moxi from Diligent Robotics (diligentrobots.com).

open doors. The high-speed Wi-Fi can integrate with the one working within a given hospital. It has a relatively roomy, secure compartment for the transport of hospital items from one location to another. It has embedded computing and cloud-based software. Sensors allow the robot to move throughout the hospital without posing any sort of safety hazard to staff, patients, or hospital infrastructure.

The face of the robot has LED lights that can configure friendly, warm, and endearing expressions that help staff and patient moral. Finally, AI within the robot systems help Moxi learn from experience. It can then utilize this information and learning to increase its effectiveness. The types of deliveries Moxi can make are quite varied. Lightweight equipment, laboratory samples, pharmacy deliveries, discharge medications, COVID-19 tests and kits, personal protective equipment (PPE), nutrition, hospitality items, bone, tissue, and blood bank supplies comprise many of its capacities. The company estimates the robot is equivalent to 2.75 full-time equivalents or up to 22 hours of work a day while the rest of the time is spent recharging. Its activities can be monitored remotely, and there is a common ledger of work actions that can be added to or subtracted from at nursing stations or other locations.

OLIVE

Olive[2] is a relatively new company that has introduced a cloud-based AI system to facilitate the interactions between providers and payors for automation that is faster, less cumbersome, and more efficient. The cloud-based system coordinates the activities of payors and providers through an AI interface that makes transactions swift and efficient. Areas addressed include reimbursement management, patient access, clearinghouse actions, payments, and population health. The vision for this company came from Sean Lane, a software engineer who worked in military intelligence and the National Security Agency as a software engineer. The company promises streamlined, faster, more efficient, and less expensive processes.

GAUMARD SCIENTIFIC

Based in Miami, Florida, Gaumard Scientific specializes in simulators and health-care provider training systems. HAL is a pediatric robotic training simulator that convincingly looks like a small boy and that can communicate feelings and responses to situations that would stress a living child (Fig. 4.2). Health-care providers can practice procedures and learn to cope with the protests and

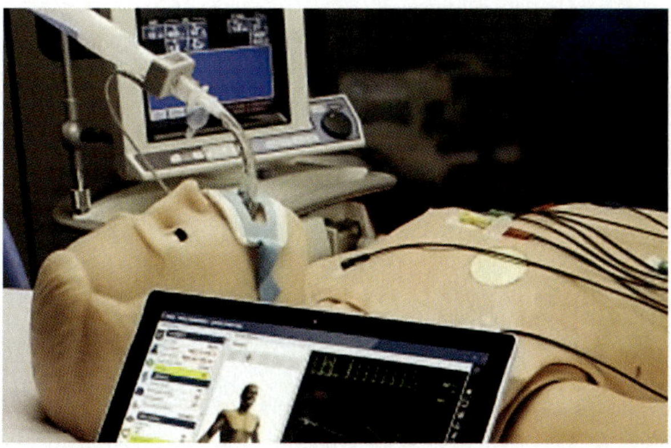

Fig. 4.2 HAL the medical robot from Gaumard Scientific.

discomfort a real child would provide. Per the company's website,[3] the wireless and tether-less simulator has the following capabilities:

Interactive eyes and active facial expressions

Dynamic lung compliance with true ventilator support

Real patient monitoring support: Spo_2, electrocardiograph, capnography, non-invasive blood pressure (NIBP), live pacing, and defibrillation

Emergency intervention: surgical airway, needle decompression, chest tube insertion

ROBOTIC SURGICAL SIMULATOR

The Da Vinci Robotic Surgery system, or RoSS,[4] is one of the most widely used for robot-guided and robot-assisted surgeries. However, to use it successfully, of course, requires training. The RoSS (Fig. 4.3) was developed through a collaboration between the Center for Robotic Surgery at Roswell Park Comprehensive Cancer Center and the University of Buffalo (UB) School of Engineering and Applied Sciences.

XENEX

Xenex,[5] a Houston-based company, has a produced a robot that employs ultraviolet light to kill microorganisms in hospitals and thus reduce the incidence of hospital-acquired infections such a *Clostridium difficile* colitis. Two epidemiologists started the company in 2008, and there has been substantial growth in their operations since then. The robot can negotiate any hospital space for disinfection and thus is highly effective in reducing toxic microorganism loads in the hospital environment.

VASCULOGIC LLC

VascuLogic LLC[6] offers the product VenousPro (Fig. 4.4). This system allows the user to operate it through a touchless screen. The patient places his or her arm into the machine, which can then identify a suitable vein for a blood draw. The system uses ultrasound to locate and assess a vein for venipuncture and once this is done the needle is placed into the vein for an accurate, one-time blood draw. The system thus promotes accuracy and comfort and avoids repeated draws due to unsuccessful attempts.

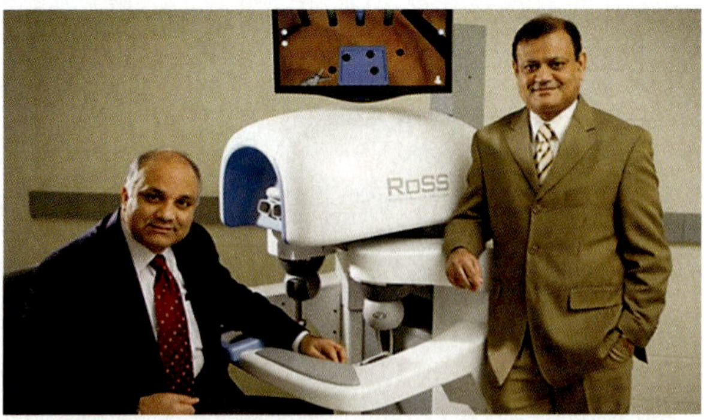

Fig. 4.3 DaVinci Robotic Surgery system; robotic surgery at Rosewell Park Comprehensive Cancer Center and University at Buffalo School of Engineering and Applied Sciences.

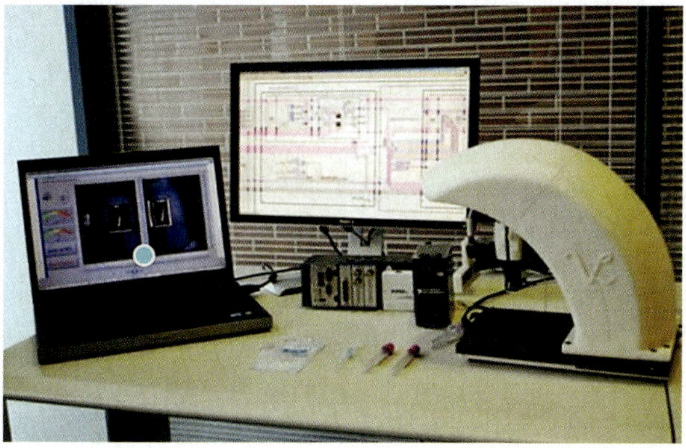

Fig. 4.4 VenousPro from VascuLogic.

ASENSUS SURGICAL

Formerly called Transenterix, this company advertises "performance-guided surgery." The Senhance minimally invasive laparoscopic surgical system boasts an eye-tracking camera, a digital interface with the patient, haptic sensing, and many other fascinating new features.

MEDROBOTICS CORPORATION

This company was founded in 2005 and is based in Massachusetts. Its main product is the Flex Robotic System, which has been Food and Drug Administration approved since 2015. The Flex Robotic System is designed to navigate with a flexible probe to tissues that do not have a linear access path such as oral access locations. There is an inner system contained within an outer one that is steered through a joystick. Rigid and flexible technologies are combined. Medrobotix obtained the worldwide licenses for technologies developed at the Carnegie Mellon University and the University of Pittsburg. The Flex Robotic System provides a high density (HD) image of anatomical structures. The company was recently acquired by the University of Kentucky.

BURT THERAPY

This company came as an offshoot of the MIT Artificial Intelligence Laboratory in 1990. It developed the WAM arm, which is the first haptic robotic arm. At its inception it was considered the most advanced robotic arm. Burt Therapy is also branching into stroke rehabilitation.

LUVOZO PBC

Luvozo PBC[7] is a start-up located at the University of Maryland with a robot named Sam to help the elderly. This robot can provide frequent check-ins and nonmedical care. It is described as a robotic concierge, and aside from remote check-ins, it can provide telehealth services and delivery of items. Luvozo also has a disinfecting robot.

Canada

Each country has its own unique needs, and in Canada delivering health care and in particular emergency care to remote towns in isolated, rural areas during warm but also more importantly extremely cold weather represents a Canadian concern. In Saskatchewan the use of such technology is already a reality. If a sick individual shows up in a clinic with a serious condition in a remote northern town, a doctor can navigate a robot to that individual and perform an assessment. The robot provides multiple opportunities for the physician who could be hundreds of miles away. Through the robot he can see the patient. He can assess breath sounds with the robot stethoscope, measure the oxygen levels through pulse oximetry, talk to the nurse, take an electrocardiograph. The telestrator allows the doctor to draw helpful pictures on a screen on the robot to get certain types of information across to the nurse or patient. Thus, skilled and expert assessment and treatment are delivered effectively across miles of distance through a robotic avatar.

The push for the development of this technology in this country is quite strong. The Canadian government[8] has applied millions of dollars to make sure academic centers keep up with the race for sophisticated and useful AI. For example, in the 2021 budget the government promises Canadian (CAD) $443.8 million over 10 years for AI development. The 2021 budget will distribute monetary support in a way that the following examples illustrate: (1) CAD $185 million for the commercialization of AI; (2) CAD $162.2 million for recruiting top talent in this area; (3) CAD $48 million for the Canadian Institute for Advanced Research; (4) CAD $40 million to increase computing capacity at AI institutes in Edmonton, Montreal and Toronto. There are other distributions as well.

EMTECH, INC

Combining robotic and AI technology Emtech[9] in Ottawa, Canada, provides consultancy solutions for multiple industries including health care. Their services cross the full network of players in Canada and include payers, providers, and business performance management. For these departments, the benefits of these systems include automation of tedious tasks, more efficiency through streamlining, coordination across platforms, predictive modeling, enhancing self-service for patients, and so forth. These sorts of innovation work toward improving practice finances, supply chains, customer satisfaction, human resource operations, medical records, cyber security, and data analytics for practice improvement, among other areas.

HOLO ROBOTS

Holo Robots[10] is a Canadian company that specializes in telepresence robots with applications across all fields including health care. Its robots boast cameras, sensors (stereo vision, ultrasound, wheel encoders, inertial measurement), microphones, a speaker, a 9.7-inch display, a battery with 4 hours of run time and 2 hours of charge time, and wireless connectivity, among other features. Multiple robots can be managed through a central portal. Surgeons have used the robot for rounding on patients when at a conference or other remote location and can manipulate the robot from virtually any platform such as a laptop or a smartphone. With the worldwide shortage of doctors and nurses, telepresence robots offer a solution that allows doctors and nurses to have a remote presence, and thus the robots serve as extenders for healthcare professionals.

Europe

Assistive robots in Europe are providing a strong and growing presence there, although companies from other regions of the world such as the United States and Japan are providing robots that are also used in the European health system. Manus made an early debut, and now another robot mounted manipulator, iArm, is offering a sophisticated robot arm that is produced through Exact Dynamics. The iArm can lift up to 1.5 kg with 6 degrees of freedom and has a reach of nearly a meter. The arm offers high dexterity and functionality.[11] Individuals with motor challenges can operate the device through a 250-kbit Controller Area Network (CAN) interface that uses both a Cartesian system of control and a velocity control.

BESTIC

An example of a more specialized robotic arm for individuals with motor challenges comes from a Swedish company and is called Bestic (Fig. 4.5). Motor challenges can vary from weakness to spastic or ataxic movements that make self-feeding difficult or impossible.[12]

The following companies represent an array of European companies that offer some interesting and cutting-edge technologies for interventional medicine. These are grouped according to the country of their home base.

Austria

TYROMOTION

Tyromotion[13] specializes in robot-assisted gait rehabilitation. It offers an array of products for both the upper extremities and lower extremities.

France

Founded in 2009 by Phillipe Bencteux and Bruno Fournier and with a valuation of several million euros, Robocath takes a lead in robotic treatments and intervention for cardiovascular conditions. R-One has received the CE mark, and it is a robotic device that has great precision and specificity and is compatible with technology already in catheterization laboratories. The operator sits at the control behind a shield and operates the robotic arm to insert cardiac stents, for example.[14] The company is targeting remote interventions for cardiovascular emergent conditions and has the potential to become a world leader in this direction.

Germany

In 2014 Stephan Nowatschin and Maximilian Krinninger founded Medineering Surgical Robotics, now a part of Brainlab Robotics, which advertises robotic surgical solutions for every subspecialty of surgery. Medineering originally targeted robotic interventions for the complex

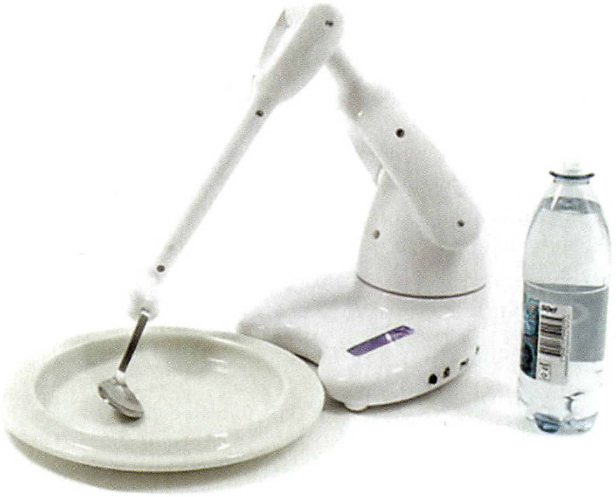

Fig. 4.5 Bestic eating device from Bestic AB, Sweden (Camanio AB, Sweden.)

anatomy involved in ear, nose, and throat surgery. However, Medineering has partnered with Brainlab to provide applications for neurosurgery. The Medineering device is modular and operates from a scalable platform. In addition to its surgical alternatives, Brainlab also has applications for radiotherapy, medical image sharing, and the digitalization of operating rooms.

KUKA ROBOTICS

This company is headquartered in Augsburg, Germany, but has branches throughout the world such as in Argentina, Brazil, Mexico, the United States, Canada, Singapore, China, South Africa, and many other locations. With sales of around €2.6 billion and about 14,000 employees, KUKA provides strong leadership in automation and robotics. It has a division devoted to robotics in health care. One of its first robotic systems in medicine was the surgical-radiation CyberKnife used for inoperable tumors in 2001.

Some of their high payload systems allow for the precise positioning of patients in coordination with other medical devices such as computed tomography scanners and the delivery of radiation treatments to precise locations for the ablation of tumors.

Kuka has now become part of Midea, a Chinese company and one of the largest in the world that has assets of around $40 billion.

Netherlands

Shiqian Wang founded Reboocon Bionics in 2016 to provide service robotic solutions for those individuals with disabilities. This type of intervention comes through lightweight, intelligent robots and ones that assist the mobility impaired in getting up and walking.

Spain

GOGOA

Founded in 2015 by Carlos F. Isoird, GOGOA Mobility Robotics[15] provides wearable robotic technology to facilitate ambulation and other mobility needs for individuals with impairments. Its products include Hank, the lower-extremity exoskeleton; Belk, the knee exoskeleton; and the Hand of Hope, which is a hand exoskeleton, as well as exoskeletons for industry. The exoskeleton Hank has a CE mark.

ABLE HUMAN MOTION

Another company providing exoskeletons such as for spinal cord injury is ABLE Human Motion.[16] Alex Garcia, Alfons Carnicero, and Josep Font founded the company in 2018. The exoskeleton allows the user with lower-limb paralysis to stand from a wheelchair and walk with the device that is relatively lightweight given that it is powered. An assistive device may be necessary but nevertheless the energy required is less than with passive knee ankle foot orthoses. The company is based in Barcelona and is dedicated to improving the life of individuals with disabilities.

Sweden

ACOUSORT

Torsten Freltoft founded AcouSort[17] in 2010. The company provides technology involved in cell separation, enrichment, and handling through acoustophoresis. Cells can be moved through acoustic vibrations (ultrasound) in a fashion that does not destroy them. Through use of ultrasound and the adjustment of various parameters, blood components can be moved through different channels and thus different blood products can be separated from the whole blood sample. Particle size, density, compressibility as well as the characteristics of the surrounding medium can be utilized to make the process accurate.

Switzerland

AOT SWISS

Founders Alfedo Bruno, Hans Florian Zeilhofer, Jurgens Philipp, and Philippe Catting created AOT Swiss[18] in 2010 based on technology that can perform bone surgeries with extraordinary precision using a robotic arm with navigation and control software that produces a laser that at the incision site and leaves bone tissue intact. The machine is called CARLO or Cold Ablation Robot-Guided Laser Osteotome. The nature of the incision allows bone to regenerate more easily at the incision site. Any desired geometric pattern can be created.

HOCOMA

Hocoma is a Swiss company started in 1996. Hocoma has a host of robotic therapies for neurologic conditions such as stroke, traumatic brain injuries, multiple sclerosis, and so on as well as low back pain. It has branches in the United States, Singapore, Slovenia, and Chile. One of its robotic gait training systems is the Andago that combines support and safety but also guidance toward improved gait for patients who have suffered gait impairing neurologic disorders. Other devices include robotic treadmill training and exoskeletons for upper-extremity retraining.

REHA TECHNOLOGY

This Swiss company also makes a robotic gait training device called the G-EO System Evolution, which has found a place in hospitals in Germany, Switzerland, and the Czech Republic. This device has applications to a pediatric population. The device employs repetition of normalized gait patterns applied to a patient's lower extremities to entrain and retrain nerve cells to gradually model normal gait through the benefits of repetition and sensory feedback on neural plasticity.

Russia

Russia also has companies to compete in the global robotics market. There are five current trends[19] in the Russian robotic market and certainly the robotic health-care market partakes of these trends. These trends concern the government support and promotion of robotics, the need and use of educational robots, the market for service sector robotics and industrial robotics, and finally robots developed for use in small and medium-sized businesses. In 2017 the Digital Economy of the Russian Federation received its launch. The Russian Association of Robotics is working in conjunction with the Ministry of Trade and Industry to strategize and promote this area. Included in these efforts is an effort on the part of the government to accelerate and extend the development of advanced robotics and AI technologies. The educational robots have taken an important role both for the economy of this sector and for its development. Thirty-one percent of all service robots in 2017 from the 10 leading companies were sold for educational purposes. Educational robots take on many different types of interfaces and programs such as drones for pilots and those with neurologic interfaces. The country provides instructional courses for robots to children and to teachers to foster the growth of this area and to fill anticipated future workforce needs. The country also has instituted compulsory computer science training since 1985, and this training has resulted in a well-trained talent bank of programmers. Another strong component in the

Russian robotic sector is the one for service robots, and there are at least 100 service robot companies providing products over a wide gamut. The top 10 companies are seeing an annual doubling of revenue and are rapidly increasing their staff to fit their needs. The companies have managed sales and profits both domestically and in a plethora of foreign countries. For example, Promobot (see later) receives sales revenue from around 33 countries that comprise 61% of its bottom line. Exports to 10 countries comprise 30% of revenues for Alpha Robotics. Similarly ROBBO, a manufacturer of educational robots, has markets in at least 12 countries.

EXOATLET

Creating exoskeletons for rehabilitation ExoAtlet has cultivated the Asian market for its product. The company markets ExoAtlet for a wide range of neurologic disorders such as spinal cord injury, traumatic brain injury, stroke, multiple sclerosis, and postsurgical arthroplasty. Research collaborations are encouraged. It has the CE mark and is ISO13485 certified with certifications and acceptance in India, South Korea, Kazakhstan, Thailand, Russian, and Vietnam. Dr. Miguel Pais-Vieira, a professor at Catolica University in Portugal, has used the device in brain-computer interface trials. The device can allow users to go up and down stairs and over uneven terrain. Data can be uploaded for storage in a cloud service.[20] The company has organized an annual symposium on exo-rehabilitation to exchange clinical and research experiences using such devices to rehabilitate people with these neurologic disorders.

PROMOBOT

Hadassah Medical, an Israeli hospital chain that has a clinic at Skolkovo Innovation Center, currently employs robotics from Promobot. These robots have AI systems and can measure a patient's blood oxygen levels, temperature, blood glucose levels, and lung volumes. Information is processed through the AI systems, which then makes recommendations.[21] Through such performance the robot can shoulder some of the doctor's duties and thus free up time for other tasks. These types of robots can to some extent alleviate the shortage of doctors and nurses in Russia and other countries such as the United Kingdom. The Ministry of Health in Russia suggests a shortfall of roughly 148,000 doctors and 800,000 nurses, and thus measures to counteract this issue take on greater significance. Promobot collaborates with clinics throughout the world and attempts to raise the level of care through its technologies and has adapted these technologies to meet the demands of the COVID-19 crisis. In addition to robots with the functions mentioned previously, Promobot offers Robo-C, a companion robot that has the capacity to mimic human emotion. It can carry on conversations, remember faces, scan and fill documents, manage a smart home, and connect with third-party applications.[22]

India

In India as in many other countries around the world, a shortage of doctors exists such that for every 1445 Indians, there is a single doctor. The World Health Organization recommends a ratio of 1 doctor per 1000 people. Hospital beds are also lacking, and the country's ratio of 0.7 beds per 1000 people falls short of the global average of 3.4. Here are some of the robotic and AI companies that currently are among those attempting to remediate this situation.[23]

ASIMOV (ADVANCED SYSTEMS WITH INTELLIGENCE MOBILITY AND VISION) ROBOTICS

ASIMOV (Advanced Systems with Intelligence Mobility and Vision) Robotics has multiple offerings that have impacted both the medical and defense sectors. Its technologies address robotic simulation and control, machine vision, virtual reality, and navigation. The company has developed KARMI-Bot to assist in the care of patients in isolation units through multiple functions. These functions would include independent navigation, delivery of food and medical supplies, video conferencing, engaging patients, and disinfection. The SEVABOT provides services such as transport of blood and ampoules to the surgical suites, intensive care unit, and pharmacy. CHHAYA provides customer assistance and information and has the capabilities through AI of showing emotion and providing gestures through prosthetics. The platform is a nonmobile torso and human appearing face. SAYABOT is another humanoid, AI-driven robot with a wide range of capabilities that include uses in health care. In addition to health care some of its functions include security, banking, hospitality, and education.

INVENTO

Invento Robotics has created Mitra, a robot with numerous capabilities. The companies advertise functions such as face recognition, autonomous navigation, AI, and fleet management where a remote human operator can manipulate the robot(s).[24] Ralaji Viswanathan founded the company in 2016. The robots are companion robots and work as medical assistants. The robots can converse with patients and have wide ranging conversational skills. The robot can act as a remote avatar and can utilize traditional examination tools such as the stethoscope. Mitra can do the initial interview with the patient and after permission take the patient's photo. It can then collect some historical information and vital signs, after which it can connect the patient to the physician who can remotely communicate and either write a prescription at that point or direct the patient to further assessment and treatment. Mitra can roam the hospital and recognize hospital personnel and patients through its facial recognition systems. Patient data are carefully protected and encrypted to meet government standards of patient privacy. The company is selling the robots in at least five countries.

SASTRA

With headquarters in Cochin, India, Sastra Robotics[25] has built up a reputation in some assessments as one of the top 50 robotic startups in the world. Its robots have a facility in mimicking human actions. The company advertises smart surgical and medical diagnostic devices for the medical field but has applications to many other fields as well. For its medical diagnostic equipment, the company has created a product with an advanced human machine interface that consists of both touch screen capabilities as well as voice commands.

India has a burgeoning sector of AI companies that have entered the health-care marketplace[26] and that are attempting to revolutionize the ways in which health care is provided. Many of these companies cover areas similar to those mentioned for other countries such as image analysis, breast cancer screening and early detection, online doctor consultation tools such as for one's smartphone, as well as health guidance systems on things like diet and exercise. Let us explore a few of these interesting startups.

LYBRATE

Lybrate joins the ranks of online doctor consultation systems and has been in operation since 2014. Its platform will link the user to an appropriate physician for assessment and advice while on the go without the limitations of having to physically go to a doctor's office. The platform provides physician services from a wide variety of specialties and allows the user to also arrange laboratory tests and receive input on weight, diet, fitness, hair, and skin issues. There is also a bot on Facebook Messenger for health consultations as well.

WYSA

Wysa is an online AI conversational bot that is aimed at improving the user's mental health. The AI conversationalist aims to help an individual with issues such as depression. Other applications include guidance for relationships, trauma, sleep, anxiety, negative moods, energy, and loneliness. The bot uses such techniques as cognitive-based therapy, motivational interviewing, and microactions to help generate more positive outlooks and feelings in users. The bot is for promotion of emotional well-being but not for diagnosis, treatment, or cure of disorders or diseases. The company advertises that people from at least 30 countries worldwide currently are using their system.

MEDA BIOTECH

Meda Biotech focuses on nanobioengineering primarily to treat cancer. The company's specific area of innovation is hybrid nanotechnology. Nanotechnology in general can facilitate the solubility and bioavailability of medications. The traditional components used in such formulations include such chemicals as surfactants, detergents, phospholipids, pegylation, and so on. Through its new technology the company improves the actions of medications that already exist primarily through increasing solubility. One of the examples provided is Nanovil versus ibuprofen, in which the solubility, efficacy, safety, and time to onset of action have been significantly improved over traditional formulations.[27]

NEXT BIG INNOVATION LABS

Certainly, 3D printing has made and continues to make many inroads into the practice of medicine and into rehabilitation medicine. Orthotic devices, prosthetic components, assistive devices, and so on have all benefited from advances in 3D printing. However, Next Big Innovation Labs[28] is in pursuit of even more lofty goals in the way of 3D printing biological tissues and organs. The company was founded in 2016 to push the limits of 3D bioprinting and is based in Bangalore, India. The company received a patent for precision bioprinting tissues in 2019. Its bioprinter Trivima can bioprint human skin or Innoskin. The ultimate goal is to help manage the ever-growing demand for transplantable organs. In addition to the creation of tissues, bioprinting can play a role in regenerative medicine as well.

GRAINPAD

GrainPad[29] proposes to support and pursue the development of a wide spectrum of fields through services such as data analytics, AI-driven roots with machine learning capabilities, automation, the creation of custom chatboxes, and drone systems. The company wants to foster research in areas such as physics, astronomy, 3D bioprinting, nanotechnology, robotics, AI, and genomics, particularly with respect to accelerating technological growth in medicine.

WELLOWISE

WellOwise promotes physical soundness through health coaching in a system that is AI based and that achieves its end through thorough data collection on an individual. Thus, recommendations are tailored to the individual and take into account genomics as well as other factors. In addition to genetics and lifestyle characteristics, the programs consider several metabolic markers as well.

RELIVA PHYSIOTHERAPY & REHAB

Not all robotic/AI systems are oriented to nursing and doctor roles. ReLiva Physiotherapy & Rehab[30] has created a system with such technology to provide expert physical therapy services through an app on one's smartphone. The company covers the full gamut of traditional conditions that can benefit from rehabilitation such as low back pain, joint replacements, fractures, neurologic and cardiac conditions, shoulder conditions, and all other conditions that a physiotherapist can design a program for and treat. The system takes a patient through an initial assessment and establishment of goals, to the treatment program, to a maintenance program, and then finally to one of prevention and maintenance of lifestyle. To accommodate the restrictions imposed by the pandemic, the com pany offers an online service that allows one to access a physiotherapist from the phone or other device.

SIGTUPLE

SigTuple is a company in India that combines the elements of AI, robotics, and data analytics to improve the speed and accuracy of health care to individuals living in areas remote from higher levels of medical care. The entire assessment of an individual can take minutes as opposed to hours and speed up the time to appropriate treatment. The company has multiple products based around advanced digital technologies. These would include Shonit, in which blood smear images are digitized and analyzed for assessments similar to what a pathologist would provide. Shrava performs the same sort of service for a urine sample. Aadi is an automated, digitized system for semen analysis. Digitizer provides more broad-based scanning of slides and digitization of images with storage on a cloud system for review by a pathologist. For diabetic retinopathy, Drishti is coupled with a fundus camera and the image is then digitized and analyzed through a cloud-based AI system that can then provide a diagnosis and flag issues such as glaucoma and macular degeneration. The company defines its journey as starting in 2015 with the digital analysis of a peripheral blood smear. Shortly after that the company obtained $740,000 in investment money for further development.

ADVANCELLS

Advancells has centered itself around stem cell therapy or regenerative medicine and directs its therapeutics to a host of disorders such as spinal cord injury, orthopedic conditions, eye conditions, skin conditions, aging, and infertility.

China

China has seen a phenomenal, recent growth[31] in its robotics and AI sectors. Health-care robotics has participated in such growth such as in the areas of rehabilitation, drug delivery, and robotic surgery. Part of the impetus for this growth in robotics, particularly for rehabilitation and home care, comes from a growing elderly population that will put great demands on the health-care workforce. Projections estimate the population over 60 in 2050 to be around 30% compared with 12% of the population in more recent times.

Surgical robotics faces more obstacles to growth as available surgical robots such as the Da Vinci Surgical System are accessible only to the wealthier hospitals and patients. Advantages such as smaller incisions, better recovery times, remote capabilities, and more precise procedures are providing the impetus for the creation and development of more local manufacturers with cheaper alternatives.

Rehabilitation robots provide a method of precisely measuring a patient's progress through sensors while also extending the therapeutic range of therapists. The market for rehabilitation robots in China has grown considerably.

Robots can also provide assistance and safety for pharmacists and pharmacy aids in the preparation of intravenous medications, particularly those with associated toxicities such as chemotherapeutic agents. The following are a few companies to illustrate these trends.

CHONGQING JINSHAN SCIENCE & TECHNOLOGY

This company was founded in 1998 and has manufactured capsule endoscopes for the assessment of the gastrointestinal tract. The company has expanded the abilities of its device by adding the capabilities for independent movement that can be controlled remotely by a physician, who can then steer the device to areas of interest for further examination, for drug delivery through silicon micro pumps, or for biopsy. In addition to the OMOM capsule robot, the company is creating the OMOM minimally invasive surgical robot.

ROBOTIC SURGICAL COMPANIES

Two companies that are aggressively pursuing the robotic surgical market include Beijing Tinavi for orthopedic systems and Beijing Bohuiweikang Technology for neurosurgery. From 2010 to around 2016, more than 2000 surgeries have been performed with the orthopedic robot. Professor Liu Da founded Beijing Bohuiweikang Technology for commercialization of the Remebot system for stereotactic neurosurgery with six axes of freedom.

MIDEA-YASKAWA

A leading Chinese appliance company, Midea, and a Japanese industrial robot company, Yaskawa, formed a joint venture, Midea-Yaskawa, in 2015 to produce rehabilitation and nursing care robots. Products include the LR2-Leg Rehabilitation Robot.

Japan

Japan represents one of the world's leaders in the development of robotics, machine learning, AI, and machine vision. In 2017 it produced 50% of the world's industrial robots and provided 297,200 robot installations in the same year. It also has a very aggressive stance in promoting startups in these areas and promoting the development of unicorns.

TELEXISTENCE

There are many interesting robotic companies in Japan, many of which have been discussed in other chapters. Telexistence or TX Inc. is a Japanese company that offers a telepresence robot with more advanced avatar abilities (Fig. 4.6). The robot provides sensory feedback to the controller who also has his movements transmitted to the robot for communication purposes and completion of physical tasks. Grasping and reaching are facilitated with AI, and the operator manipulates the robot through a VR platform.

HONDA MOTOR

With revenues of around $142.4 billion, Honda Motors is perhaps the largest robotics company in the world. It is well known for its humanoid robot called ASIMO or Advanced Step Innovative Mobility. Honda has cultivated the Walking Assist Device, which can provide walking

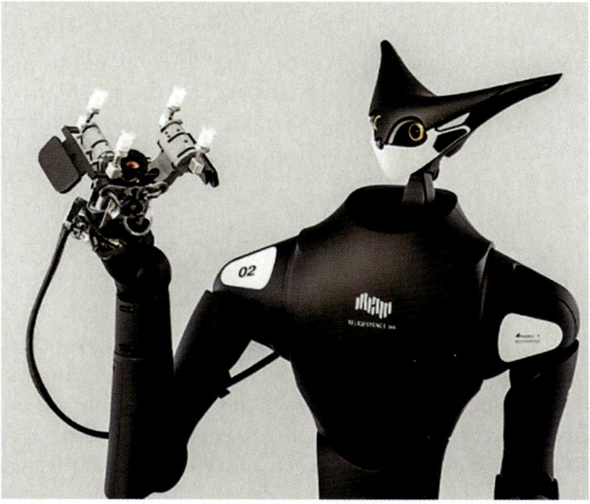

Fig. 4.6 Robot from Telexistence.

and mobility support to individuals with weakness, paralysis, or coordination deficits that impede the ability to walk. The device has received Food and Drug Administration clearance. Clinical trials were carried out in 2014 at the Shirley Ryan Ability Lab in Chicago, Illinois. Applications to individuals with stroke, Guillain-Barré syndrome, spinal cord injury, cerebral palsy, and lower-extremity amputation have been reported.[32–34]

Latin America

In some respects, this area of the world is considered somewhat lagging in the development of robotic companies. Of all the countries in Latin America, Mexico has probably made the most progress as evidenced by progress in industrial robots. The projected sales are $314 million (US dollars) by 2021. Second to Mexico is Brazil, with a figure of $36 million (US dollars). For other countries in this entire region, the combined value is $24 million (US dollars). Robot use per worker in Mexico is 36 robots per 10,000 workers compared with over 200 for the United States. Cost efficiency improvements underscore the value of utilizing robots as a workforce. In 2010 the cost of a robot was about 5.3 years of a worker's salary, but in 2016 this number had improved to 1.5 years. Medical robots in this region have primarily focused on AI for diagnosis, robots centered around neurologic issues, and robots employed in laparoscopic procedures. Brazil currently is the largest exporter of pharmaceuticals to its Latin America neighbors and has the largest pharmaceutical industry in this region. Certainly, advances in robotics and AI would benefit this industry. Overall, Latin America is poised for rapid growth in the area of medical robotics and AI.

EIDOS

Located in Montevideio, Uruguay, Eidos.ai has found itself among the top 10 AI companies in Latin America according to Clutch, an online resource for finding companies relevant to your needs. This company provides multiple types of AI intervention but with respect to health care has created an AI system for interpreting sign language. This project involves the development of a web-based platform for teaching sign language to the hearing impaired to increase inclusion for this group of people with hearing disabilities.

ROOSTRAP

Also located in Montevideo, Uruguay, Roostrap provides AI solutions for many areas of our culture including health care. One example of the latter deals with the analysis of DNA information for optimal health counseling on diet, exercise, and activity modifications based on genetic markers. The user uploads their DNA data into an app that then provides individualized advice through AI algorithms.

Africa

At this point the development of AI and robotics in Africa has lagged other areas of the world due to a lack of skilled technicians. Nevertheless, there is evidence of a burgeoning industry here. With nearly half a billion dollars in funding, robot startup companies are forging a new future on this continent. Let us look at a few of these.[35,36] Keeping in the spirit of African technology, AFRON, or African Robotics Network, sponsored a $10 robotic challenge whereby participants attempted to design a robot with parts costing under $10. In Monrovia, which is the capital of Liberia, in 2014 a robot was utilized in the missionary hospital ELWA. Called Tru-D, the robot could disinfect and decontaminate its surroundings of dangerous microorganisms that included the Ebola virus.

ENOVA ROBOTICS

Enova Robotics[37] has roughly $1.6 million in funding at this point and provides robotic and AI support for the development of technical solutions for its customers. It is based in Tunisia. With mobile robotic and AI technology, the company attempts to provide solutions in education, health care, marketing, and security. It has a European branch in France. One of its products includes Veasense, which was designed to meet the care needs of an aging population (Fig. 4.7). This robot can monitor the health status of individuals and provide a telepresence for doctors or nurses whereby preliminary diagnostic impressions can be made on patients—even those in remote locations.

RYONIC ROBOTICS

Located in South Africa and founded in 2014, Ryonic Robotics provides robotic solutions for a variety of industry and business applications and currently has about half a million dollars in funding as of 2021.

Australia and New Zealand

Both these countries have experienced a boom in the development of AI/robotics, and the investment capital pouring into this kind of technology in these two countries clearly underscores that fact. From 2011 to 2016 this capital has surged from $32 million to $96 million. The New Zealand Ministry of Health has identified the health-care and service assistance sector as the largest employer in the country. Robots are targeted as assisting in supplying the necessary workforce especially for repetitive types of tasks. Several promising companies are bearing the fruit of this level of investment. The first social robot to be trialed in Australia was Pepper, which is produced by a Tokyo-based company. Pepper served the patient population through answering simple questions such as about the influenza vaccine and providing a friendly interface. Robot-assisted

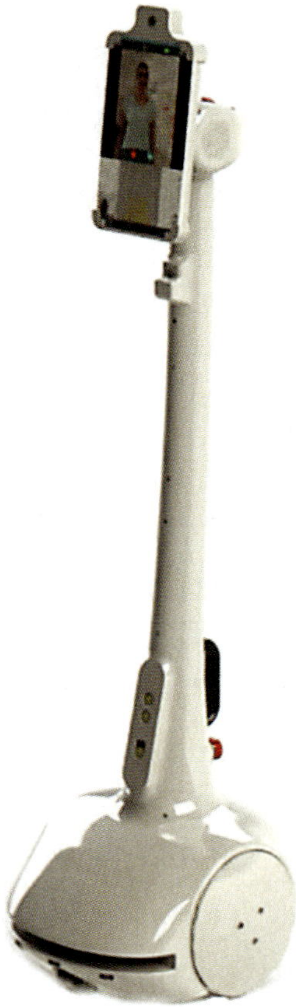

Fig. 4.7 Veasense from Enova Robotics.

surgery has also made its entrance into the New Zealand hospital systems and currently exists in at least three hospitals. The first robot-assisted surgery with the Da Vinci system occurred at Grace Hospital in Tauranga.

MAXWELL PLUS

The company has headquarters in Brisbane and started in 2016 with initial funding of $2.7 million. The company has developed an AI program for diagnostic imaging that can detect prostate cancer. Breast cancer, lung diseases, and neurodegenerative conditions have lined up as future targets for their system. Maxwell Plus Cloud provides physicians the assistance for the diagnostic imaging.

VIRTUAL BLUE

Mercy Radiology and Clinics in collaboration with Virtual Blue[38] created Matilda, which is a robotic process automation system that prepares invoices for scans and tests. The virtual worker is faster, more efficient, and less prone to error than the human counterpart. To better process patient appointments, Mercy Radiology and Clinics utilized Rob-e, a Blue Prism intelligent digital worker, also from the New Zealand company Virtual Blue. This company uses robotic process automation for human resources (HR) services, finance and accounting, supply chain and information technologies services through several programs—Blue Prism intelligent digital worker, UiPath, Smart Capture, Smart Routing, Smart Search, and replikr.

Although the technology did not originate in Australia, RoboFit touts itself as the first Cyberdyne[39]-certified rehab clinic and uses HAL (Hybrid Assisted Limb) to provide rehabilitation for those suffering from paralysis, whether from stroke, spinal cord injury, multiple sclerosis, or some other disabling condition. HAL is an exoskeleton that reads the user's intent to move through the sensing of bioelectric signals. The goal is to create new neural pathways that result in improved strength and motor function. Located in Tsukuba, Japan, Cyberdyne produces HAL, which the company designates as the first wearable cyborg.

References

1. Diligent Robotics. https://www.diligentrobots.com
2. Olive. https://oliveai.com
3. Pediatric HAL S2225—Advanced pediatric patient simulator—Gaumard. https://www.gaumard.com/s2225
4. Simulator for robotic surgery training. Jacobs School of Medicine and Biomedical Sciences. University at Buffalo. https://medicine.buffalo.edu/research/research_highlights.host.html/content/shared/smbs/research_highlights/rossimulator.detail.html
5. DePuy Synthes. J&J. Medical Devices. https://www.jnjmedtech.com/en-US/companies/depuy-synthes
6. VascuLogic. VenousPro. https://vasculogic.com/venouspro.html#learnMore
7. Luvozo PBC. RBR staff. Robotics Business Review. Published April 5, 2016. https://medicine.buffalo.edu/research/research_highlights.host.html/content/shared/smbs/research_highlights/rossimulator.detail.html
8. Kelly É. Canada makes multi-million dollar bets on green tech, quantum and AI in annual budget. Published April 20, 2021. https://sciencebusiness.net/climate-news-technology-strategy-board/news/canada-makes-multi-million-dollar-bets-green-tech#:~:text=From%20the%20government's%202021%20budget,will%20aim%20to%20bolster%20computing
9. Emtec Business. Technology Empowered Oracle. https://www.emtecinc.com/technology/oracle/
10. Holo Robots About Us. https://holorobots.com/about-us/
11. iARM. http://www.iarmrobot.com/index.shtml
12. Reeler Working Paper Series. Responsible Ethica Learning with Robotics. https://reeler.eu/fileadmin/user_upload/REELER/WP02_Feeding_Assistive_Robotics.pdf
13. Advanced Rehabilitation Technology. Tyromotion Austria. https://tyromotion.com/en/
14. Robocath. https://www.robocath.com/product/
15. Know us. GOGOA. https://en.gogoa.eu/conocenos
16. ABLE Human Motion start-up. About ABLE Human Motion. https://www.ablehumanmotion.com/able-human-motion-about/
17. AcouSort. https://acousort.com/
18. AOT We Laser Bone. https://aot.swiss/
19. Konuikhovskaia A. Five trends in Russian robotics. International Federation of Robotics. Publishe2d August 2, 2019. Accessed September 19, 2022. https://ifr.org/post/five-trends-in-russian-robotics
20. ExoAtlet I. https://exoatlet.lu/product-page-exoatlet-i/
21. Russian Robotics. An Israeli Clinic's Answer to Diagnostics. Sk. Published October 5, 2020. https://sk.ru/news/russian-robotics-an-israeli-clinics-answer-to-diagnostics/
22. Robo C-2. PROMOBOT. https://promo-bot.ai/robots/robo-c/
23. Chadha A. India's healthcare has a new best friend: robots. Fortune India. Published January 13, 2021. Accessed September 19, 2022. https://www.fortuneindia.com/opinion/indias-healthcare-has-a-new-best-friend-robots/105028
24. Invento Robotics. https://mitrarobot.com/.
25. Sastra Robotics. https://sastrarobotics.com/?s=sr+scara+pro
26. Top Robotics Companies in India. iNurture. Published March 6, 2019. Accessed September 19, 2022. https://inurture.co.in/top-robotics-companies-in-india/

27. Nano Meda. http://www.nanomeda.com/index.php.
28. About NBIL—Next Big Innovation Labs. https://nextbiglab.com/about-nbil/
29. Grainpad. https://grainpad.in
30. Physiotherapy Specialist de Hospital. Home. ReLiva. https://reliva.in/home/aboutus/
31. Soh S.T. The rise of China's medical robotics sector—Robohub Sanbot humanoid robot. Published December 22, 2016. Accessed September 19, 2022. https://robohub.org/the-rise-of-chinas-medical-roboticssector/#:~:text=Medical%20robots%20are%20used%20by%20Chinese%20hospitals%20and,used%20in%20both%20soft%20and%20hard%20tissue%20surgeries
32. Kakou H, Shitama H, Kimura Y, et al. [Walking assist robot and its clinical application]. *J UOEH.* 2009;31(2):207–218. Japanese.https://doi.org/10.7888/juoeh.31.207.
33. Kawasaki S, Ohata K, Yoshida T, Yokoyama A, Yamada S. Gait improvements by assisting hip movements with the robot in children with cerebral palsy: a pilot randomized controlled trial. *J Neuroeng Rehabil.* 2020;17(1):87. https://doi.org/10.1186/s12984-020-00712-3.
34. Koseki K, Yozu A, Takano H, et al. Gait training using the Honda Walking Assist Device® for individuals with transfemoral amputation: a report of two cases. *J Back Musculoskelet Rehabil.* 2020;33(2):339–344.https://doi.org/10.3233/BMR-191726.
35. Robotics startups in Africa. https://startuplist.africa/industry/robotics
36. Itebu J. Robots in Africa. What does this mean for the continent? Swali Africa. Published October 12, 2015. http://blog.swaliafrica.com/robots-in-africa/
37. Enova Robotics. Pguard the autonomous mobile security robot. https://www.enovarobotics.eu/
38. Virtual Blue. Leave the Robotic Processes to the Robots. https://www.virtualblue.co.nz/
39. Corporate identification—Cyberdyne. https://www.cyberdyne.jp/english/company/index.html

5

Medical Robotics in Acute Care Medicine (Urgent Care, Pain Management, and Robot-Assisted Surgery)

Denise D. Lester

KEY POINTS

- Many different types of robotic technologies are enhancing acute medicine.
- Humanoid robots outfitted with artificial intelligence can help patients and put them at ease.
- Small, friendly robots can reduce pain and anxiety in children undergoing painful procedures.
- Robotic surgical systems extend the skills of surgeons for better outcomes.
- Micro- and nanorobots hold a bright future for acute medical care.

Acute care medicine can be defined as acute care that is not associated with a chronic illness. This would include medical interventions provided in settings such as emergency rooms, urgent care clinics, pre- and postprocedural areas, and environments specifically providing acute and subacute pain management such as inpatient, hospice, and nursing home facilities.

Recently medical robotics have entered the acute care algorithm for assistance with many medical services such as social roles (augmented human interaction), work roles (augmented work efficiency and accuracy), and even acute care prediction roles. For example, medical robots with "social" functions have been shown to augment psychosocial support using artificial intelligence (AI) to effectively distract and reduce fear, anxiety, and stress during intravenous insertion in pediatric emergency room patients.[1] Medical robots with primarily "work" functions such as the well-known robot-assisted surgery (RAS) device da Vinci system have enabled surgeons to perform complex surgeries that would have required extensive incisions for adequate exposure. These RAS devices have been shown to have less bleeding complications compared with all other forms of surgery,[2] as well as better visualization, more precise technique, advanced vascular repair, and less anastomotic leak rates.[3] Lastly, we will review a third class of "predictive" acute medical care assistive robot. This group of AI robots may utilize gene mapping to predict a variety of medical care outcomes such as a patient's potential opioid requirement and which patients will benefit from a preoperative acute pain service consultation.[4–6]

Adult Population Acute Care Medicine Robotic Pain Management Health Care

Founded by David Hanson, PhD, over 2 decades ago, Hanson Robotics has engineered humanoid robots of all ages, ethnicities, and specialties. These robots appear genuinely alive and utilize extensive AI to socialize and respond appropriately to human interaction. These humanoid robots utilize AI to appear to express and perceive human emotions and can communicate with humans using high level dialogue as well as natural visual cues. The robots have over 48 major "muscles" in their face, thus they can do a variety of human facial expressions such as gaze and gestures of surprise, sadness, or profound elation.[7] These robots were developed for several goals including AI platforms for research, education, medical and health care, sales, service, and entertainment applications. Hanson robotics has reported that the use of their robots will make human life more autonomous and fuller.

Although their most known robot is Sophia the humanoid robot (who was the only robot to ever receive a citizenship), our chapter will discuss her "cousin" Grace (Figs. 5.1, 5.2A–B, 5.3), the health care humanoid robot.[8]

Grace assists the burden of frontline health-care workers in a variety of ways . She provides social interaction especially for the elderly. Using her AI data bank, she can provide high-level dialogue with the patients about the things that are important to them such as their family and friends. She can do guided meditation and talk therapy. This social interaction can improve mood, pain, and altered thinking especially in the elderly. Her advanced robotics allows for processing and gathering accurate data in real time. She can recognize and respond to seven human emotions and can mirror her patient's facial expressions, appearing empathetic and compassionate.

Robots are unique in that they can provide this human socialization without bathroom breaks or fatigue or boredom. The attention provided is continuous and at the same level as they do not extinguish or decline during the visit. Another health-care feature Grace provides is increased physical activity. This may be individualized to the patient ranging from activities as simple as dancing with Grace or as advanced as a formal prescribed physical therapy session. Many clinicians utilize Grace as a biodata monitor. Her chest holds a thermal camera that can assess temperature, pulse, blood pressure, level of wakefulness, awareness, and response to verbal commands. She can be programmed to deliver medications and provide feedback during and after her visit

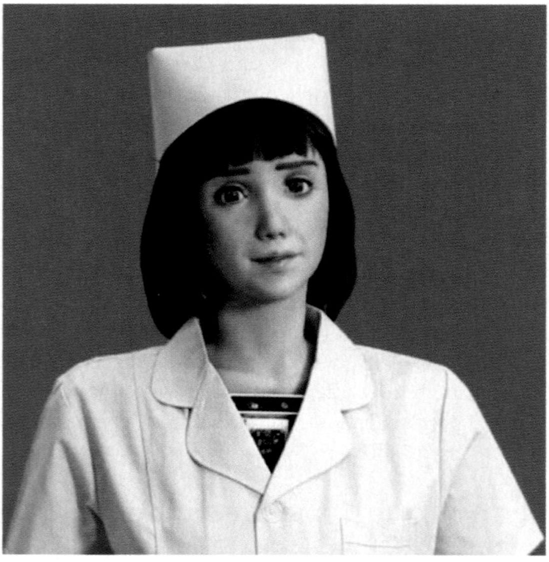

Fig. 5.1 Grace the robot @ Robot, Hanson Robotics. Grace was created by Awakening Health Ltd. of Hong Kong to serve the global medical industry, in particular the elderly care sector, as the world first humanlike nurse assistant. (From Hanson Robotics. https://www.hansonrobotics.com/Awakening Health Ltd. https://awakening.health/.)

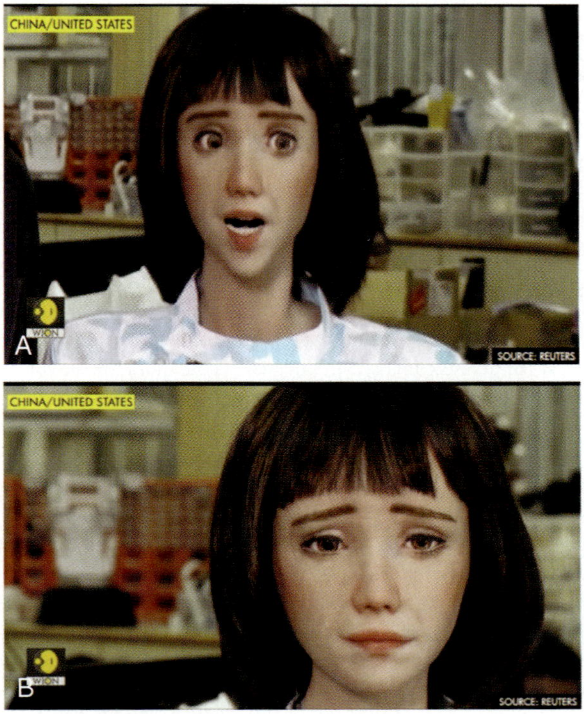

Fig. 5.2 (A, B) Grace displays different emotions.

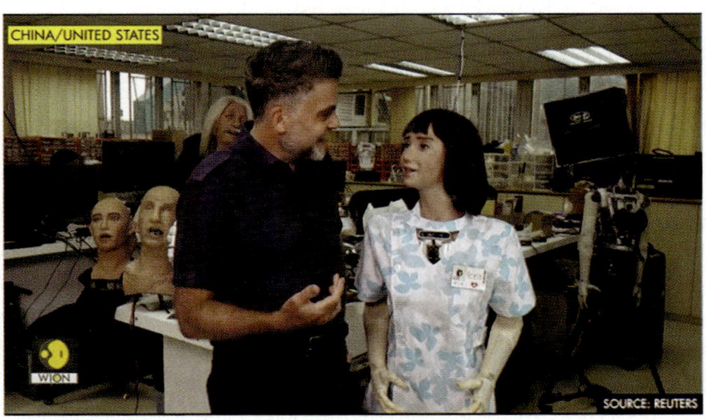

Fig. 5.3 Grace and her creator, Mr. Hanson.

to the clinician group. An interesting fact is her language skill set. Since language is one of the most powerful connectors between clinicians and their patients, Grace connects with her Asian patient population by speaking and listening in native quadrilingual fluency (English, Cantonese, Mandarin, and Korean).

So why would a medical system require a robotic nursing assistant? Recent years have put strains on our current health-care system with many unfilled positions for health-care workers in the face of higher numbers of patients needing care. This leads to more patients using emergency room services for their routine care, and downstream delay of emergency resources for true emergencies. In addition, patients who have no home care available are alone, develop more advanced mood disorders such as depression and anxiety, and may become less compliant with their home schedule treatment regimen. Having a robot to assist with this growing health-care need is beneficial. Although Grace is not meant to replace the skill set of a trained clinician or the warmth of a family member's hug, she is a new solution for a new need with the potential to fill the health-care gap.

Pediatric Population Acute Medicine Robotic Pain Management Health Care

We discussed one humanoid AI robot that is used in adult acute medicine. This section will discuss two humanoid AI robots that are used in pediatric acute medicine—Mediport and NAO. 2.2 MEDiPORT cognitive-behavioral arm MEDiPORT is a 3-foot-tall humanoid robot (NAO© hardware produced by Softbank Robotics© and MEDi® software produced by RxRobots©; Figure 1)[9]. NAO is also a humanoid robot produces by Aldebaran Robotics. They both stand 3 feet tall and can walk, grip things with their hands, speak, and listen. They have several microphones for sound projection. They are versatile robots because they can be programmed well ahead of a scheduled painful pediatric procedure. This allows the provider to simply push a button to start the robot's schedule. Its speech and its movements can be preset based on the individual child's age, intellect, and level of speech. They can be programmed to deliver jokes, blow bubbles with the child, dance, hug, tell stories, play games, ask specific preprogrammed questions, give praise and confirmatory feedback, empathize with facial expressions and vocalizations, and provide more advanced social interactions before during and after painful pediatric procedures. The provider can "click and drag" a multitude of options from a digital library into the robot prior to the child arriving. The only robot maintenance is recharging the battery.

Several randomized controlled studies have been performed to see if there is a difference in pain and distress in pediatric procedures when adding these humanoid robots.[10,11] In 2013, Beran and her team noted that flu vaccinations were a source of distress in millions of children throughout the United States.[10] Most of these children and their families attempted distractions with some form of electronic technology such as a cell phone or laptop computer. Dr. Beran knew that children enjoy the reciprocity of interacting bidirectionally with robots and wanted to test her theory by randomizing 57 children to receive either the robot programmed to socially interact and distract or the nurse using their traditional methods during administration of the flu vaccine (Fig. 5.4).

In 2011, 57 children between the ages 4 and 9 years old who were either admitted to or in an outpatient clinic at Alberta's Children's Hospital in Alberta, Canada, were randomized to receive the robot-assisted distraction or the nurse traditional distraction during the flu vaccine procedure. Parents rated their children's level of pain at prior vaccinations and completed all demographic information prior to the vaccination. Computer randomization then took place, and each child in the treatment group sat in a parent's lap next to the nurse and directly across from the robot. The robot was among an assortment of toy blocks on the table and a container containing a few of the blocks. The robot was programmed to participate in three phases. The first phase was when the child walked to his or her seat to sit down. During that time the researcher pushed a button on the robot discreetly and the robot introduced himself to the child and asked the child's interests, such as favorite movie or music. The robot might also have given the child a high five depending upon the child's age. The nurse used this time to begin preparing the vaccination. The second phase involved the researcher discreetly pressing the robot again and the robot asking the child to help put the blocks in the container. The robot then remarked that the blocks looked "pretty dusty" and suggested that they both blow the dust off the blocks before putting them into the container. At this point the nurse prepared the arm with alcohol and then provided the vaccination while the child continued

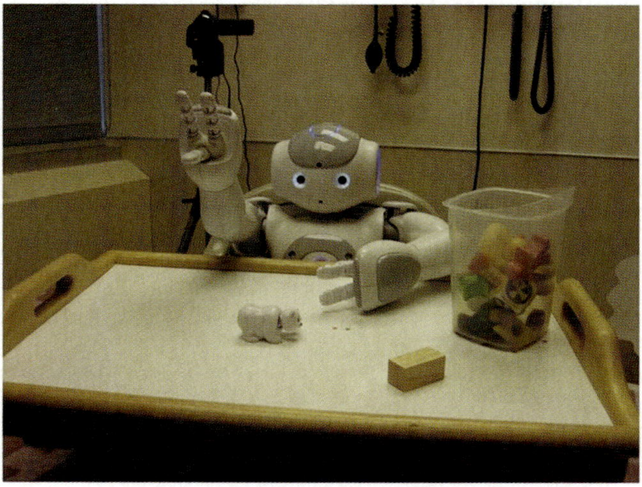

Fig. 5.4 Robots used to reduce the pain of vaccinations. (From Beran TN, Ramirez-Serrano A, Vanderkooi OG, Kuhn S. Reducing children's pain and distress towards flu vaccinations: a novel and effective application of humanoid robotics. *Vaccine*. 2013;31(25):2772–2777. https://doi.org/10.1016/j.vaccine.2013.03.056.)

to blow off the blocks with the robot and put them into the container. The second stage continued for a long as the nurse needed to complete the vaccination. In the third stage the researcher again activated the robot and the robot thanked the child for helping clean up the blocks, gave a positive statement about bravery or encouragement, and then waved goodbye as the patient left the area.

The control arm of the study involved the nurse providing the vaccination in a traditional manner without a robot intervention. The nurse used minimal distraction—asking the child to look at the animals on the wallpaper. The outcomes demonstrated a significant reduction in pain and distress as reported by children, nurses, and parents as compared with the control. This effect was seen across genders and across ages. The effect was still present in the children who reportedly had prior painful difficult vaccinations as well. Of the children in the robot-assisted group, 85% (n = 24) reported they would like the robot when they get injections in future, and 3% (n = 1) reported "not sure."

The second humanoid robot randomized controlled study in pediatrics was performed using the robot Mediport to decrease pain and distress for children with cancer undergoing subcutaneous port access. It was primarily a pilot feasibility study to see if traditional cognitive distraction therapy with the robot was as effective or less effective compared with the robot being more active (robot dancing, singing, etc.). This study was conducted by Jibb et al. in 2018 (Table 5.1).[11] Forty children from an outpatient hematology oncology clinic of a pediatric tertiary care center in Canada were selected to participate. Demographics included children who were 4 to 9 years old, English speaking, at least 1 month from diagnosis, and actively receiving treatment for cancer and who had had at least one subcutaneous port accessed in the past. End-of-life children were excluded. All children received a standard dose of EMLA cream prior to accessing the port. The children in the control arm of the study had the robot only provide cognitive assurance to child. The stages have very specific language in this arm.

The differences in outcome in this study were primarily the outcomes for distress. The children, parents, and nurses all reported outcomes that were much improved in the treatment limb for distress, although both robot techniques were equally effective when asked about pain. Technical difficulties were significantly more common in the cognitive behavioral arm of study. Acceptability ratings were listed as "satisfactory" in all three groups of responders both in the control arm and

TABLE 5.1 ■ **Using Robots During Painful Procedures**

Mediport Cognitive-Behavioral Arm (Robot Using Evidence-Based Cognitive-Behavioral Interventions)		
Stage Control	**Nurse and Researcher Action**	**Robot Action**
1	Nurse prepares needle. Researcher uses tablet to begin. Mediport begins dialogue.	Robot: "Hi my name is . . . What is your name?"
2	Nurse turns toward child to let him know its time to begin injection.	Robot: "I will be here with you to help you feel brave."
3	Nurse begins to remove EMLA patch.	Robot: "Time to take off your patch. The nurses are so gentle, and you are doing a great job."
4	Nurse inserts needle into subcutaneous port.	Robot: "Now is when we get to practice our belly breathing. Breathe in . . . now hold that air in the belly while I count to two!"
5	Nurse applies sterile dressing.	Robot: "You are very brave! Here's a high five."
Mediport Active Distraction Arm (Robot Dancing and Singing)		
Stage Intervention	**Nurse and Researcher Action**	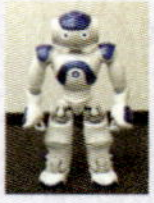 **Robot Action**[11]
1	Nurse prepares needle. Researcher uses tablet to begin. Mediport begins dialogue.	Robot: "Hi my name is . . . What is your name?" Robot starts dancing and singing loudly.
2	Nurse turns toward child to let him know its time to begin injection.	Robot continues dancing and singing loudly.
3	Nurse begins to remove EMLA patch.	Robot continues dancing and singing loudly.
4	Nurse inserts needle into subcutaneous port.	Robot continues dancing and singing loudly.
5	Nurse applies sterile dressing.	Robot: "Here's a high five."

the cognitive behavioral arm. Parents and children both reported "liking" the dancing robot and hoping he would return for the patient's next scheduled port injection. There was no difference in postprocedural pain score in either robot group.

Surgical Robotics

The field of RAS is so large that it fills up a series of textbooks, and a comprehensive review is not feasible in this chapter. Instead, we will focus on one system, the da Vinci Surgical System by Intuitive. Da Vinci Surgical Systems are very common in surgical practices. We mentioned in the introduction that RAS devices have benefits greater than traditional open incisional surgeries and even greater benefits when compared with closed laparoscopic surgeries. (See the introduction for the benefits of RAS.)

DA VINCI SYSTEM

The da Vinci system (Fig. 5.5A–C) is made of three components: (1) the surgeon console, (2) the patient side cart, and (3) the vision cart. The surgeon sits in the surgeon console and has 3D,

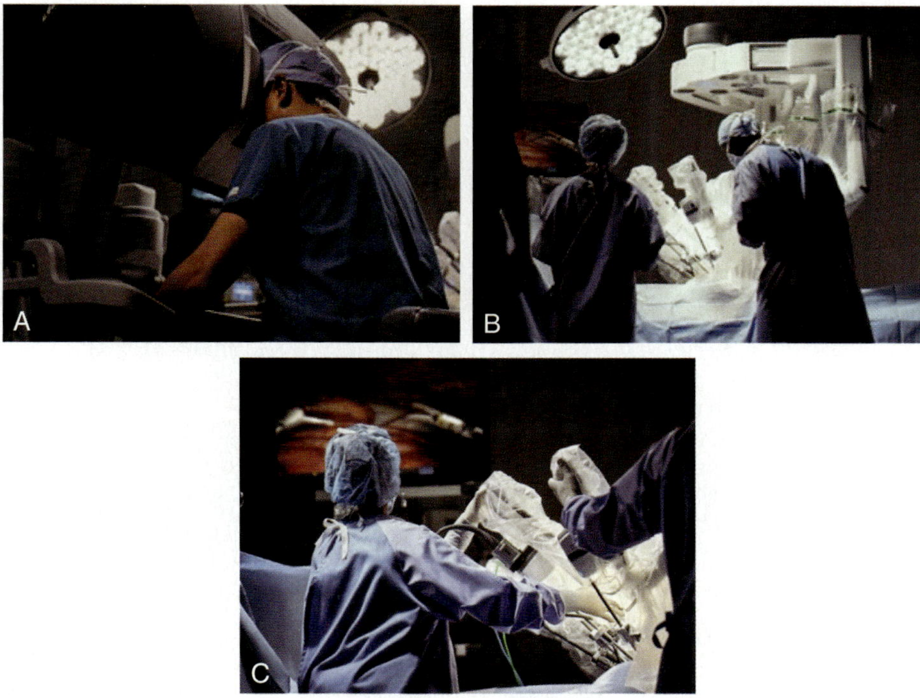

Fig. 5.5 Da Vinci Surgical System consists of (A) surgeon console, (B) patient side cart, and (C) vision cart. Cardiac robot-assisted surgery. (From Intuitive. Intuitive for Cardiac Patients. https://www.davincisurgery.com/procedures/cardiac-surgery.)

high-definition views of the anatomy and instruments. It is reported that the surgeon will see 10 times the magnification using the console compared with normal vision. The instruments are controlled while sitting at this location even though the patient is across the room. The surgeon is essentially moving the robotic limbs in his surgical console, which is then moving the actual instruments inside the patient's body. The construct of the instruments in the console moves like a human hand but provides a much greater range of motion and a better ability to maneuver around technically challenging areas of tissue (Fig. 5.6A–B).

The side cart is placed near the patient and contains the instruments that are completing the surgery. The vision cart is the screen that is displaying the surgical procedure. RAS is not new, and it is reported that the first RAS was in 2001 with the introduction of a specialized robot arm to perform surgery on patients at Children's Hospital Boston,[10] and now almost every type of surgery is utilizing some form of RAS option (cardiac surgery, colorectal surgery, general surgery, gynecologic surgery, head and neck surgery, thoracic surgery, urologic surgery). To reinforce the benefits again, the da Vinci RAS system has enabled surgeons to perform complected surgeries that would have required extensive open incisions that may have still had inadequate exposure. The da Vinci can look "around corners" and allows vision in ways that the natural eye could never accomplish. RAS devices have been shown to have less bleeding complications compared with all other forms of surgery[2] (Fig. 5.7A–B), as well as better visualization, more precise technique, advanced vascular repair, and less anastomotic leak rates.[3]

There is much debate as to whether the benefits of RAS are solely linked to the technique itself or the idea that there is a "captain of the ship" phenomenon. This phenomenon suggests that the environment preparing and performing the RAS is much "cleaner" and more disciplined

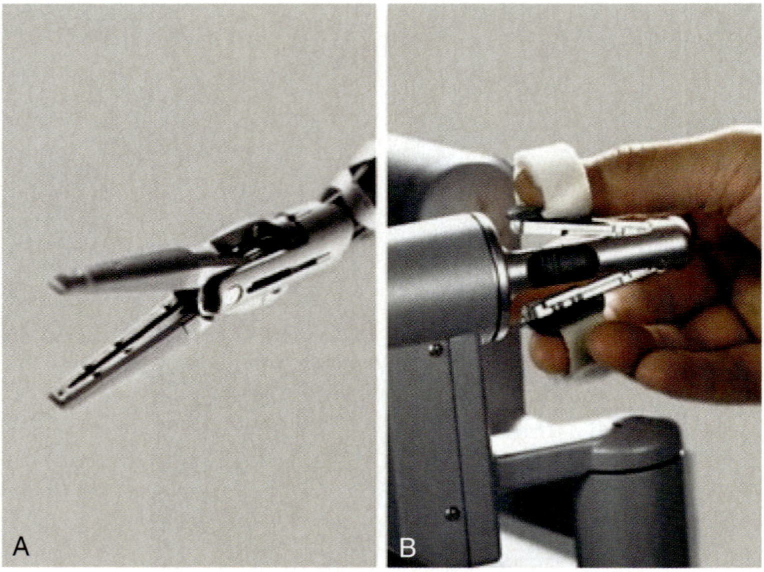

Fig. 5.6 (A, B) Tiny instruments that the surgeon uses to perform the surgery using Da Vinci System robotic-assisted surgery for patients. (From Intuitive. Da Vinci Robotic-Assisted Surgery. https://www.intuitive.com/en-us/patients/da-vinci-robotic-surgery.)

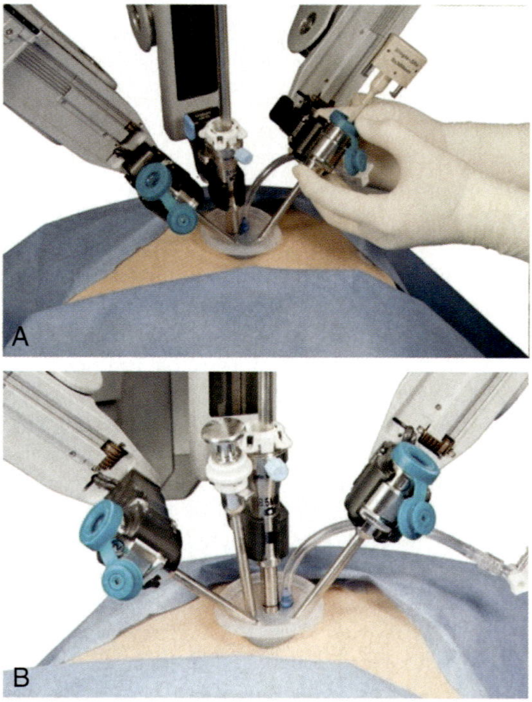

Fig. 5.7 (A, B) Da Vinci Single-Site platform for gallbladder and gynecologic procedures. (From Matanes E, Lauterbach R, Boulus S, Amit A, Lowenstein L. Robotic laparoendoscopic single-site surgery in gynecology: a systematic review. *Eur J Obstet Gynecol Reprod Biol*. 2018;231:1–7. https://doi.org/10.1016/j.ejogrb.2018.10.006. ©2018 Intuitive Surgical, Inc.)

compared with a traditional open procedure. Alverdy wrote that there are "multiple positive elements that contribute to the improved outcomes being observed with robotic surgery inclusive of 1) more stringent patient selection, 2) mandated procedure rehearsal, 3) a greater attention to operating bloodlessly, 4) a smoother anastomotic construction beyond the technical aspects of the connection itself, and 5) a higher demand on oneself to operate at peak performance."[9] Either way, it is always difficult to tease out cause and effect but it is easier to support its use when your outcomes are improved over tradition open and laparoscopic techniques.

Artificial Intelligence in Pain Management

GENE MAPPING ARTIFICIAL INTELLIGENCE TO PREDICT TREATMENT OUTCOME IN OPIOID DEPENDENCE

It is known that genetic differences may explain variability in treatment outcomes. The mapping of genomes is facilitated by AI (Fig. 5.8). This molecular-level diagnostic intervention can affect a patient who is attempting to remain abstinent from an opioid use disorder. There may be a benefit from having genetic testing prior to deciding if you should augment opioid use disorder recovery with buprenorphine versus methadone. In a study by Crist et al., pharmacologic analysis was performed of the effects of genetic variants in *OPRD1* (the gene encoding the delta opioid receptor) on the prevalence of opioid-positive urine tests in 77 African Americans and 566 European Americans undergoing treatment for opioid use disorder. Patients were then randomly assigned to treatment with either methadone or buprenorphine/naloxone (Suboxone) over 24 weeks. Illicit drug use was monitored by weekly urine assessments. In African Americans the Ionic SNP rs678849 predicted treatment outcomes for both medications. Patients with CC genotype receive methadone treatment were less likely to have opioid-positive urine samples than those in the combined CT and TT genotypes. However, individuals with CC genotype in the buprenorphine/naloxone group were more likely to have positive opioid drug screens than individuals in the combined CT and TT genotype groups.[5]

GENE MAPPING ARTIFICIAL INTELLIGENCE NOT YET ABLE TO PREDICT OPIOID REQUIREMENTS IN CANCER PAIN

When researchers attempted to use the information learned in the genetic buprenorphine versus methadone study, they had difficulty reproducing the same results using genetic profiling. In 2018, Olesen et al. used AI in the form of a vector support learning machine program to attempt to predict required doses of opioid in patients with cancer and pain using their genetic profiles.[4] They chose 18 single nucleotide polymorphisms within the delta and mu opioid receptor genes and the catechol-o-methyltransferase gene for analysis. Twelve hundred thirty-seven patients with cancer were analyzed. No predictive value was found. The authors listed several reasons why there may still be a connection that was not found during the study. Reasons ranged from not enough

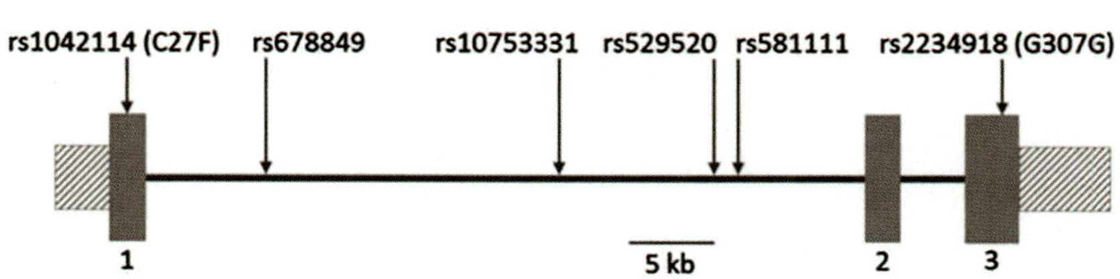

Fig. 5.8 Gene mapping.

selected single nucleotide polymorphisms to the phenomenon of epistasis, which is the interaction between genes that can alter the effect of the genes studied. More work is needed before the answers are sufficient.

ARTIFICIAL INTELLIGENCE MACHINE PREDICTING ACUTE PAIN CONSULTATION NEEDS

The last example of AI being used in acute medicine includes the predictive value of patients requiring an acute pain consult preoperatively. Tighe et al. demonstrated that machine learning classifiers could effectively predict which patients would require a preoperative acute pain service consultation (Fig. 5.9).[6] This took place at the University of Florida. All in-hospital surgical cases performed between January 1, 2010, and June 30, 2010, were reviewed if they were posted on the operating room list. Current Procedural Terminology codes were reviewed. Eleven points of data were collected (operating room location; patient status, either inpatient, outpatient, or postoperative; admission; surgeon; anesthesiologist; primary and secondary Current Procedural Terminology codes). The primary outcome was the preoperative acute pain service (APS) consultation request. Machine-learning classifiers correctly predicted preoperative requests for APS consultations in 92.3% (95% confidence intervals [CI], 91.8–92.8) of all surgical cases. This may be a new method to screen for preoperative acute pain interventions rather than trying to less effectively provide pain management after surgery is completed.

Conclusion (Future of Robotics in Acute Medicine)

What can we expect to see more of in the future of robotics in acute medicine? Everything we discussed in this chapter is continuing to be refined. Robots are more readily entering homes and households, and just like the little floor-sweeping robot that many of you have, robots are going

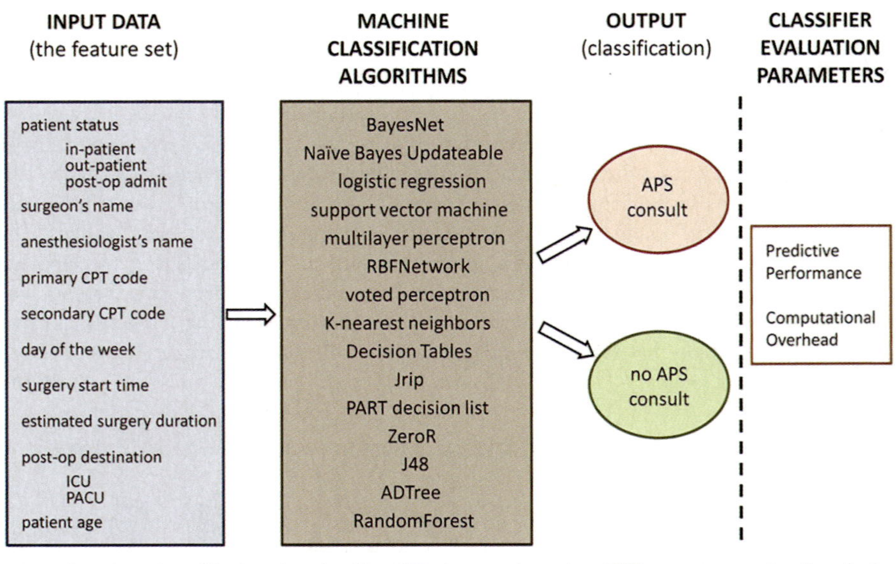

Fig. 5.9 Overview of machine learning classifier. APS, Acute pain service; CPT, current procedural terminology; ICU, intensive care unit; PACU, post anesthesia care unit. (From Tighe PJ, Lucas SD, Edwards DA, Boezaart AP, Aytug H, Bihorac A. Use of machine-learning classifiers to predict requests for preoperative acute pain service consultation. *Pain Med*. 2012;13(10):1347–1357. https://doi.org/10.1111/j.1526-4637.2012.01477.x.)

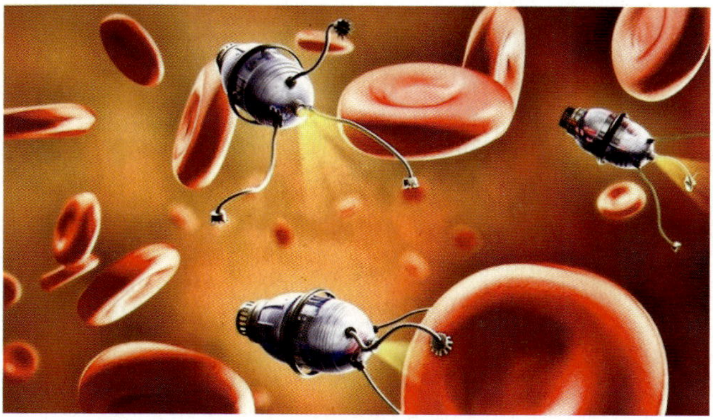

Fig. 5.10 Technology Innovation Today . Nanobots wade through blood to deliver drugs. (From https://techinnovationtoday.org/medicaltech/nanorobots-wade-through-blood-to-deliver-drugs/.)

to remain available to do the repetitive but important tasks within our health-care system. One interesting future improvement in robotics is their size. Micro- and nanorobotics will be entering the health-care system very soon. Plans are being developed to have nanorobots befitted with an antibiotic and then "steered" directly to the tissue in our body that requires the drug (Fig. 5.10). Even using *Escherichia coli* and liposomes to target drug deliveries throughout the body is being developed. There is so much that robots can do in our health system as they can go the places we cannot (think pandemic) and they do not exhaust or fatigue. The opportunity exists to use robots in those areas that are especially hard to fill, hard to reach, and hard to sustain.

References

1. Ali S, Manaloor R, Ma K, et al. A randomized trial of robot-based distraction to reduce children's distress and pain during intravenous insertion in the emergency department. *CJEM*. 2021;23:85–93.
2. Kamarajah SK, Bundred JR, Marc OS, et al. A systematic review and network meta-analysis of different surgical approaches for pancreaduodenectomy. *HPB (Oxford)*. 2020;22(3):329–339.
3. Wang Y, Liu Y, Han G, Yi B, Zhu S. The severity of postoperative complications after robotic vs laparoscopic surgery for rectal cancer. A systematic review, meta-analysis and meta- regression. *PLoS One*. 2020;15(10):e0239909.
4. Olesen AE, Gronlund D, Gram M, et al. Prediction of opioid dose in cancer pain patients using genetic profiling: not yet an option with support vector machine learning. *BMC Res Notes*. 2018;11:78.
5. Crist RC, Clarke T, Ang A, et al. An intronic variant in OPRD 1 predicts treatment outcome for opioid dependence in African Americans [published correction appears in Neuropsychopharmacology. 2014 Mar;39(4):1039]. *Neuropsychopharmacology*. 2013;38(10):2003–2010.
6. Tighe PJ, Lucas SD, Edwards DA, Boezaart AP, Aytug H, Bihorac A. Use of machine-learning classifiers to predict requests for preoperative acute pain service consultation. *Pain Med*. 2012;13(10):1347–1357.
7. Fosch-Villaronga E, Drukarch H, eds.
8. *AI for healthcare robotics*. Eduard Fosch-Villaronga. Hadassah Drukarch. 2022. CRC Press; 441.
9. Jibb LA, Birnie KA, Nathan PC, et al. Using the MEDIPORT humanoid robot to reduce procedural pain and distress in children with cancer: a pilot randomized controlled trial. *Pediatr Blood Cancer*. 2018;65(9):e27242.
10. https://www.hansonrobotics.com
11. Beran TN, Ramirez-Serrano A, Vanderkooi OG, Kuhn S. Reducing children's pain and distress towards flu vaccinations: a novel and effective application of umanoid robotics. *Vaccine*. 2013;31(25):2772–2777.

6

Robotics in Rehabilitation Medicine: Prosthetics, Exoskeletons, All Else in Rehabilitation Medicine

Riya Fukui ■ William Lovegreen

KEY POINTS

- Robots assist with upper- and lower-extremity physical rehabilitation.
- This technology can also provide therapies for social and emotional concerns.
- Safety in design is a primary concern.
- Robots can help meet the needs of a growing aging population.
- The integration of robotics into prosthetic and orthotic devices follows a natural historic progression.
- Patients can expect greater restoration of the function of lost limbs through robotic prostheses.
- Improvements in these devices restore not only function but also a more natural appearance and motion.
- Advances in the brain-computer interface and osseointegration promise encouraging new potentials.

Robotics has fascinated us since its conception. In popular culture, robots have been portrayed as helping with chores, as fighting alongside soldiers in battles, or as true friends with real emotional connections. It is clear that robots could assist humanity through integration into various different areas of our lives. Rehabilitation is one area in which robots could excel. A robot is potentially strong and durable and can automate tasks with exact reproducibility in situations where humans might otherwise become fatigued, leading to errors and variances. Robotic devices could capture and record data through sensors, then process and analyze those data and provide dynamic feedback to the end users.[1–5] These features could be used for therapeutic, adaptive, and assistive purposes.[1]

In rehabilitation, we can classify robots into two major categories: robots used for therapy, such as physical or occupational therapy, and robots used for assistance in daily living to increase independence and/or decrease caregiver burden. Robots designed to be used for therapy are used to improve an individual's function by assisting in supervised professional therapy sessions such as strengthening and neurorestorative or cardiopulmonary conditioning therapies.[1] Robots designed for assistance in daily living can support and augment a patient's function or even replace their disabilities and limitations, ultimately to enhance a person's independence and/or decrease dependence on others.[1] However, robotics in rehabilitation is not limited to just these two broad categories. There are also robots that are designed to fulfill social interactions and emotional support.[1]

Robotic rehabilitation therapies began in the early 1900s with a machine invented by Theodor Budigen to support stepping movements for patients with heart disease.[6] By the 1930s, Richard

Scherb had created early prototypical exoskeletons[6] with cables and mechanical joints that aided in orthopedic therapy, mechanically helping to increase range and to stretch the patient's limbs.[7] Similarly, later industrial manipulator robots helped in therapies incorporating repetitive dynamic movements, where the robot would hold on to pads and move the pad according to the preplanned therapy regimen.[7] Powered exoskeletons were invented around the 1970s utilizing pneumatic, hydraulic, and electromagnetic actuators for limb movement.[7]

It was not until the 1980s that scientists first started designing robots for neurorehabilitation.[7] In 1989, Dr. Krebs and his team at the Massachusetts Institute of Technology designed the robot MIT-Manus to allow finer control over the force and movements of the upper extremity.[8,9] Lokomat, first introduced in 1994, is another pioneer robot in lower-body rehabilitation that supports body weight during treadmill training[10] (see Fig. 6.1). In 2002, Reading University (UK) developed a robot that allows patients to train with virtual reality.[9] Since then, there has been a proliferation of developments, many designed with neurorehabilitation in mind, that interact with patients through passive movements, as well as assisted-active and actively resisted movements, virtual reality, and sensory feedback[7] (see Fig. 6.2).

Neurorehabilitation is a method in rehabilitation where neurorestorative therapies are employed with the goal of neurorecovery: the restoration of neurologic functions after a neurologic injury or insult. Neurorestorative therapies help patients who have lost sensorimotor control and function after neurologic injuries such as stroke, brain injury, and spinal cord injury.[15] These therapies attempt to take advantage of neuroplasticity, based on the theory that the nervous system can be retrained.[15,16] To reestablish neural pathways, therapy consists of sensory and motor stimulation through a passive range of motions, functional exercises, and strengthening programs.[7,15,17] These types of therapy are often high intensity and repetitive, since a very high dose of these tasks is necessary to achieve meaningful gains.[7,16,18] During a traditional therapy session, patients typically perform about 30 repetitions in a 45-minute session.[19] However, robots are capable of consistently delivering a reproducible experience, and each session can consist of as much as 1000 repetitions.[16,17,20,21] With the help of robots, therapists are able to offload highly repetitive and tiring tasks, and instead are able to focus more on finer nuances, overall therapeutic goals, and/or more efficiently seeing higher volumes of patients.[2,5,17,22]

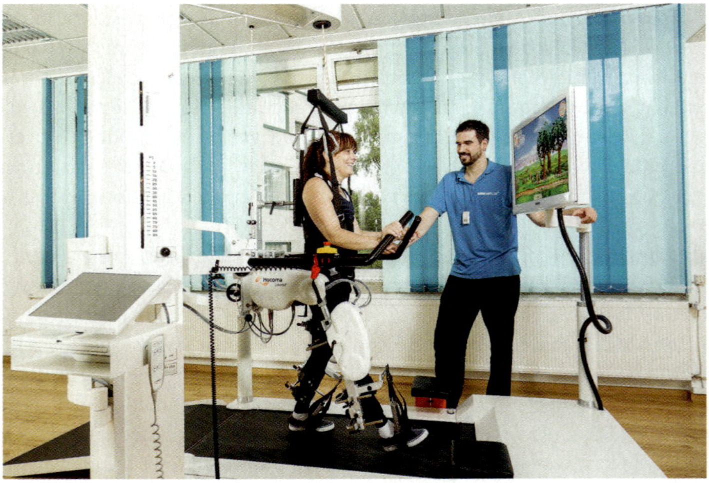

Fig. 6.1 Lokomat: an adjustable body weight support system with treadmill and robotic legs that allows and aids in physiologic movement of legs through the gait cycle.[1,11] Patients can be challenged through tasks on the monitor and receive real-time feedback.[11] (From Hocoma, Switzerland.)

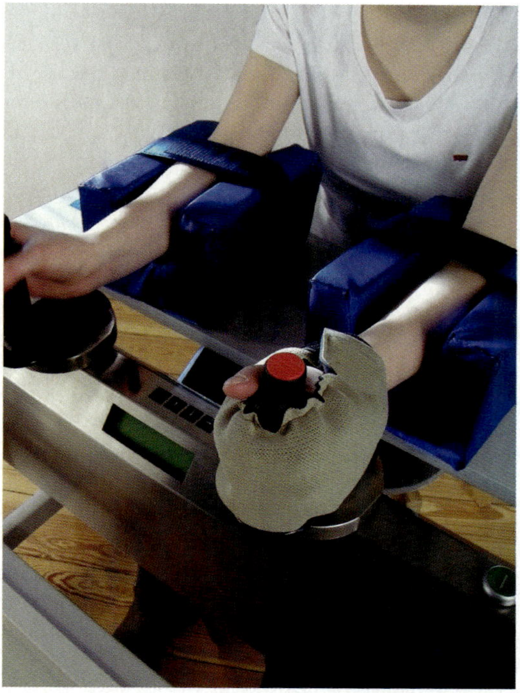

Fig. 6.2 Bi-Manu-Track. A robot for pronation/supination and wrist flexion and extension exercises through bimanual mirrored exercises.[12,13] The unaffected arm is able to actively drive the affected arm and perform exercises through simple games.[12,13] It also has a selection of passive, active, or assist-as-needed modes.[14]

Robots are not just limited to repetitive tasks. Equipped with onboard sensors, robots can gather objective data, such as limb position, velocity, and force, to estimate muscle activation, as well as other physiologic states of the user such as cardiac output and respiratory effort. These data could be processed and analyzed in real time or stored in memory for clinicians to monitor progress and augment clinical decision-making to potentially enhance neurorecovery.[1–5,14] Additionally, data can be analyzed through computational models for the robot to adapt to fluctuations in the patient's performance and to make real-time changes to treatment.[2–4] By providing direct feedback to patients and providers, robots enhance neurorecovery through optimal synchronization between patient motivation and their motor output.[7,23]

One highly effective neurorestorative approach is called constraint-induced movement therapy.[7] After one limb becomes less functional, the other limb compensates for the loss of function, thereby patients are unable to recover much function of the affected limb due to prolonged disuse.[16,17] Constraint-induced movement therapy was developed to prevent learned disuse and maximize functionality of the affected limb. However, providing the right amount of assistance while maximizing patient effort to complete the tasks are difficult and depends on the severity of the impairment.[24] Incorporating robotic therapies allow for fine-tuning and adapting as the patient fatigues or, conversely, recovers more strength.

In addition to motor impairments, sensory and cognitive impairments also contribute to decline in function. Sensory function is necessary in providing feedback to the brain, for example in maintaining appropriate strength while grasping an object or positioning the limb in space right before taking a step.[25] Patients often rely on visual compensation; however, they also suffer from cognitive impairments, and these compensations could be limited.[26]

Despite every effort for neurorecovery, not all patients recover completely. Even those who obtain partial function most rarely achieve over 70% to 80% of the previous baseline.[27–29] To compensate for residual impairments, assistive robots can help maximize independence during activities of daily living and minimize caregiver burden. For example, some patients may benefit from exoskeletons that provide gravity support and movement assistance, allowing them to regain control of the surrounding environment.[7]

This chapter will present basic concepts in designing robots for rehabilitation, how therapy robots are used for upper- and lower-limb recovery, as well as social and emotional domains and how assistive and other robots are contributing to rehabilitation.

Basic Concepts in Robotic Design for Rehabilitation

There are two major types of robotic design for rehabilitation, end-effector types and exoskeleton types. End-effector robots control and guide the most distal part of the patient's body, such as a hand or foot, through the endpiece of the robot, and thus the whole system is mostly independent of the patient.[7,9,18] Due to this independence, these robots have a greater degree of freedom, a larger field of space, and higher motion dynamics.[7,9] In contrast, exoskeleton robots control one or more joints and are either integrated or attached directly to the patient's limb.[18] As exoskeleton robots are constrained by human joints, they have less freedom of movement but are more compact and better able to assist motion.[9] Further discussion of exoskeleton robots will be presented later in the chapter.

The most important robotic design feature is safety[1,2,16] (see Table 6.1). Often, excessive tensions can cause injuries to muscle, tendons, ligaments, and bones, therefore robotic devices should monitor and prevent any tissue damage while working within reasonable ranges of motion, speed, and force.[9] These safety measures should be enforced through both mechanical constraints and software limiters.[9] Furthermore, it is critical that all machines have prominent and easily accessible stop buttons.[9,30] Despite all these precautions, patient safety ultimately lies with the machine operator who must set reasonable parameters for the robot and monitor and control the situation.[9]

Before the design phase, it is important to understand rehabilitation physiology and have a standardized therapy method that the robot could model.[2,7] Without a standardized treatment

TABLE 6.1 ■ **Possible Safety Mechanisms**[30]

Safety Mechanism	Description
User initiated	
Emergency button	Button provides an easy method for patient to override control unit for immediate stop.
Voice command	Robot listens for a "stop" voice command.
Unactuated digit detection	Patients control the unit through voluntary movement of digits that are not being actuated.
Sensors	
Strain sensor	Sensor measures joint bending and stress on joint and shuts off if threshold strain is exceeded.
Pressure sensor	Sensor measures pressure in areas directly in contact with patient and shuts off if a threshold pressure is exceeded.
Mechanical limiters	
Rotation limiter	Spools that guide cables are intrinsically limited in rotation to avoid hyperflexion or hyperextension of the limb.
Magnetic coupling	Cables are connected to magnetic ends and mechanically detach when tension exceeds the magnetic strength threshold.

plan, the robot and patient could begin repetitive motions in a slightly wrong position or trajectory, which could lead to learned mal-use and worse outcomes.[2,16] In addition, robots must be able to recreate and reproduce intended motions according to the treatment plan while detecting for deviations and provide corrective measures or sound an alert.[16]

The rehabilitation robot must be able to adapt to varying degrees of impairment in strength, range of motion, mobility, and coordination. Robots must be able to provide full assistance for a weak limb, including anticipating the patient's intended motions or movements, which would be most helpful in adaptive robots assisting in daily living activities.[16,30] However, robots must also be able to provide varying degrees of resistance for strength training.[16] To achieve both these facets, the robotic actuators, or devices that convert control signals into mechanical motions, should have low impedance or resistance to change but a high capacity in delivering motion.[16,17] Depending on specific therapy goals, the device should be able to change its focus between different parameters, such as range of motion, strength, speed, and coordination; be able to detect muscle spasms, while concomitantly adapting to varying inputs, patients, and environments; and be able to avoid collisions with other objects.[1,9,16] The robotic system should be able to process the environment through its onboard sensors and adjust any limb malpositioning or trajectory deviation, and perhaps even individualize the treatment depending on the circumstance or the patient.[1,16]

Another critical design factor is ease of use and maintenance.[1] Many of the robotic devices are quite complex to use, with long setup procedures that may take up valuable allotted therapy time.[1,7,31] To remedy this challenge, an effective design team should be represented by engineers, therapists, physicians, and patients.[31] Similarly, physical aesthetics may play a large role in minimizing emotional barriers of use and should also be strongly considered in design decisions.[2] Other development concerns include use of different materials such as soft and fluid material as opposed to traditional rigid structures,[15,30] software security of the robots to prevent malicious hacking, and financial cost of the robotic system. Another important consideration is the ethics of robot use.[1] To what extent do users have control over the robot? What about privacy of the data collected by the robots? These questions are universal as we adopt more robotics and computer systems in our lives.

Upper-Extremity Robotic Therapy

Hand and arm impairments are common sequelae of neurologic and musculoskeletal insults such as stroke, spinal cord injuries, Parkinson's disease, and arthritis. Particularly after a stroke, there are a number of established physiotherapeutic approaches including Bobath, Brunnstrom, Proprioceptive Neuromuscular Facilitation, and task-specific training.[32] Although none of these approaches show any significant advantages over the other, task-specific training has been the most common, sometimes used in combination with constraint-induced movement therapy.[30,32,33] The goal of task specific training, also known as functional task practice, is to facilitate relearning of the appropriate motor skill to improve task performance.[33] Given its acceptance and effectiveness, many of the upper-extremity therapy robots are based on repetitive task-specific motions.

Designing for upper-extremity therapy robots poses its own challenges. Shoulder joints are very complex, with 3 degrees of freedom and movement of the center of rotation while a shoulder is mobilized.[9] The wrist also has three degrees of freedom and the hand with one to 2 degrees of freedom depending on the joint. Hand function, with the hand's numerous joints, is usually one of the last places to recover, if at all, after a neurologic insult.[7] Another difficulty is that upper extremities exhibit strong synergistic muscle contractions after a stroke, often leading to dystonic upper-extremity posturing, thus isolating individual muscle groups for exercise is challenging.[34] Due to these concerns, conventional therapy focuses first on training the proximal limb such as shoulder and elbow.[17]

Evidence for the use of upper-extremity therapy robots is mixed. Some findings imply that robotic-assisted therapy can facilitate motor recovery with meaningful changes in activities of daily living, but others suggest no difference from usual care.[18] One important factor to consider is that the timing at which robot therapy is done also affects outcome. After a stroke, most of the recovery happens in the first 3 months.[18,33] Studies demonstrate robotic therapy increases motor control in the chronic phase (beyond 3 months postinjury), whereas studies looking at acute/subacute phase (less than 3 months postinjury) cannot differentiate therapeutic intervention recovery from natural recovery.[18,35]

For dose-matched trials that were performed for poststroke rehabilitation, when conventional therapy and robotic therapy with the same intensity and repetitions were compared, the outcome for robotic therapy appeared to be as effective as that of conventional therapy.[20,36–39] Similarly, in robotic therapy after a distal radial fracture, there were no significant differences in outcome between robotic therapy and conventional therapy.[40] As these robots were designed to simulate and reproduce therapists' manual exercises, the comparable effectiveness is an argument for the implementation of robotic devices to offload therapist's taxing tasks and allow the clinician to focus on functional rehabilitation.[40]

Above all, there are no reported significant adverse events, and robot-assisted therapy appears to be safe.[16,18,40,41] A limitation to the overall recommendation for robots in therapy is the heterogeneity of studies using different robots with different doses. Despite this variability, the evidence indicates that outcomes are independent of the use of a specific robot, but rather from the use of robots in general.[42] This evidence has led the American Heart Association to announce that robotic therapy can be considered in delivering more intensive therapies.[33]

Recent studies have shown that the use of robotics with botulinum toxin in spastic arm conditions has synergistic effects in improving upper-limb function.[14] Additionally, some robotic therapy showed reduction in neuropathic pain in the shoulder and hands.[14] These findings demonstrate that there may be other unexplored benefits to robotic therapy in the upper extremity.

Lower-Extremity Robotic Therapy

Gait dysfunction is another common sequela of neurologic and musculoskeletal injuries. Especially after a stroke, the ability to walk independently is one of the major determinants for home discharge, and walking speed is an indicator of functional community ambulation.[43,44] Such as in upper-extremity rehabilitation, patients usually start their therapy course with passive range of motion, then move on to active exercises with assistance, active exercises without assistance, and active exercises with resistance.[4] Conventional therapy for gait training involves varying combinations of strengthening, task-oriented exercises, functional electric stimulation, biofeedback, and treadmill exercises requiring many repetitive motions and many iterations of practice[33,43,45]; thus, gait training is a good candidate for robotic therapy.

For lower-extremity gait training, there are several different types of robots, including tethered and nontethered exoskeleton machines and end-effector type machines.[46] In tethered exoskeleton systems such as Lokomat and LOPES, patients are usually suspended in a harness with robotic legs attached to their legs so that the exoskeleton supports and guides limb motion on a treadmill.[1,46] There are untethered exoskeleton systems such as the ReWalk, Indego, and Ekso that allow for the most realistic walking experience.[46] Details of exoskeleton devices will be mentioned later in this chapter. Examples of end effector–type robots include Gait Trainer, G-EO System, and GAR[1,46,47] (see Fig. 6.3). These robots guide the patient's feet through a gait cycle, imitating stance and swing phases with less friction and motor interference than exoskeleton devices.[48] As such, they have greater variability in motion, which allow for balance training and stair climbing in addition to gait retraining.[46,47]

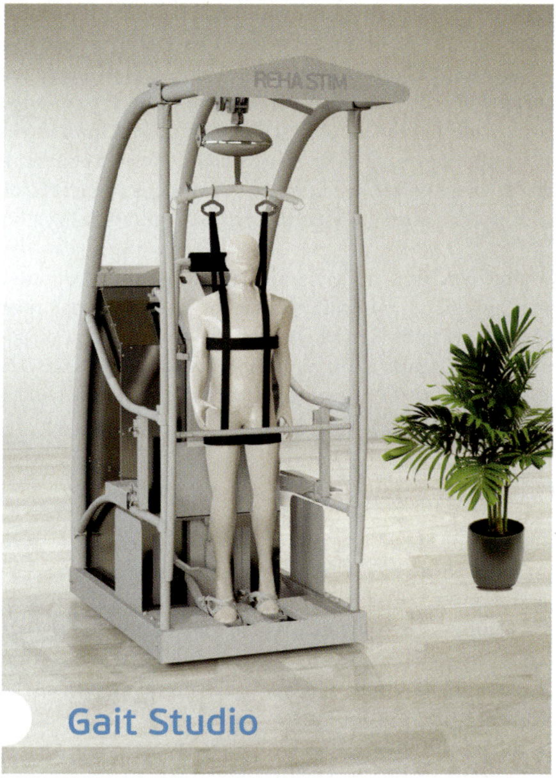

Fig. 6.3 Gait Trainer II. An end effector–type gait training device that modulates feet movement during the gait cycle through foot plates.[47] It has a quick and easy setup with intuitive user interface to allow optimal use of therapy time.[49] (From Reha-Stim.)

For patients who are wheelchair bound, there are significant advantages to treadmill training with a system that supports body weight.[47,48,50] Typically, two or three therapists are required to assist such patients not only to help support their weight, but to control trunk and limb movement.[7,48] Replacement with a robotic system allows for early verticality, which improves cardiorespiratory rehabilitation and also stimulates wakefulness, an important goal especially in patients with severe cognitive neurologic impairment.[47] Although gravity could be mostly eliminated through a body weight support mechanism, these robotic machines still require patients to have adequate endurance and the ability to stand.[4] For those without those residual facilities, there are robots that allow training in a seated or lying position to work on building endurance and strength, mobility, and coordination.[4]

As with upper-extremity robotic therapy, the evidence of robotic therapy over conventional therapy is mixed. For positive findings, patients who had stroke and who received robotic therapy in combination with conventional therapy seemed to have a higher likelihood of achieving independent walking.[7,44,46–48,51,52] However, it is not clear whether exoskeleton devices or end effector–type devices are more effective or whether robotic therapy is effective for patients with subacute or chronic condition. Currently the strongest evidence is for robotic therapy with end effector–type devices, in conjunction with conventional therapy for patients with subacute condition after a stroke.[43,47,53] Nevertheless, a number of studies did not show any significant benefit.[43,50] Critics have noted that robotic devices like Lokomat are restricted in the coronal and axial planes, focusing only on movement in the sagittal plane and reducing training for postural stabilization.[50] Additionally, although robots support patients and reduce cardiopulmonary load, this may inhibit the aerobic stimulus required for gait relearning.[53,54] Finally, because robots assist in limb trajectory, there is little cognitive component, which is essential for neuroplasticity.[50] Despite these mixed findings, the American Heart Association recommends considering robotic devices for poststroke therapy in patients who have limited ambulation or are nonambulatory.[33]

For patients with spinal cord injury, a meta-analysis showed that robotic-assisted gait training improved endurance and mobility and decreased spasticity, but did not change the level of their pain.[55] Authors proposed that rhythmic passive exercises from gait training could stimulate neuroplastic reorganization in the spinal cord, leading to decreased spasticity.[55] Alternatively, critics also note that passive motion leads to degeneration of motor neurons with no patient's cognitive input.[7]

Virtual Reality in Rehabilitation

As mentioned previously, neurorecovery requires active engagement to promote neuroplasticity and motor relearning.[7,56–58] However, the level of patients' participation during therapy depends on their motivation and interest.[59] One method of increasing popularity is to engage patients via virtual and augmented reality.[57] Virtual reality technology creates an immersive environment for the patients beyond what is possible in the physical world.[15] This technology has previously been used in other areas such as flight simulation, surgical training, treatment of phobias, and post-traumatic stress disorder.[56]

There are many benefits from integrating virtual reality into therapy. First, patients describe the immersive environment as more interesting and thus encouraging higher intensity and repetitions during therapy.[56,60] This can also be combined with games.[56,57] Second, virtual reality could allow patients to practice daily activities beyond the hospital environment, such as in supermarkets and in the street, and individualize the training environment for the patient.[56,58] And lastly, there are data that show virtual reality induces cortical reorganization and neuroplasticity.[61,62]

With virtual reality, patients have reported greater motivation, less fatigue, improved visuospatial awareness, and overall better quality of life.[58,60] This technique is especially helpful for patients with impaired cognition and reduced visuospatial awareness.[58] Although particular task exercises may not be generalizable, improved visuospatial awareness will allow patients to adapt and participate in activities of daily living.[58] Further, the visuospatial training for return to automobile driving could be done in a safe virtual environment.[58] Virtual and augmented realities could also become another important tool for therapist assessment of patient performance, such as for automobile driving after stroke or for fall risks in those with Parkinson disease.[3,60] In addition, pain management is another area that utilizes virtual reality by creating an illusion of the patient's body, which may help with phantom limb pain.[58]

Evidence for the use of virtual reality in therapy is still under investigation. There is some evidence to suggest a better ability to manage activities of daily living and better gait and balance after therapy utilizing virtual reality.[3,56,57,63] Although virtual reality combined with robotic machines interfaces and tactile feedback could provide immersive and synchronized experience, many of the current technologies are too slow, causing a delay between responses in motor output and sensory feedback, which leads to increased task difficulty and motion sickness.[9,64] The true effectiveness of virtual reality in rehabilitation is yet to be established and awaits better advancements in technology.

Social and Emotional Therapy Robots

Mental health is another area where robotic therapy can help. Patients with social anxiety or developmental disorders often have difficulty engaging with others and expressing and communicating emotions appropriately.[1] Patients with autism spectrum disorders are naturally drawn to robots that have predictable behavior.[1] There are robots that are socially interactive, participating in simple games with the patient for simple cognitive and physical exercises.[65] One robot, Facial Automation for Conveying Emotions (FACE), is able to display and express lifelike human emotion to help patients with autism to identify and practice emotional expressions to improve communication skills.[1,66] Other robots may look like a stuffed animal or a cute toy to increase interaction and companionship[1] (see Fig. 6.4). Although these robots are specifically designed for social and emotional support, the concepts could also be applied to other therapy and assistive robots that are approachable and provide support to patients.

Assistive Robots

Despite intense rehabilitation, many patients still require long-term assistance,[7] and with an aging population increasing demand for professional caregivers has led to a shortage.[68] Fortunately, robots could fill this gap and moreover provide consistent and reliable care at any time of the day, whereas caregivers are limited by their working hours, as well as physical and mental fatigue. These assistive robots could decrease caregiver burden while improving patient autonomy and independence, thereby possibly delaying transition into nursing homes.[68]

Assistive robots are designed to aid across various aspects of activities of daily living, including transfer and mobility, dressing, eating, hygiene, bathing, and toileting. Mobility aide robots such as nonanchored rolling frame robots can dynamically support the body and maintain a stable posture while allowing patients to walk around.[46] Other robots have guidance system for ease of

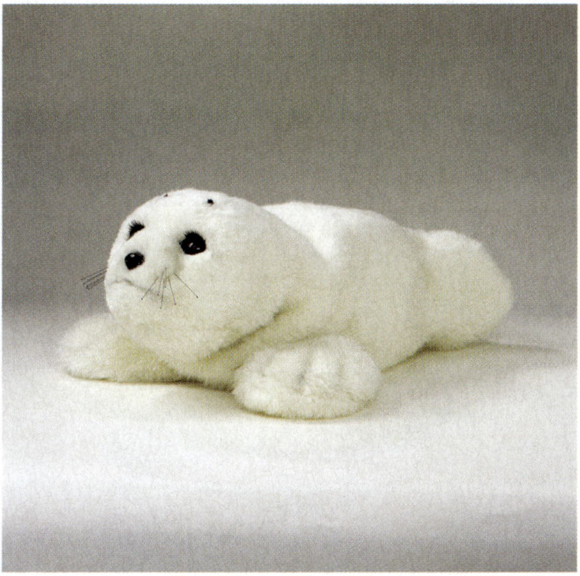

Fig. 6.4 PARO, a soft seal robot used for animal therapy.[1,67] PARO can detect whether it is being stroked and respond in ways users prefer.[1,67] This therapeutic environment reduces stress and enhances psychological well being.[1] (Courtesy of AIST.)

navigation, some with fully autonomous robotic wheelchairs that can drive patients around their house or even in the community[68]. Transfers to and from beds to chairs are frequent and often lead to back pain in caregivers,[68] but machines like the Robot for Interactive Body Assistance can provide assistance in carrying patients[68] (see Fig. 6.5). Other tasks requiring more fine motor control such as feeding, bathing, and toileting are better facilitated by articulated manipulator arm robots with 3 or more degrees of freedom.[63,69] These manipulators can be mounted on a surface, and through artificial intelligence, patients can command the arm to do tasks such as grasping, pushing, and brushing.[63,69] A particular commercialized robot, Obi, is specifically designed for feeding[70] (see Fig. 6.6).

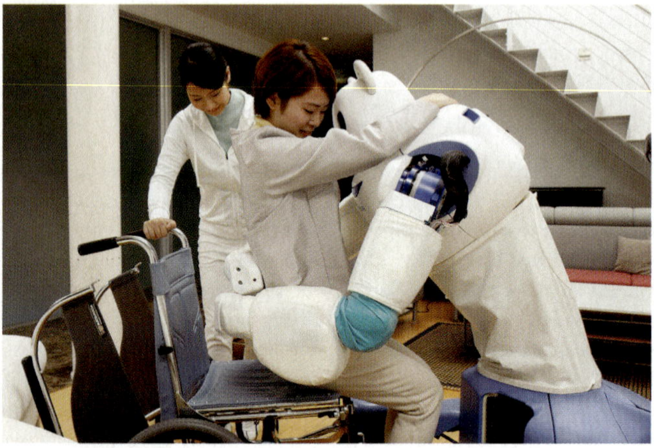

Fig. 6.5 Robot for Interactive Body Assistance (RIBA). A robot shaped like a polar bear designed to safely pick up and transfer patients.[72] It can respond to verbal commands and recognize faces and voices.[72] (From Riken, Japan.)

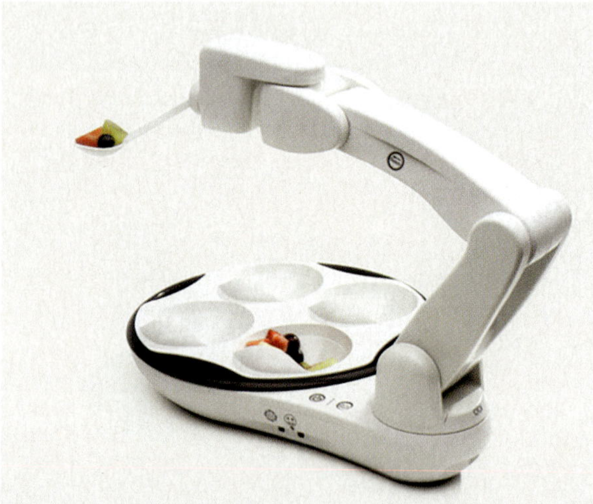

Fig. 6.6 Obi is a dining service robot that aids in independent feeding.[70] Obi can deliver food at optimal portions without unwanted drips and splashes and can provide intuitive animated gestures through its arm with 6 degrees of freedom.[70]

In addition to physical assistance, augmentative and alternative communication systems help patients interact with other people and with their surroundings.[63] These devices accept a number of different routes for information input, through arm or leg movement or even just with eye movement. The information is processed, often using predictive algorithms, into either voice or text outputs or into commands for phone, computer, or home appliances.[63] Combined with articulated manipulators and artificial intelligence, assistive robots are being continuously developed into dynamic and integrated machines to help patients achieve independence.

Other Topics

Widespread implementation and acceptance are some of the biggest issues facing robotics in rehabilitation. There are several reasons for this, such as efficacy, usability, and cost. Substantiated evidence for clinically meaningful advantages of robotic therapy is still lacking,[14,73] and still there are no standardized protocols for robotic therapy such as dosage, frequency, or modes of integration into conventional therapy plans.[14,73] There have been some efforts to integrate robotic therapy as a "robotic array" system to efficiently use different types of robots, but further studies are needed for the efficient use of robots.[22]

There has been a lack of attention to the sensory and cognitive components of motor recovery.[14,74] Much of the literature on robotic rehabilitation excludes patients with cognitive comorbidities such as aphasia, apraxia, or other deficits.[73,74] Many patients requiring rehabilitation have varying degrees of cognitive deficits that affect their daily living.[73] Cognition is crucial in motor relearning and neuroplasticity, and without cognitive attention, patients have difficulty forming new motor memory.[14,74] Recent investigations have focused on how robotic therapy could facilitate motor recovery through sensory stimulation and modulating the cognitive state.[15] But without studies that include patients with cognitive deficits, much of the literature on robotic rehabilitation may not be generalizable to daily clinical practice.[73]

As mentioned previously, neuroplasticity relies on patient engagement and active participation, when simply increasing repetition and intensity may be insufficient for therapeutic gains.[7,14,74] However, patient attitudes toward the robotic devices are not always favorable.[68] Interestingly, patients have reported quite different emotional responses from a robot with identical movements, depending on how the individual patient perceives the robot's "intention."[68] A patient's perception on the robot may affect motivation and emotional response to therapy, which could affect neuroplasticity.[74] Therefore, robotic therapy is not meant to replace human touch and the expertise of therapists but rather as a tool to augment therapy by generating complex and controlled therapy plans.[74]

And lastly, cost will always be a major factor to implementation. Some available commercial robots for therapy cost from several thousand to close to a half a million US dollars.[75,76] Initial investment costs might be too much for many small rehabilitation facilities or individuals. Additionally, the machines must be maintained and the users trained.[1] Nevertheless, one analysis demonstrated that patients who underwent robotic therapy consumed less overall health-care costs.[77] More investigation is needed to explore cost efficiency and cost benefit of robotic therapy systems, with consideration of overall health-care cost rather than just the cost of the machine.[73]

Conclusion

Although the idea of the use of robotics for rehabilitation and assistance in daily activity has been around since the early 20th century, it is nevertheless still in its infancy. With an aging population that requires more rehabilitation and more assistance, compounded by the shortages of younger caregivers and ever-increasing work pressure on therapists, the need for robotics is evident. This is especially true for low-resource areas that have high demand but lack qualified workers. Robots will not only be able to reduce repetitive, fatiguing, and injury-prone work, but also increase independence for patients and improve efficiency for therapists. However, there are still many areas requiring improvement, from technological maturity to cost and social acceptance. Advances in artificial intelligence technologies would eventually allow robots to process various signals and commands from individuals, and then predict and perform the desired outputs. Many therapies could potentially become virtual, which could be useful for remote areas. As robots become less cumbersome, more relatable, and cost-effective, robotic-assisted therapy will become more accessible, useful, and integrated into our society.

Prosthetics: The Merging of Humans With Robotics

The intervention of prosthetics and orthotics in humankind has a very long history. There are two definitions for "prosthetics" as defined by the *Oxford Languages* dictionary: (1) an artificial body part; a prosthesis; (2) an artificial feature or piece of flexible material applied to a person's face or body to change his or her appearance temporarily. The definition of "orthotics" according to the *Oxford Languages* dictionary is: a support, brace, or splint used to support, align, prevent, or correct the function of movable parts of the body. This part of the chapter will be dealing with just prosthetics, past, present, and possible future state, with a possible new definition of "prosthetics": the merging of advanced robotics to replace or enhance human body segments.

PAST

The early history of prosthetics shows humanities attempt to both replace and enhance a person's limb loss. The "Cairo Toe" (see Fig. 6.7), dating back to around 950 BCE, is one of the earliest examples of functional replacement and cosmesis. It allows the user to maintain foot balance and still wear sandals.

Another example of early prosthetics is the "Capua Leg," which dates around 300 BCE (Fig. 6.8). The original was original thought to be made of bronze and had both functional and cosmetic use. However, achieving both cosmetic form and function was usually reserved for the very

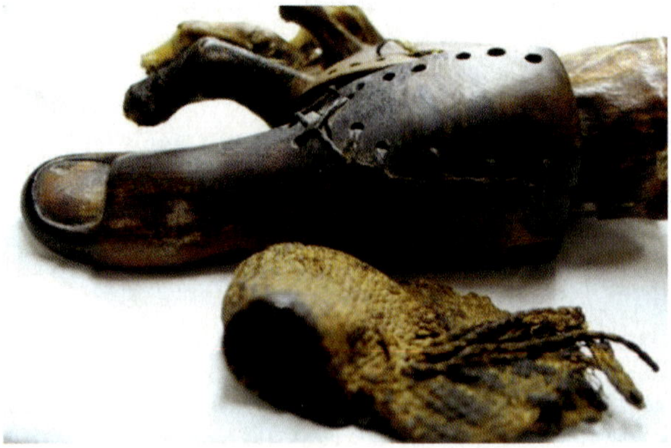

Fig. 6.7 Cairo toe. (From www.world-archaeology.com.)

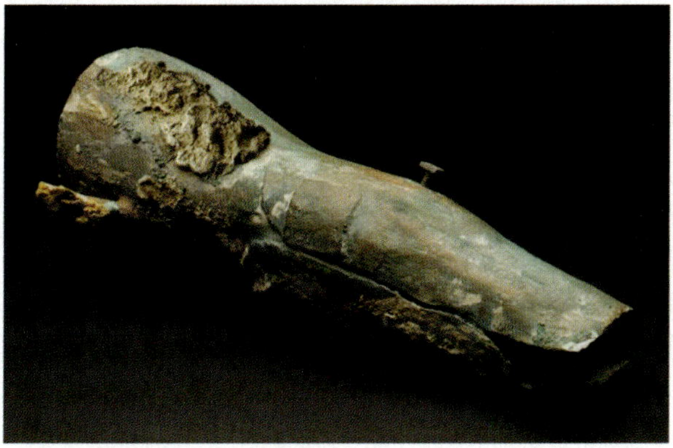

Fig. 6.8 Capua leg. (From London Science Museum.)

wealthy. Most limb loss in the early days of humankind was due to trauma, warfare, and early industrial development. Of course, people still had limb loss due to congenital reasons and disease. The survival rate to the actual amputation surgery were very low, and the early surgeons had to be very quick due to the lack of anesthesia and blood loss.[78]

Although both the field of prosthetics and the surgeons doing the amputation progressed as time went on, it was not until the early 1500 s AD that major advances in both prosthetics and surgery occurred. This was done by Ambroise Paré, a Parisian barber surgeon who advance the field of amputation surgery and prosthetics.[79]

The next big step for the actual amputation surgery came in the 1800s with the introduction of antisepsis by Joseph Lister[80] and anesthesia by Joseph Long.[81] These two simple techniques saved countless lives; who knew washing your hands, keeping dirt out of the surgical field, and providing the patient with pain relief and a nontraumatizing surgery would be one of the largest benefits to the field of surgery.

In the meantime the field of prosthetics made very slow gains in form and function. The elaborate prosthetic devices were left to the rich and famous. Most prosthetic devices concentrated on replacing basic functions like ambulation and use of tools and eating utensils, thus allowing the person with limb loss to perform basic activities of daily living and return to a somewhat normal life. As with everything else advancement in technology, which includes prosthetics, came after a war.

The melding of humans and artificial components especially for people with upper-extremity limb loss became popular after World War I and advanced after World War II and the Korean War.[82] The procedure was called a tunnel cineplasty (Fig. 6.9), which utilized a portion of a person's remaining musculature and looping it proximally with flaps of skin inside the tunnel. This created an attachment point and active external pulley. The prosthesis was then made, and a cable looped through the tunnel would control the terminal device (hook or hand) (Fig. 6.10), thus creating the human-machine interface and freeing the wearer the additional harnessing and control systems that is required for an upper-extremity prosthesis (Fig. 6.11).

During the same period, developments were happening with creating a powered upper-extremity prosthesis, starting in 1915 with a German pneumatic hand, which continued into the 1960s.

The myoelectric prosthesis was first reported in the 1940s by a physicist named Reinhold Reiter.[83] A myoelectric prosthesis is one that utilizes an electromyogram (EMG) signal produced by a muscle, which is picked up by an electrode placed inside the prosthesis touching the skin. That signal is then boosted to control an electrical hand or hook terminal device. The earliest

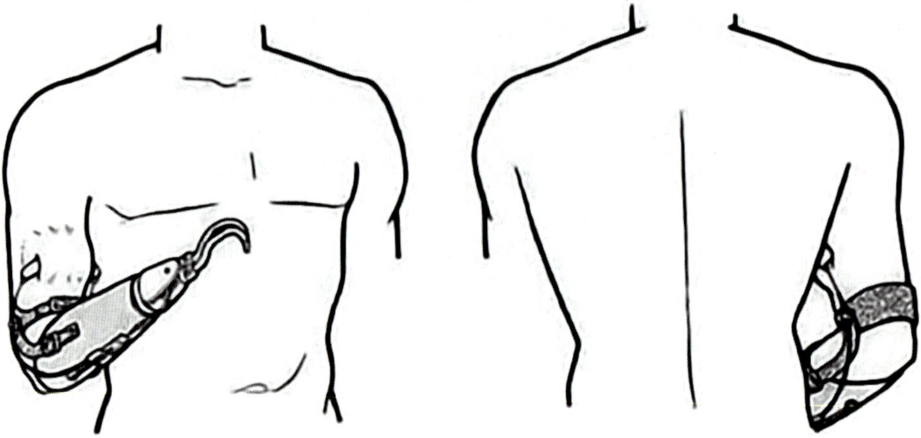

Fig. 6.9 Biceps cineplasty. (From OandPLibrary.org.)

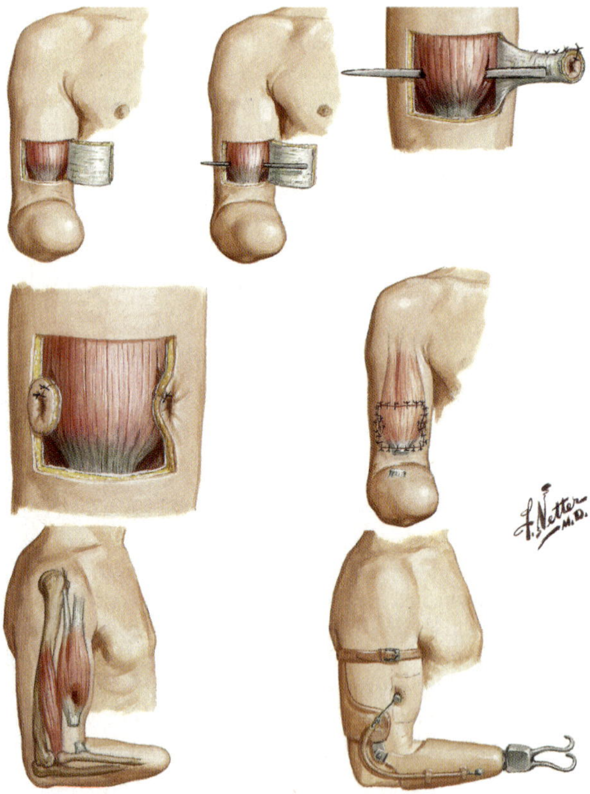

Fig. 6.10 Externally powered transradial prosthesis. (From rehab.research.va.gov.)

models provided a hand that would open and close and an elbow that would flex and extend. As time move forward, the hand became stronger, providing up to 30 pounds of pinch force in a three-jaw chuck pinch pattern (normal human pinch is about 12 pounds). This is a far cry from the "Six Million Dollar Man" with his bionic limbs. The early electric elbows for trans humeral and shoulder disarticulation were barely able to move their own weight with terminal device. As technology advanced, refinement in the use of the EMG signals increased and proportion control of the prosthesis became possible. In other words, a stronger EMG signal from the muscle group in the residual limb used to control the ability to close your hand (finger flexors) led the prosthetic hand closing more quickly or with more force, thus giving the user the ability to develop light grasp patterns (think picking up an egg or a potato chip) (Fig. 6.12).

Even the with the advancements in electronics and microprocessors that are incorporated into the upper-extremity prosthesis, the researchers and prosthetists have not been able to duplicate the intricacies of the human arm and hand. The freedom of movement combined with the sense of touch is the holy grail for prosthetics.

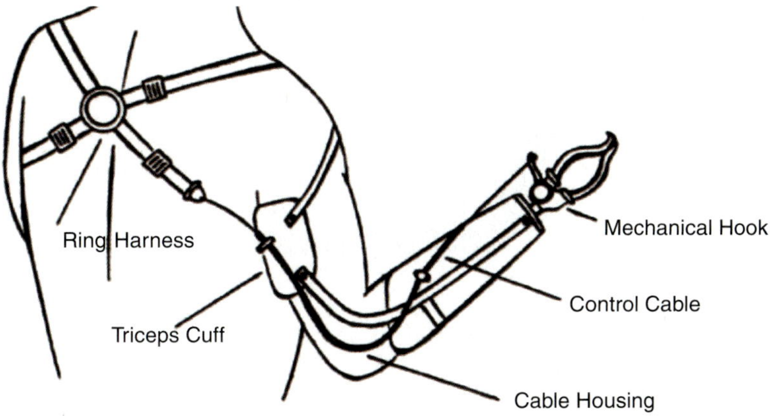

Fig. 6.11 Bowden cable body-powered prosthesis. (This is a work of the U.S. Government and is not subject to copyright protection in the United States.)

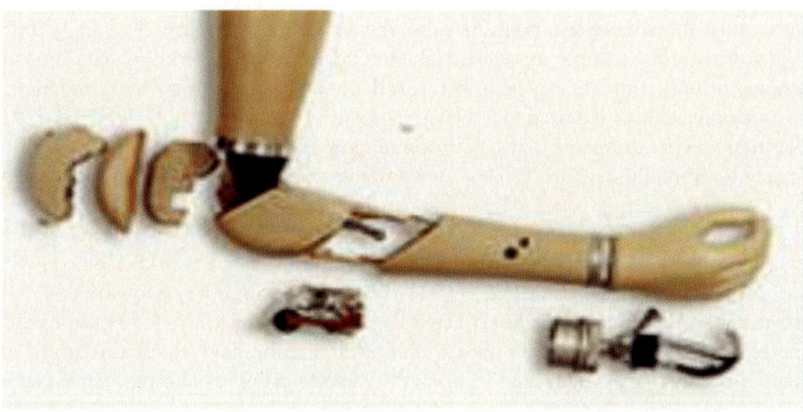

Fig. 6.12 Utah Arm, motion control. (From Fillauer Inc.)

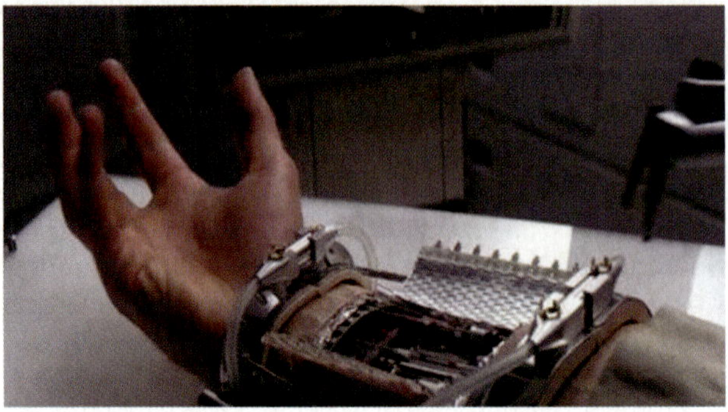

Fig. 6.13 Luke Skywalker arm.

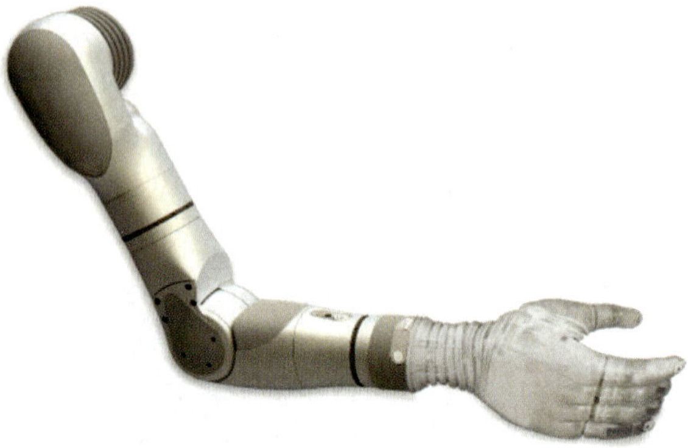

Fig. 6.14 LUKE Arm. (From Mobius Bionics Inc.)

The LUKE Arm named after the famous *Star Wars* scene in which Luke Skywalker gets a new arm and hand (Fig. 6.13). The prosthesis was developed in cooperation with Mobius Bionics and Department of Defense and the Veterans Administration and is the first device for upper-extremity amputees that starts to come close, with multiple degrees of freedom, tactile feedback (provided by a vibratory motor), and proportional control (Fig. 6.14).

However, this all comes with a price, literally. The device for a shoulder disarticulation weighs in at 4.7 kg and requires multiple inputs to make the device work, including EMG sensors, inertial measurement units that are typically worn on the user's shoes, and switches mounted to the extensive harnessing that is required to keep the prosthesis on.

Unlike upper-extremity prosthetics, advancements in lower-extremity prosthetics is moving much slower even though there are 150,000 new lower-extremity amputation a year in the United States.[84]

Since War World II there have been some major engineering designs in lower extremity in both the function and control of the prosthesis and even how they attach to a person with limb loss. Prior to these developments people with lower-extremity limb loss had very few choices in how a prosthesis worked. Prosthetic knees acted like a hinge, and prosthetic feet were made from rubber, both incorporating wood. The new materials and technology that came from war gave the industry a boost. Lightweight aluminum and hydraulic cylinders allowed better control of a transfemoral (above knee) prosthesis. The Hydra-Cadence Knee provided fluid control of both the knee and the foot both during the swing and stance phases of gait (Fig. 6.15).

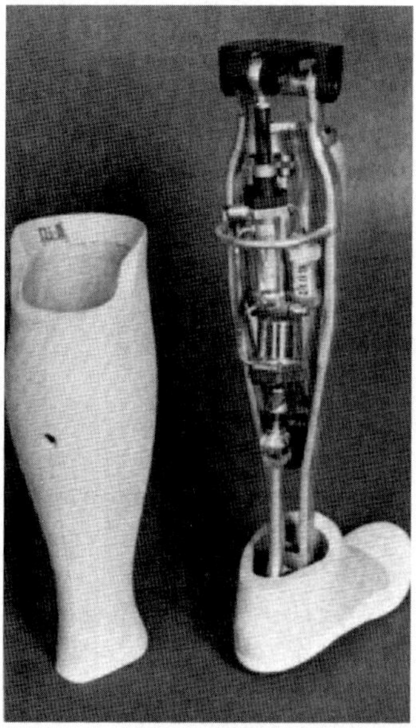

Fig. 6.15 Hydra-Cadence Knee. (Reproduced with permission from the Prosthetics Research Program, Veterans Administration.)

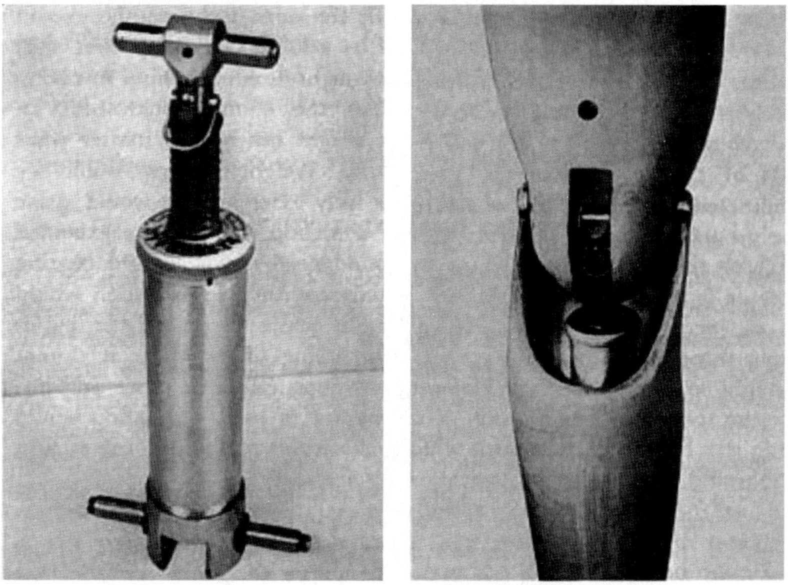

Fig. 6.16 Swing and Stance knee. (Mauch S-N-S Hydraulic Knee Veterans Administration Bulletin of Prosthetics research – Fall 1968.)

In the 1960s Hans Adolph Mauch, a German engineer known for his work during the war on jet engines and the V-1 flying bomb, was also involved in prosthetic developments and was brought to the United States by the US Army Air Forces to work on their many projects. In 1959 he left their service, formed his own company, and developed the Mauch S-N-S (Swing and Stance) control prosthetic knee (Fig. 6.16). This became a big game changer for people with transfemoral limb loss. It allowed them to walk with confidence down steps, inclines, and uneven terrain, and it is still widely used today.

Besides the developments with prosthetic knees, the next big development came with feet, with biggest breaks coming when the Seattle Foot was launched. This was developed by Ernest Burgess, the Veterans Administration, and Dupont, who invented Delrin plastic. This was groundbreaking because the material's ability to store and release energy allowed a more natural gait pattern.[85] The other advancement with foot prostheses was the life cast foot shell. In other words, a prosthetic foot that looked like a foot right down to a split between big toe and second toe allowing a person to wear a sandal or flip flop (Fig. 6.17A–B).

The next big advancement in feet came in 1992 by Van Phillips, who used carbon graphite to create the Flex-Foot (Fig. 6.18). This applied energy storing and release to a whole new level. With its unique J shape design, the carbon strut, which attached just below the socket (portion of the prosthesis that fit onto the person), went all the way to the toe portion. This created a large lever arm and area to store and then release energy—sort of like a diving board at a pool. The harder you loaded this spring, the more it pushed back, allowing the user to run.[86]

Although endoskeletal components have been around since the 16th century, this type of structure did not become widely used until the 1970s. Prior to this most prostheses were made

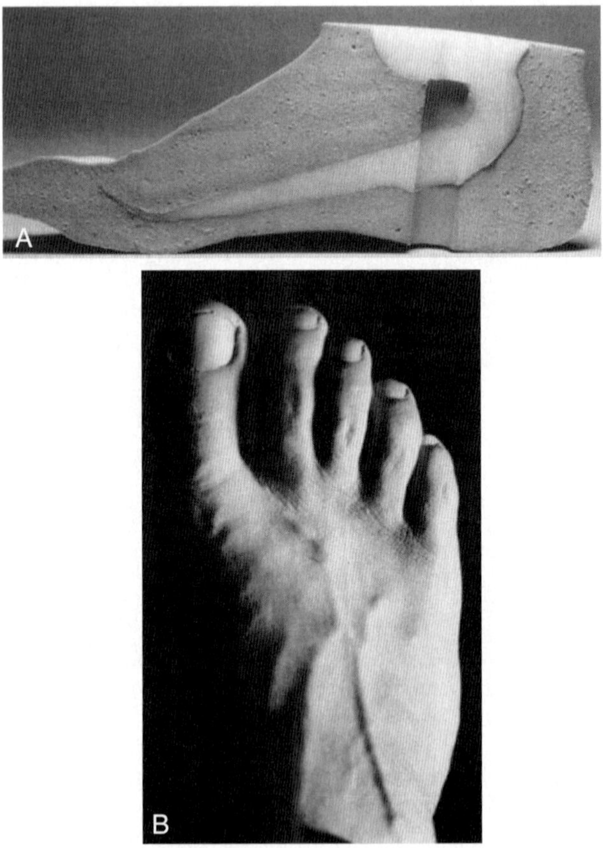

Fig. 6.17 (A, B) Seattle Foot. (History of the VA in 100 Objects March 24,2022; Seattle Foot Energy storing keel producing a spring like effect – History of the VA in 100 Objects March 24,2022.)

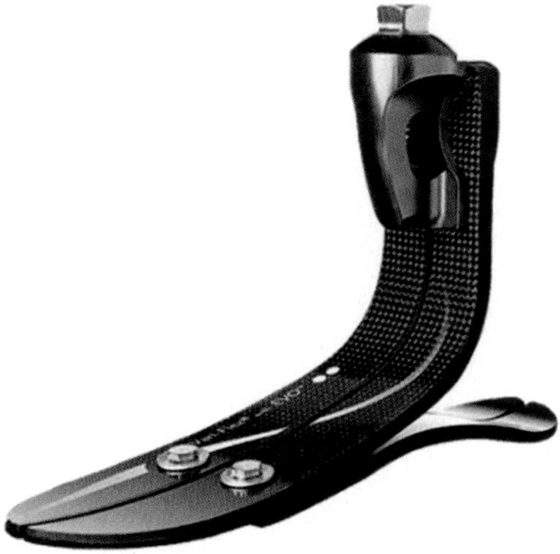

Fig. 6.18 Vari-Flex Foot®. (From Ossur Inc.)

with an exoskeletal construction. So what is the difference between the two? When you think of endoskeletal construction, think of the boney structure within the human body. We have a skeleton with muscle, soft tissue, and skin covering all of this, leaving the hard support structure inside. An exoskeletal support structure exists on the outside. With lower-extremity prosthetics the current norm includes endoskeletal parts with many types of components (knees and feet) that can be switched out as people progress through their rehabilitation after limb loss. The norm for the upper extremity is exoskeletal construction. Even with the most sophisticated components, such as myoelectric with microprocessors, the components are contained inside the exoskeletal shell for protection and durability. However, currently very few advanced electronic prosthetic components are completely waterproof and thus do not permit a person with limb loss to swim or even do the dishes with their prosthesis on.

So as lower-extremity prosthetic components advance with new materials and designs, which include powered knees (Fig. 6.19) and feet that will push off and propel a person forward (Fig. 6.20), there is still a major disconnect between amputees and their prostheses.

FUTURE

So the biggest challenge for a person with lower-extremity limb loss is the environment. What do I mean by this? Imagine driving into work and parking in a lot that is far from the front door. You get out of the car, grab your stuff, and start walking in. You step over curbs, avoid numerous obstacles, step over fallen branches from trees, and cross a couple of streets. You perform these actions while simultaneously looking at your phone or listening to your favorite podcast and drinking your morning coffee. If you were to watch that person walking in from ground level, you would notice that their feet barely clear the ground. The human mind has an incredible capacity to process vast amounts of data from all your senses. Sight, sound, smell, taste, and touch are essential to navigate the world. Lose one of these senses and you must rely on the others to help pick up the slack. The person with lower-extremity limb loss loses part or all the sense of touch. So even with the most high-tech components, gyroscopes, microprocessors, and force sensors that

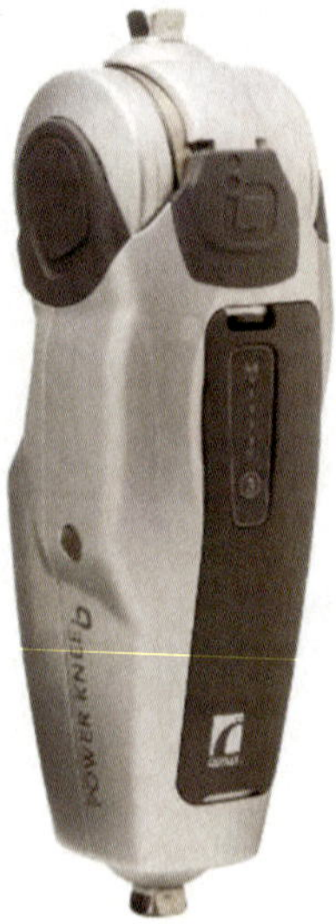

Fig. 6.19 Power Knee. (From Ossur Inc.)

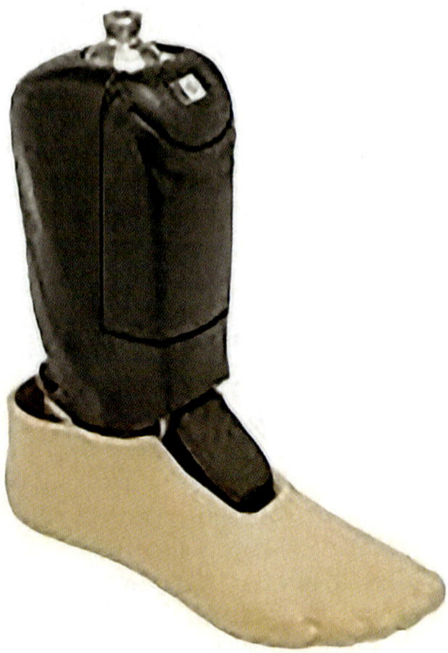

Fig. 6.20 Empower foot/ankle. (From Otto Bock Inc.)

are built into the components, people with limb loss have to overcompensate or exaggerate their movement. They must rely on their other senses to guide them over the obstacles in the way. If they are physically fit, they might be able to multitask and deal with their prosthesis. However, in most people with lower-extremity limb loss, the amputation was caused by disease.[84] Their other senses could be slightly impaired. Although they can be physically fit, they now need to really concentrate on walking, trying not to trip on a twig or a crack in the sidewalk. Their prosthesis can be well fitting and state of the art, however, it cannot react to the surrounding environment. The energy expenditure just walking into work, doing household choirs, or taking an afternoon hike increase dramatically for a person with lower-extremity limb loss. For someone with a transtibial amputation (below knee), there is a 30% energy expenditure increase such as the increase with walking up a hill. Transfemoral (above knee) amputation increases energy expenditure to 70% to 100% (like walking up a set of stairs all day).[87]

So what is the answer to this loss of a sense? Brain-computer interface (BCI), which is the direct communication between the brain and an external device for the general purpose of restoring lost cognitive or sensorimotor functions.

There are three types of BCI: (1) targeted muscle reinnervation, (2) a chip implanted directly into the brain, and (3) surface electrodes that detect electroencephalographic waves.

In 2016 a team of researchers at the Richmond Veterans Administration took the first step in providing a control system that provided transfemoral amputees with the ability through BCI-surface electrodes to control their prosthetic knee.[88] During this study, a person with a transfemoral limb loss was asked to unlock his prosthetic knee using BCI. The knee was a manual locking knee, basically a single pivot hinge that locked when the knee was fully straight. The only way to unlock it was by pulling a lever. In this study the release was attached to a device that through the person's electroencephalographic signal would unlock the knee when the patient thought it. Several trials were done with person walking and then sitting down. The person was successful throughout the clinical trial. The real breakthrough came after the trial. The subject had thrown his keys on the ground to get them out of the way. A the end of the trial while still hooked up to the BCI unit, he knelt down and picked up the keys without thinking about unlocking his prosthetic knee. Total control of his environment without hesitancy. It was reproduceable and not an artifact (Fig. 6.21).

In people with upper-extremity limb loss, the research has been steady and continuous. The goal is to restore not only muscle function but the ability to touch and feel something, hot, cold, soft, hard, smooth, or rough. At this point the systems that are commercially available only provide vibratory feedback with no real neurologic sense.

Once again we look to the surgeons for advancements in both upper- and lower-extremity prosthetics. Osteointegration of a prosthesis is a surgical procedure that implants a metal piece into the bone, which then comes through the muscle and skin and attaches directly to the components of the prosthesis. This eliminates the need for an external socket that fits over the residual limb and provides direct attachment and feedback from the prosthetic components, recreating the endoskeletal portion of the human body.

Osteointegration sounds strange; however, it has been done since the mid 1960s by a professor P.I. Brånemark from the University of Gothenburg in Sweden, who was an oral surgeon and pioneered dental implants and then went on to limb implants.[89]

At this point in time there are multiple studies and several types of implants, all with goal of restoring a person's limb (Fig. 6.22). This includes the ability of the implant in a person with upper-extremity limb loss to have bidirectional communication with the prosthesis and the implanted electrodes in the muscle and nerve endings. This would allow more dynamic control and feedback system that simulates the normal pathways.[90]

There have been major breakthroughs as recently as December 2020 by the researchers at RMIT University in Melbourne, Australia. They have made a synthetic skin fabricated from silicone that can feel pain.[91] The original intent for this artificial skin was to use it for skin grafting

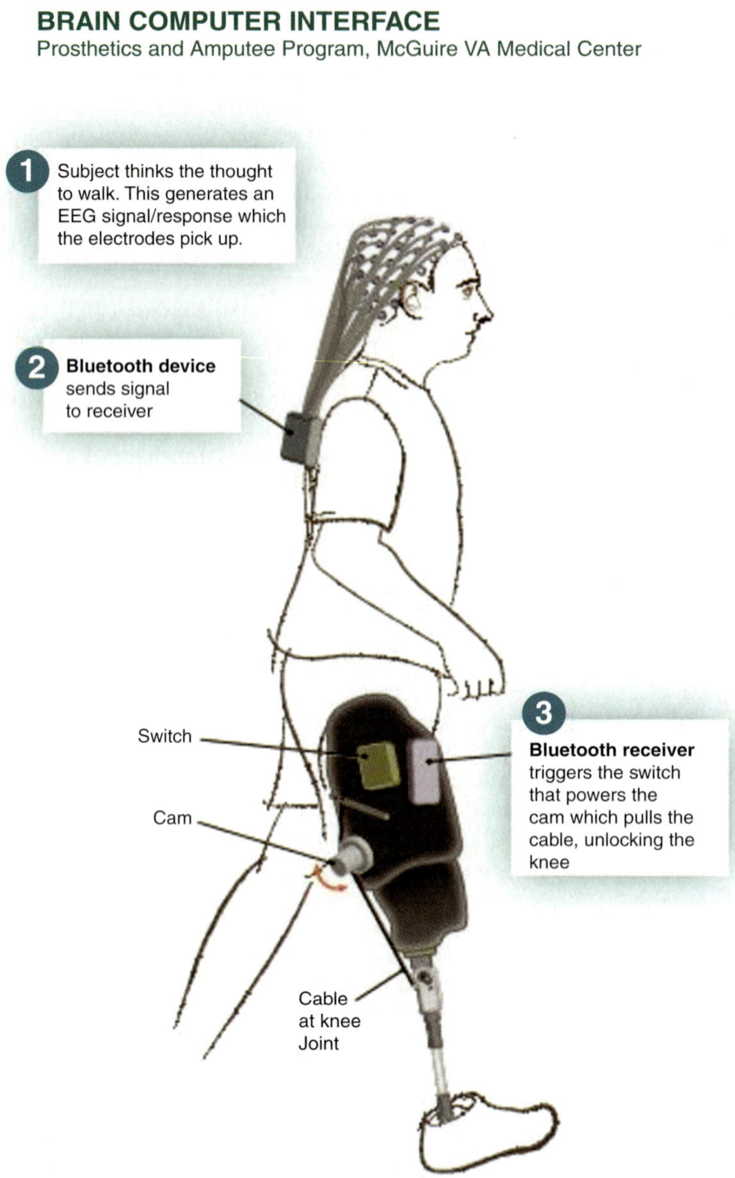

Fig. 6.21 Brain Computer Interface Richmond VAMC Mary Beatty-Brooks. EEG, electroencephalographic.

when real skin was not available; however, it has implications for prosthetic use, allowing the person with upper-extremity limb loss the ability to feel a pain stimulus. However, this dramatic invention is a going to take some time before it is used in the general population.

So what are the real advances in prosthetics? These will come from newer, lighter, stronger materials to fabricate and possibly power the devices such as carbon nanotubes.[92,93] Creating artificial muscles would allow the integration of powered mobility and upper-extremity dexterity.[94]

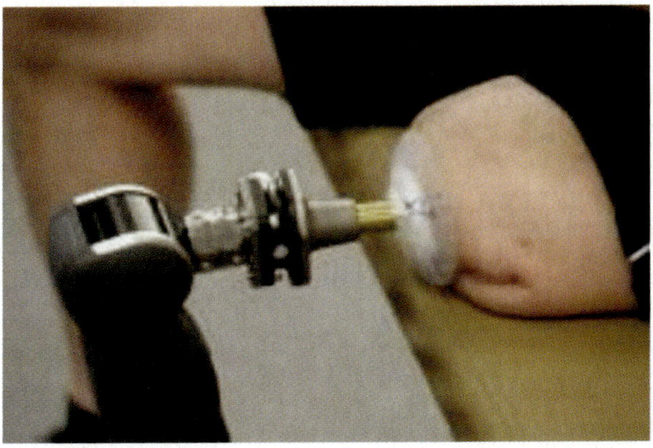

Fig. 6.22 Osseointegration. (https://www.researchgate.net/publication/341892383_Technological_Advances_in_Prosthesis_Design_and_Rehabilitation_Following_Upper_Extremity_Limb_Loss August 2020.)

Included in this will be the ability to 3D print new biologic gels and skinlike materials to be used in the prosthesis.[95]

In addition to BCI systems that will allow people with limb loss to control their prosthesis, new and advanced artificial intelligence will be added to the system. This will allow a more intuitive control of the prosthesis.[84]

So as the field of prosthetics slowly merges with surgery, neuroscience, and robotics, the hope of replacing a limb with something that is functional and cosmetically acceptable is becoming a reality. What at one time took generations to achieve is leaping forward with new breakthroughs coming every day. So when will we achieve the goal of totally replacing and/or enhancing a limb loss like in the *Six Million Dollar Man* TV show of the 1970s? Only time will tell.

References

1. Yakub F, Md Khudzari AZ, Mori Y. Recent trends for practical rehabilitation robotics, current challenges and the future. *Int J Rehabil Res*. 2014;37(1):9–21. https://doi.org/10.1097/MRR.0000000000000035
2. Alvarez-Perez MG, Garcia-Murillo MA, Cervantes-Sánchez JJ. Robot-assisted ankle rehabilitation: a review. *Disabil Rehabil Assist Technol*. 2020;15(4):394–408. https://doi.org/10.1080/17483107.2019.1578424
3. Asakawa T, Sugiyama K, Nozaki T, et al. Can the latest computerized technologies revolutionize conventional assessment tools and therapies for a neurological disease? The example of Parkinson's disease. *Neurol Med Chir (Tokyo)*. 2019;59(3):69–78. https://doi.org/10.2176/nmc.ra.2018-0045
4. Eiammanussakul T, Sangveraphunsiri V. A lower limb rehabilitation robot in sitting position with a review of training activities. *J Healthc Eng*. 2018;2018:1927807. https://doi.org/10.1155/2018/1927807
5. Yang J, Zhao Z, Du C, Wang W, Peng Q, Qiu J, Wang G. The realization of robotic neurorehabilitation in clinical: use of computational intelligence and future prospects analysis. *Expert Rev Med Devices*. 2020;17(12):1311–1322. https://doi.org/10.1080/17434440.2020.1852930
6. Khalili D, Zomlefer M. An intelligent robotic system for rehabilitation of joints and estimation of body segment parameters. *IEEE Trans Biomed Eng*. 1988;35(2):138–146.
7. Gassert R, Dietz V. Rehabilitation robots for the treatment of sensorimotor deficits: a neurophysiological perspective. *J Neuroeng Rehabil*. 2018;15(1):46. https://doi.org/10.1186/s12984-018-0383-x
8. Krebs HI, Hogan N, Aisen ML, Volpe BT. Robot-aided neurorehabilitation. *IEEE Trans Rehabil Eng*. 1998;6(1):75–87.
9. Zhang K, Chen X, Liu F, Tang H, Wang J, Wen W. System framework of robotics in upper limb rehabilitation on poststroke motor recovery. *Behav Neurol*. 2018;2018:6737056. https://doi.org/10.1155/2018/6737056
10. Colombo G, Joerg M, Schreier R, Dietz V. Treadmill training of paraplegic patients using a robotic orthosis. *J Rehabil Res Dev*. 2000;37(6):693–700.

11. Lokomat. Hocoma. Published 2021. https://www.hocoma.com/us/solutions/lokomat/
12. Hsieh YW, Wu CY, Liao WW, Lin KC, Wu KY, Lee CY. Effects of treatment intensity in upper limb robot-assisted therapy for chronic stroke: a pilot randomized controlled trial. *Neurorehabil Neural Repair*. 2011;25:503–511. https://doi.org/10.1177/1545968310394871
13. Bi-Manu-Track. NeuroRehab Directory. Published 2021. https://www.neurorehabdirectory.com/rehab-products/bi-manu-track/
14. Morone G, Cocchi I, Paolucci S, Iosa M. Robot-assisted therapy for arm recovery for stroke patients: state of the art and clinical implication. *Expert Rev Med Devices*. 2020;17(3):223–233. https://doi.org/10.1080/17434440.2020.1733408
15. Nizamis K, Athanasiou A, Almpani S, Dimitrousis C, Astaras A. Converging robotic technologies in targeted neural rehabilitation: a review of emerging solutions and challenges. *Sensors (Basel)*. 2021;21(6):2084. https://doi.org/10.3390/s21062084
16. Krebs HIgo. Twenty + years of robotics for upper-extremity rehabilitation following a stroke. *Rehabilitation Robotics*. Elsevier; 2018:175–192.
17. Krebs HI, Volpe BT, Williams D, et al. Robot-aided neurorehabilitation: a robot for wrist rehabilitation. *IEEE Trans Neural Syst Rehabil Eng*. 2007;15(3):327–335. https://doi.org/10.1109/TNSRE.2007.903899
18. Veerbeek JM, Langbroek-Amersfoort AC, van Wegen EE, Meskers CG, Kwakkel G. Effects of robot-assisted therapy for the upper limb after stroke. *Neurorehabil Neural Repair*. 2017;31(2):107–121. https://doi.org/10.1177/1545968316666957
19. Lang CE, Macdonald JR, Reisman DS, et al. Observation of amounts of movement practice provided during stroke rehabilitation. *Arch Phys Med Rehabil*. 2009;90(10):1692–1698.
20. Lo AC, Guarino PD, Richards LG, et al. Robot-assisted therapy for long-term upper-limb impairment after stroke. *N Engl J Med*. 2010;362:1772–1783.
21. Burgar CG, Lum PS, Scremin AM, et al. Robot-assisted upperlimb therapy in acute rehabilitation setting following stroke: Department of Veterans Affairs Multisite Clinical Trial. *J Rehabil Res Dev*. 2011;48(4):445–458.
22. Jakob I, Kollreider A, Germanotta M, et al. Robotic and sensor technology for upper limb rehabilitation. *PM R*. 2018;10(9 Suppl 2):S189–S197. https://doi.org/10.1016/j.pmrj.2018.07.011
23. Ada L, Dorsch S, Canning CG. Strengthening interventions increase strength and improve activity after stroke: a systematic review. *Aust J Physiother*. 2006;52(4):241–248.
24. Rowe JB, Chan V, Ingemanson ML, Cramer SC, Wolbrecht ET, Reinkensmeyer DJ. Robotic assistance for training finger movement using a Hebbian model: a randomized controlled trial. *Neurorehabil Neural Repair*. 2017;31(8):769–780.
25. Johansson RS. How is grasping modified by somatosensory input. *Motor Control: Concepts and Issues*. 1991;14:331–335.
26. Carey L, Macdonell R, Matyas TA. SENSe: study of the effectiveness of neurorehabilitation on sensation: a randomized controlled trial. *Neurorehabil Neural Repair*. 2011;25(4):304–313.
27. Prabhakaran S, Zarahn E, Riley C, et al. Interindividual variability in the capacity for motor recovery after ischemic stroke. *Neurorehabil Neural Repair*. 2008;22:64–71.
28. Kwakkel G, Kollen B, Lindeman E. Understanding the pattern of functional recovery after stroke: facts and theories. *Restor Neurol Neurosci*. 2004;22(3–5):281–299.
29. Winters C, van Wegen EE, Daffertshofer A, Kwakkel G. Generalizability of the proportional recovery model for the upper extremity after an ischemic stroke. *Neurorehabil Neural Repair*. 2015;29(7):614–622.
30. Chu CY, Patterson RM. Soft robotic devices for hand rehabilitation and assistance: a narrative review. *J Neuroeng Rehabil*. 2018;15(1):9. https://doi.org/10.1186/s12984-018-0350-6
31. Oña ED, Cano-de la Cuerda R, Sánchez-Herrera P, Balaguer C, Jardón A. A review of robotics in neurorehabilitation: towards an automated process for upper limb. *J Healthc Eng*. 2018;2018:9758939. https://doi.org/10.1155/2018/9758939
32. Langhammer B, Stanghelle JK. Can physiotherapy after stroke based on the Bobath concept result in improved quality of movement compared to the motor relearning programme. *Physiother Res Int*. 2011;16(2):69–80. https://doi.org/10.1002/pri.474
33. Winstein CJ, Stein J, Arena R, et al. Guidelines for adult stroke rehabilitation and recovery: a guideline for healthcare professionals from the American Heart Association/American Stroke Association. *Stroke*. 2016;47(6):e98–e169.

34. Irmady K, Jabbari B, Louis ED. Arm posturing in a patient following stroke: dystonia, levitation, synkinesis, or spasticity? *Tremor Other Hyperkinet Mov (NY)*. 2015;5:353. https://doi.org/10.7916/D8222TBH
35. Zhang C, Li-Tsang CW, Au RK. Robotic approaches for the rehabilitation of upper limb recovery after stroke: a systematic review and meta-analysis. *Int J Rehabil Res*. 2017;40:19–28.
36. Kutner NG, Zhang R, Butler AJ, Wolf SL, Alberts JL. Quality-of-life change associated with robotic-assisted therapy to improve hand motor function in patients with subacute stroke: a randomized clinical trial. *Phys Ther*. 2010;90:493–504. https://doi.org/10.2522/ptj.20090160
37. Abdullah HA, Tarry C, Lambert C, Barreca S, Allen BO. Results of clinicians using a therapeutic robotic system in an inpatient stroke rehabilitation unit. *J Neuroeng Rehabil*. 2011;8:50. https://doi.org/10.1186/1743-0003-8-50
38. Chien WT, Chong YY, Tse MK, Chien CW, Cheng HY. Robot-assisted therapy for upper-limb rehabilitation in subacute stroke patients: a systematic review and meta-analysis. *Brain Behav*. 2020;10(8):e01742. https://doi.org/10.1002/brb3.1742
39. Lo K, Stephenson M, Lockwood C. Effectiveness of robotic assisted rehabilitation for mobility and functional ability in adult stroke patients: a systematic review. *JBI Database System Rev Implement Rep*. 2017;15:3049–3091
40. Picelli A, Munari D, Modenese A, et al. Robot-assisted arm training for treating adult patients with distal radius fracture: a proof-of-concept pilot study. *Eur J Phys Rehabil Med*. 2020;56(4):444–450. https://doi.org/10.23736/S1973-9087.20.06112-2
41. Mehrholz J, Pohl M. Electromechanical-assisted gait training after stroke: a systematic review comparing end-effector and exoskeleton devices. *J Rehabil Med*. 2012;44(3):193–199. https://doi.org/10.2340/16501977-0943
42. Coscia M, Wessel MJ, Chaudary U, et al. Neurotechnology-aided interventions for upper limb motor rehabilitation in severe chronic stroke. *Brain*. 2019;142(8):2182–2197. https://doi.org/10.1093/brain/awz181
43. Dickstein R. Rehabilitation of gait speed after stroke: a critical review of intervention approaches. *Neurorehabil Neural Repair*. 2008;22(6):649–660. https://doi.org/10.1177/1545968308315997
44. Ada L, Dean CM, Vargas J, Ennis S. Mechanically assisted walking with body weight support results in more independent walking than assisted overground walking in non-ambulatory patients early after stroke: a systematic review. *J Physiother*. 2010;56(3):153–161. https://doi.org/10.1016/s1836-9553(10)70020-5
45. English C, Hillier S. Circuit class therapy for improving mobility after stroke: a systematic review. *J Rehabil Med*. 2011;43(7):565–571. https://doi.org/10.2340/16501977-0824
46. Esquenazi A, Talaty M. Robotics for lower limb rehabilitation. *Phys Med Rehabil Clin N Am*. 2019;30(2):385–397. https://doi.org/10.1016/j.pmr.2018.12.012
47. Cho JE, Yoo JS, Kim KE, et al. Systematic review of appropriate robotic intervention for gait function in subacute stroke patients. *Biomed Res Int*. 2018;2018:4085298. https://doi.org/10.1155/2018/4085298
48. Bruni MF, Melegari C, De Cola MC, Bramanti A, Bramanti P, Calabrò RS. What does best evidence tell us about robotic gait rehabilitation in stroke patients: a systematic review and meta-analysis. *J Clin Neurosci*. 2018;48:11–17. https://doi.org/10.1016/j.jocn.2017.10.048
49. Gait Trainer GT. II. Reha-Stim. Published 2021. https://reha-stim.com/gt-ii/
50. Hornby TG, Campbell DD, Kahn JH, Demott T, Moore JL, Roth HR. Enhanced gait-related improvements after therapist- versus robotic-assisted locomotor training in subjects with chronic stroke: a randomized controlled study. *Stroke*. 2008;39(6):1786–1792. https://doi.org/10.1161/STROKEAHA.107.504779. Erratum in: *Stroke*. 2008;39(8):e143.
51. Mehrholz J, Elsner B, Werner C, Kugler J, Pohl M. Electromechanical-assisted training for walking after stroke: updated evidence. *Stroke*. 2013;44(10):e127–e128. https://doi.org/10.1161/strokeaha.113.003061
52. Mehrholz J, Thomas S, Werner C, Kugler J, Pohl M, Elsner B. Electromechanical-assisted training for walking after stroke. *Cochrane Database Syst Rev*. 2017;5:CD006185.
53. Macko RF, Ivey FM, Forrester LW, et al. Treadmill exercise rehabilitation improves ambulatory function and cardiovascular fitness in patients with chronic stroke: a randomized, controlled trial. *Stroke*. 2005;36:2206–2211.
54. Macko RF, Ivey FM, Forrester LW. Task-oriented aerobic exercise in chronic hemiparetic stroke: training protocols and treatment effects. *Top Stroke Rehabil*. 2005;12:45–57.
55. Fang CY, Tsai JL, Li GS, Lien AS, Chang YJ. Effects of robot-assisted gait training in individuals with spinal cord injury: a meta-analysis. *Biomed Res Int*. 2020;2020:2102785. https://doi.org/10.1155/2020/2102785

56. Laver KE, George S, Thomas S, Deutsch JE, Crotty M. Virtual reality for stroke rehabilitation. *Cochrane Database Syst Rev*. 2011(9):CD008349. https://doi.org/10.1002/14651858.CD008349.pub2
57. Mekki M, Delgado AD, Fry A, Putrino D, Huang V. Robotic rehabilitation and spinal cord injury: a narrative review. *Neurotherapeutics*. 2018;15(3):604–617. https://doi.org/10.1007/s13311-018-0642-3
58. Tieri G, Morone G, Paolucci S, Iosa M. Virtual reality in cognitive and motor rehabilitation: facts, fiction and fallacies. *Expert Rev Med Devices*. 2018;15(2):107–117. https://doi.org/10.1080/17434440.2018.1425613
59. Fukui R, Gutierrez C, Frontera J. How does motivation to therapy contribute to functional recovery: a case report. Paper presented at: Association of Academic Physiatrists/International Society of Physical and Rehabilitation Medicine Annual Meeting; March 2020; Orlando, FL.
60. Moreira MC, de Amorim Lima AM, Ferraz KM, Benedetti Rodrigues MA. Use of virtual reality in gait recovery among post stroke patients—a systematic literature review. *Disabil Rehabil Assist Technol*. 2013 Sep;8(5):357–362. https://doi.org/10.3109/17483107.2012.749428
61. You SH, Jang SH, Kim YH, et al. Cortical reorganization induced by virtual reality therapy in a child with hemiparetic cerebral palsy. *Dev Med Child Neurol*. 2005;17:628–635.
62. You SH, Jang SH, Kim YH, et al. Virtual reality-induced cortical reorganization and associated locomotor recovery in chronic stroke: an experimenter blind randomized study. *Stroke*. 2005;36:1166–1171.
63. Reyes F, Niedzwecki C, Gaebler-Spira D. Technological advancements in cerebral palsy rehabilitation. *Phys Med Rehabil Clin N Am*. 2020;31(1):117–129. https://doi.org/10.1016/j.pmr.2019.09.002
64. Leung AK, Hon KL. Motion sickness: an overview. *Drugs Context*. 2019;8. https://doi.org/10.7573/dic.2019-9-4.2019
65. Fitter NT, Mohan M, Kuchenbecker KJ, Johnson MJ. Exercising with Baxter: preliminary support for assistive social-physical human-robot interaction. *J Neuroeng Rehabil*. 2020;17(1):19. https://doi.org/10.1186/s12984-020-0642-5
66. The FACE robot from Research Center "E. Piaggio" casted by the 20th Century Fox. UNIPINEWS. https://www.unipi.it/index.php/english-news/item/8261-the-face-robot-from-research-center-e-piaggio-casted-by-the-20th-century-fox
67. PARO therapeutic robot. PARO. Published 2021. http://www.parorobots.com/
68. Maalouf N, Sidaoui A, Elhajj IH, Asmar D. Robotics in nursing: a scoping review. *J Nurs Scholarsh*. 2018;50(6):590–600. https://doi.org/10.1111/jnu.12424
69. Gordon R. Getting dressed with help from robots. MIT News. Published 2021. https://news.mit.edu/2021/getting-dressed-with-help-from-robots-0714
70. Obi—the first dining robot of its kind. Obi. Published 2021. https://meetobi.com/
71. Smart Cane for blind and visually impaired people, Smart Cane manufacturer and seller. Phoenix Medical Systems. Published 2021. https://www.phoenixmedicalsystems.com/assistive-technology/smartcanes/
72. RIBA robot for interactive body assistance: science fiction in the news. Technovelgy.com. Published 2021. http://technovelgy.com/ct/Science-Fiction-News.asp?NewsNum=2500
73. Mehrholz J, Pohl M, Platz T, Kugler J, Elsner B. Electromechanical and robot-assisted arm training for improving activities of daily living, arm function, and arm muscle strength after stroke. *Cochrane Database Syst Rev*. 2018;9(9):CD006876. https://doi.org/10.1002/14651858.CD006876.pub5
74. Molteni F, Gasperini G, Cannaviello G, Guanziroli E. Exoskeleton and end-effector robots for upper and lower limbs rehabilitation: narrative review. *PM R*. 2018;10(9 Suppl 2):S174–S188. https://doi.org/10.1016/j.pmrj.2018.06.005
75. Project Lokomat | Help individuals with neurological injury walk again. Projectlokomat. Accessed August 18, 2021. www.projectlokomat.com/
76. There's no cure for Covid-19 loneliness, but robots can help. Wired. www.wired.com/story/covid-19-robot-companions/
77. Wagner TH, Lo AC, Peduzzi P, et al. An economic analysis of robot-assisted therapy for long-term upper-limb impairment after stroke. *Stroke*. 2011;42(9):2630–2632.
78. Sachs M, Bojunga J, Encke A. Historical evolution of limb amputation. *World J Surg*. 1999;23:1088–1093. https://doi.org/10.1007/s002689900628
79. Hernigou P, Amproise Paré II. paré contributions to amputation and ligature. *Int Orthop*. 2013;37(4):769–772.
80. Kennedy M. *A brief history of disease, science and medicine*. Asklepaid Press; 2004.
81. Porter R. *The greatest benefit to mankind: a medical history of humanity*. W.W. Norton; 1999.

82. Hueston J. Biceps cineplasty for forearm Amputees. *Aust N Z J Surg*. 1959;28:280–285.
83. Childress DS. Historical aspects of powered limb prosthesis. *Clinical Prosthetics and Orthotics*. 1985;9(1):2–13.
84. Molina CS, Faulk J. Lower extremity amputation. In: StatPearls. Published January 2021. Updated August 26, 2021. https://www.ncbi.nlm.nih.gov/books/NBK546594/
85. Burgess EM. Development and preliminary evaluation of the VA Seattle Foot. *J Rehabil Res Dev*. 1985;22:76–77.
86. Supan TB. Motion analysis of SACH vs. Flex-Foot(tm) in moderately active below-knee amputees. *Clinical Prosthetics and Orthotics*. 1987;1:55–62.
87. Miller MS, Newgent EW, O'Connell SM, Broadus C. A comprehensive scoring system to evaluate patient-centred risk factors regarding lower extremity amputation. *J Wound Care*. 2017;26(Suppl 10):S20–S28.
88. Murphy D. Electroencephalogram based brain computer interface and lower limb prosthesis control: a case study. *Front Neurol*. 2017;8.
89. Buser D, Sennerby L, De Bruyn H. Modern implant dentistry based on osseointegration: 50 years of progress, current trends and open questions. Periodontol 2000. 2017;73:7–21. https://doi.org/10.1111/prd.12185
90. Mastinu E, Doguet P, Botquin Y, Hakansson B, Ortiz-Catalan M. Embedded system for prosthetic control using implanted neuromuscular interfaces accessed via an osseointegrated implant. *IEEE Trans Biomed Circuits Syst*. 2017;11(4):867–877.
91. Prisco J. New artificial skin can feel real pain. CNN Health Report. December 2, 2020. https://www.cnn.com/2020/12/02/health/artificial-pain-sensing-skin-spc-intl/index.html
92. Melissa Paradise TG. Carbon nanotubes—production and industrial applications. *Materials & Design*. 2007;28(5):1477–1489.
93. Desai SB, Madhvapathy SR. Sachid AB, et al. MoS2 transistors with 1-nanometer gate lengths. *Science*. 2016;354(6308):99–102.
94. Duduta M HE, Hajiesmaili E, Zhao H, Wood RJ, Clarke DR. Realizing the potential of dielectric elastomer artificial muscles. *Proc Natl Acad Sci U S A*. 2019;116:2476–2481.
95. Shifeng N, Jinchang Z, Haozhe Z, et al. Three-dimensional printable, extremely soft, stretchable, and reversible elastomers from molecular architecture-directed assembly. *Chem Mater*. 2021;33:2436–2445.

7

Neuroprosthesis Applications of Robotic Exoskeletons

Ashraf S. Gorgey ■ Hope Jervis-Rademeyer

KEY POINTS

- Using a robotic exoskeleton for exoskeleton-assisted walking has improved quality of life and mental health for individuals with spinal cord injury according to self-report measures.
- For individuals living with spinal cord injury, adding exoskeleton-assisted walking to rehabilitation has translated to improvements in motor and autonomic function.
- Robotic exoskeletons are a feasible approach to enhance task-specific training for locomotion.
- In animal and human trials, a robotic exoskeleton has demonstrated efficacy as a stand-alone intervention and in combination with other neuromodulatory approaches to enhance neuroplasticity.
- These positive changes in neuroplasticity (e.g., improved neural connectivity) due to exoskeleton-assisted walking have been demonstrated in several clinical populations (e.g., stroke, muscular dystrophy) with improved outcome measures, such as gait speed.

Overground locomotion is a dream goal for more than a million survivors with spinal cord injury (SCI). Today, advances in medical research findings through tissue engineering, stem cell research, and the development of neuroprostheses have paved the scientific road to achieve this goal.[1] A key neurophysiological principle that has evolved over the last 3 to 4 decades and strengthened these findings is that task-specific training is highly important to restore standing and stepping in persons with SCI.[2–8] Task-specific training relies on repetitively administering afferent influx to the nervous system to modulate specific behavioral or functional motor output.[4–6] This volley of afferent influx is likely to be integrated at the central pattern generators to generate a pattern of flexion-extension oscillation (i.e., fictive locomotion) and ultimately result in a motor behavior similar to walking.[9] Lovely et al. were among the first to demonstrate the effects of task-specific training on cats with completely transected cords (T12–T13). After 5 to 7 months of training, the paralyzed cats were capable of full weight-bearing and regained control of hind limb stepping.[10,11]

Task-specific training resulting in neuroplastic adaptations of the injured spinal cord has emerged as a potential rehabilitation intervention that may restore overground locomotion in persons with SCI.[12–18] Neuroplastic pathways may effectively integrate neural, neurochemical, metabolic, and muscular systems to enhance functional adaptions after SCI.[5,8] In 2006, Dobkin et al. published the first multicenter randomized clinical trial that demonstrated the efficacy of task-specific training on overground mobility in persons with incomplete SCI.[4] The authors implemented body weight supported treadmill training (BWSTT) for 12 weeks and compared it to overground training. The findings suggested that task-specific training using either BWSTT or overground ambulation is equally effective in the rehabilitation of persons with incomplete SCI.[4]

These outcomes intrigued several other groups, causing them to explore the effects of task-specific training on restoring overground locomotion in persons with SCI. This has sequentially resulted in the development of the Reeve Foundations NeuroRecovery Network clinical centers that deliver extensive rehabilitation for persons with SCI.[11] The NeuroRecovery Network provides locomotor training combined with functional electrical stimulation (FES) to enhance motor recovery after SCI.[6] The goal of the program is to provide continuous training to enhance neuroplasticity of the injured cord.

Recently, the robotic exoskeleton has emerged as a potential successful rehabilitation tool that can provide immediate overground ambulation for persons with SCI.[19–26] An introductory editorial suggested that robotic exoskeletons encompass the future of rehabilitation in persons with SCI.[26] Several exoskeleton devices have been developed to allow overground stepping with varying efforts, including some that are approved by the Food and Drug Administration, such as, the ReWalk, Indego, Ekso Bionics, and others that remain experimental.[19,24,27,28] Unlike strenuous task-specific training, robotic exoskeleton ambulation does not require the same number of trained staff that are typically involved in BWSTT.[23,25,29] It is common to have three or four therapists involved in the training of one person during BWSTT compared with only one or two therapists when using the exoskeleton for overground ambulation.[4,6,7] We have previously contrasted different brands of exoskeletons and highlighted the potential indications for each brand after SCI.[19] A thematic review also has detailed several of the pros and cons that need to be considered when prescribing robotic exoskeletons for the rehabilitation of persons with SCI.[24] The purpose of this chapter is (1) to review recent accomplishments in the applications of robotic exoskeletons for the rehabilitation of persons with neurologic disabilities and (2) to develop the hypothesis that robotic exoskeletons can be used as an effective neuroprosthesis for task-specific training in persons with SCI. This is important because several research investigators are still debating the efficacy of the robotic exoskeleton to enhance neuroplasticity and to facilitate overground ambulation.

Definition of Lower Limb Robotic Exoskeleton

For the purpose of this chapter, a lower limb robotic exoskeleton or exoskeleton-assisted walking (EAW) will be defined as a computerized unit that involves sensors, actuators, algorithms, a structural framework, and control strategies capable of processing information to execute functional movements.[19,24] The structural framework involves external robotic legs joined at the hip and knee joints and pelvic-hip support with or without trunk support. Furthermore, the robotic exoskeleton field has increased to involve rehabilitation of the upper extremities, trunk control, balance, lower extremity training, and gait reeducation.[19] In this chapter, we are going to focus on gait reeducation in persons with neurologic disabilities and primarily persons with SCI (Table 7.1). We should also point the reader's attention to another Chapter 33 that was dedicated for a similar purpose.[19]

Major Indications and Accomplishments of Robotic Exoskeletons

EXOSKELETON AND QUALITY OF LIFE

A current multicenter cooperative study has furnished the road to investigate the effects of the robotic exoskeleton on quality of life (QOL) and other comorbidities after SCI.[30,32] Preliminary evidence indicated that EAW remarkably enhanced QOL and increased independence in persons with SCI.[32] Although the trial was limited to one brand of robotic exoskeleton and only targeted veterans with SCI, striding benefits have been inferred from the trial that will shape future rehabilitation programs and enhance our understanding of the design of future exoskeletons and the interface between humans with physical disabilities and robotics.

TABLE 7.1 ■ **Benefits of Using EAW for Persons With Neurologic Disabilities and SCI**

Indication	Benefits of USING EAW
Physical activity—locomotion	• Increased gait speed*[30,31] • Increased endurance*[28,30,32]
Pulmonary function	• Increased VO_2[23,25,33] • Increased forced vital capacity[34] • Increased predicted forced vital capacity percent • Increased forced expiratory volume in 1 second
Lower extremity motor function	• Increased strength in some participants[31,35,36] • Increased leg circumference due to muscle hypertrophy[4,37] • Decreased leg circumference due to reduction in edema
Seated balance	• Improved endpoint excursion[38] • Improved maximal excursion • Improved seated balance control[39]
Spasticity	• Decreased severity of spasticity in majority of participants[37,40] • Decreased frequency of spasticity[40]
Bowel function	• Improvement in the frequency of the bowel evacuations[41] • Fewer bowel accidents • Reduced laxative and stool softener • Reduced time to complete bowel management[42]

EAW, Exoskeleton-assisted walking; SCI, spinal cord injury.
*Benefits noted for individuals with SCI and stroke; all other benefits apply to SCI only.

Earlier studies have also taken a cursory look at QOL for individuals living with SCI using subjective outcome measures. In a pre-post study including 45 participants, there was a slight increase in the Satisfaction with Life Scale; however, this increase was not significant.[37] Despite these findings, Juszczak et al. observed that some participants had the potential to operate an exoskeleton in the community thus facilitating increased participation and theoretically altering QOL. In one case study, an individual living with SCI noted that using an exoskeleton had a positive effect on QOL as shown by significant improvements in six out of eight thematic areas of the Short Form 36 Health Survey.[43]

A Canadian study provided home use of robotic EAW for the purpose of indoor exercise and outdoor activities.[44] Fourteen participants with SCI were asked to complete the Dutch version of the Quebec User Evaluation of Satisfaction With Assistive Technology scale (1–5 scale) and the System Usability Scale (0–100 scale) questionnaires at the beginning and at the end of a 2- to 3-week period. Participants reported that EAW was used for individual exercise for 74% of all sessions and for 48% of outdoor activities. The Quebec User Evaluation of Satisfaction With Assistive Technology scale showed dissatisfaction regarding the weight of the exoskeleton, ease of use, and safety. The participants reported mixed signs of positive (mental health [n = 5], decreased spasticity [n = 3], neuropathic pain [n = 1] and increased range of motion [n = 1]) and negative (muscle or joint pain [n = 1], skin damage [n = 2], increased spasticity [n = 1] and fecal incontinence problems [n = 1]) health outcomes.[44]

EXOSKELETON AND PHYSICAL ACTIVITY

The first observation showed that using a robotic exoskeleton resulted in a 30% increase in walking speed after longitudinal training of eight individuals with SCI. This study showed a reduction in temporal parameters including stride time, stance time, and double-support time. The findings may suggest enhancement of the motor learning curve after more than 100 hours of EAW.[45]

Another case report noted that the level of physical activity increased in a participant with C4 complete SCI.[29] The participant, using a platform roller walker, demonstrated that both standing time and walking time increased within two sessions. These findings may collectively suggest that despite the level of injury and severity of injury, EAW may be capable of increasing the level of physical activity in persons with SCI. Anecdotally, most participants with SCI reported enjoyment of the training session and trained up to 120 minutes without reporting any signs of fatigue. This anecdotal evidence may support earlier findings that noted reduced metabolic cost during robotic training and may explain the lower rate of fatigue during EAW compared with other training modalities.[8,25]

EXOSKELETON AND PULMONARY FUNCTION

Enhancement in the level of physical activity is also accompanied by increased oxygen uptake. A recent study demonstrated that 60 sessions of EAW resulted in increased gait speed by 94%, decreased rate of perceived exertion by 46%, and increased VO_2 by 30%.[33] Another recent study from our laboratory showed that following 12 weeks of exoskeleton training, twice weekly, there was no effect on peak VO_2. Compared with resting sitting and resting standing, VO_2 increased 2 and 1.11 times during EAW, respectively.[46] These findings were previously confirmed in two different studies using other brands of exoskeletons.[23,25] However, in a recent study, EAW training also showed a decrease in peak VO_2 by 17%.[46] In a case report, the authors noted no difference in 6-minute VO_2 when using Canadian crutches compared with a standard roller walker.[25]

In a randomized controlled pilot study, Xiang et al. found that EAW positively affected pulmonary function in individuals living with SCI.[34] Participants underwent 1 hour of EAW training or conventional training (i.e., strength and aerobic exercise) 4 days per week for a total of 4 weeks (16 sessions). After training, the EAW group showed significantly higher values of forced vital capacity (FVC) (3.8 ± 1.1 L) predicted FVC% ($94.1\% \pm 24.5\%$) and forced expiratory volume in 1 second (FEV_1) (3.5 ± 1.0 L) in comparison with the conventional group (FVC: 2.8 ± 0.8 L; $FVC\%_{predicted} = 65.4\% \pm 17.6\%$; FEV_1: 2.4 ± 0.6 L). Similar to the findings by Knezevic et al.[33] and Sutor et al.,[46] these results show that EAW has the potential to improve pulmonary function in individuals with SCI.

EXOSKELETON AND LOWER EXTREMITY MOTOR FUNCTION

Another pilot study clearly demonstrated that EAW enhanced motor function in persons with acute SCI. The study showed lower extremity motor scores and the Functional Independence Measure increased 3.1 and 1.4 times, respectively, more than controls who did not undergo EAW.[35] These findings were confirmed in a multicenter trial that showed that 36 sessions of EAW resulted in 80%, 82%, and 84% completion of the 10-m walking time (10-MWT; ≤40 seconds), distance during 6-minute walking time (6-MWT; ≥80 m), and time up to go (≤90 seconds) criteria.[30] A similar observation was noted in 50 participants with a stroke who completed single-blinded randomized parallel trial for 6 to 8 weeks. EAW resulted in improvement in walking speed (0.24 m/s), walking endurance (11%), balance (17.9%), and corticomotor excitability (145%) compared with controls in persons with hemorrhagic stroke.[47]

An observational study with 28 participants with SCI also showed positive improvements in gait parameters.[31] Over 2 weeks (10 sessions) there was an increase in participants' walking speed during the 10-MWT (≥0.03 m/s) and distance during the 6-MWT (≥11 m) while wearing the exoskeleton. Interestingly, individuals with complete injuries ASIA Impairment Scale (AIS A) showed more improvement in both gait speed and distance than those classified as AIS B.[31] The same findings were true for individuals with higher injuries compared with those with lower injuries. Unfortunately, there was no improvement in lower extremity motor scores across participants; however, in a study by Aach et al.,[36] lower extremity motor scores improved significantly (21.75 ± 8.3 to 24.38 ± 7.6) in all participants with chronic SCI (n = 8) in addition to an increase in leg circumference (5–50 mm) in seven participants and a reduction in leg circumference (25 mm) due to edema in the remaining participant.[36]

Nine participants with stroke were enrolled in a quasicontrolled trial with 12 weeks of twice weekly therapy using the REX exoskeleton (Auckland, New Zealand).[48] The primary outcomes were measured by using the five-item motor assessment scale. The five-item scale includes supine to side lying, supine to sitting, balanced sitting, sitting to standing, and walking. Other batteries of motor outcomes were included. Overall, there was no change in motor function; however, five out of the nine participants had changes that indicated improvements in their motor scores. Four out of these five participants had the lowest motor scores at the time of enrollment in the study. Other improvements were observed in the grip strength of the affected limb, the electromyography of the affected quadriceps, and independence with activities of daily living.[48] These findings suggest that EAW may result in both spinal and cortical neuroplasticity that act to improve functional outcomes.

EXOSKELETON AND SEATED BALANCE

Developing effective training strategies, such as using a robotic exoskeleton to reactivate trunk muscles, are needed to facilitate independence during seated balance activities in individuals with SCI. In a pilot study, Tsai et al. showed that EAW training transferred to improvements in seated balance for eight individuals with SCI.[38] After a median of 30 (range 7–90) sessions, a significant improvement was found in endpoint excursion and maximal excursion. Median endpoint excursion scores increased from 37.2 to 48.7, and median maximal excursion scores increased from 58.0 to 78.3. Other improvements were noted in the modified Functional Reach Test and subscales of physical functioning and role limitations; however, these improvements were not significant.[38]

Furthermore, a case report by Chisholm et al. showed that overground compared with stationary (i.e., treadmill) EAW produced a larger improvement in postural stability.[39] Three individuals with motor complete SCI underwent 30 sessions of robotic gait training. They completed a randomized trial using one of two alternating treatment designs beginning with either a stationary or an overground EAW intervention. Results showed that overground EAW actively recruited trunk muscles through postural control mechanisms. Although both groups showed improved seated balance control, as evidenced by reduced time taken during the T-Shirt Test and increased distance on the modified Functional Reach Test, the overground group improved slightly more than the stationary EAW group.

EXOSKELETON AND INDICES OF SPASTICITY

Frequency and severity of spasticity have been positively affected though overground EAW. In a pre-post study by Stampacchia et al.,[40] 21 individuals with SCI showed improvements in spasticity after completing only one overground walking session using a powered exoskeleton. The session lasted 40 minutes with 7 to 25 minutes of active walking time. Participants subjectively evaluated perceived spasticity using a 0- to 10-point numerical rating scale. Using this scale, the median score decreased from 2.0 to 0.0 after the walking session. Objective assessments of spasticity were measured using the Modified Ashworth Scale (MAS) and the Penn Spasm Frequency Scale (PSFS). Scores on these scales improved from a median score of 4.0 to 2.0 on the MAS and 1.0 to 0.0 on the PSFS.[40]

Another pre-post intervention, across five rehabilitation institutes, showed mostly positive effects of EAW on spasticity.[37] Forty-five participants living with SCI engaged in three to four EAW sessions per week for 8 weeks, completing a total of 26 sessions. These individuals reported a significant reduction in spasticity from the start (1.6 ± 0.9) to the end of the study (0.9 ± 1.7). Although most participants experienced a decrease (n = 12) or no change (n = 28) in spasticity, as evidenced by the MAS, few participants' (n = 5) spasticity increased.[37]

EXOSKELETON AND BOWEL FUNCTION

An observational study noted improvements in bowel function following 25 to 63 sessions of EAW. Participants (50%–80%) reported an improvement in the frequency of the bowel evacuations, fewer bowel accidents, reduced laxative and stool softener use, and improved overall satisfaction and related QOL.[41] The reduction in the use of laxative and stool softener is considered important finding because they negatively impact the beneficial gut microbiome. The disruption in gut microbiome is likely to increase the risks of other comorbidities including obesity, insulin resistance, and type II diabetes in persons with SCI.[49] The findings were just recently confirmed in a randomized controlled trial that demonstrated that EAW plays a major role in overcoming bowel dysfunction in persons with SCI. The time to complete bowel management decreased in 24% of the EAW participants in this study.[42]

Exoskeleton as a Platform for Neuromodulation Techniques to Enhance Neuroplasticity

Growing evidence suggests that robotic exoskeletons can be used as a neuroprosthesis for sensorimotor rehabilitation in persons with SCI.[50] Several animal and human trials have demonstrated the efficacy of robotic exoskeleton use in conjunction with neuromodulatory approaches such as trans-spinal stimulation (TS) or implanted epidural stimulation (ES) as well as brain-computer interfaces.[46,51–57] A brain-computer interface integrates the user's volitional intention with the operation of a robotic exoskeleton.[58] It has the potential to achieve this integration between devices in persons with different neuromotor disorders.[58] Myoelectric control is another example of using either electromyography to control exoskeleton ambulation or integrating FES with a robotic exoskeleton.[59] A previous editorial described the combinatory approach of EAW with neuromodulation techniques as promising for gait rehabilitation in persons with SCI.[50] This integrative approach provides the opportunity to augment the automaticity of the spinal circuitries to enhance volitional stepping. Eventually, it can be translated into overground locomotion in persons with SCI. Furthermore, it provides sensorimotor integration of the spinal and supraspinal networks.

Although the major focus of these studies was to provide an alternative approach for task-specific training, there remains an important question of whether EAW can be used as an alternative to the labor-intense BWSTT approach. EAW has been recognized as an effective approach to enhance neuroplasticity.[54,55] EAW is characterized by a lower metabolic cost[8,25,60] and enhancement of QOL[1] and has the capability to offer full overground weight-bearing on day one in completely paralyzed persons with SCI.[25,46] Multiple studies have demonstrated improvement in electromyography activities of the paralyzed muscles following EAW training in persons with SCI.[20,55] In this section, we are going to review the evidence that may support developing the hypothesis that EAW can be used for enhancing neuroplasticity after SCI. We will start with animal studies and then follow with human trials.

In the journal *Science*, van den Brand et al. showed that a robotic postural interface combined with ES resulted in recovery of voluntary movements in completely transected rats.[53] Using both paradigms, rats were capable of initiating and sustaining full weight-bearing bipedal locomotion following daily training for 30 minutes for 5 to 6 weeks. The authors suggested that this multisystem neuroprosthetic training resulted in the formation of intraspinal detours that relay supraspinal information.[53] This was accompanied by an increase in the number of neurons after continuous locomotion in the overground trained rats compared with the nontrained rats. This paradigm of combining a robotic interface with ES has been adopted in number of other research studies that were conducted by the same group.[52,53]

Gad et al. demonstrated that combining EAW with noninvasive TS resulted in positive synergistic effects as demonstrated by increasing the effort of walking, interlimb coordination, and smoothened stepping in a person SCI.[54] In this case report, an individual with motor complete SCI completed overground stepping using an exoskeleton enhanced with TS and/or a pharmacologic intervention (i.e., buspirone). Using the exoskeleton, after overground baseline training for 4 weeks, the participant engaged in 1 week of training using TS only followed by 1 week using the drug therapy only. The last week of stepping training combined TS and drug therapy. Sessions took place 5 days per week for 1 hour using the variable assist mode. When used, noninvasive TS was delivered at the spinous process between T11 and T12 and at a frequency of 30 Hz.[54] Average subjective scores on the participant's perception of improved muscle tone, sensation, early morning sensation, body perspiration, and hand-to-leg coordination were highest in the TS only and TS + drug conditions. The TS-only condition reduced mean step cycle duration from 2.13 seconds to 2.03 seconds and 2.07 seconds in the drug-only condition. The mean step cycle duration decreased the most in TS + drug condition (2.00 seconds). Higher levels of assistance from the exoskeleton were needed when TS was not present. Delivering assistance as needed resulted in the participant engaging the lumbosacral spinal networks to control the swing phase in one leg while the opposite leg remained in stance. The use of TS with EAW resulted in a remarkable decrease in the provided robotic assistance and an increase in the integrated activities of rectus femoris and tibialis anterior muscles. TS also supported the stimulation of standing and stepping through modulating the excitability of the spinal neural networks to reestablish connections from cortical networks to spinal networks. Thus, a high level of agonist-antagonist coordination was established through these highly excitable network projections to the motor pools. Furthermore, the variable assist mode in this study provided an opportunity to engage the central pattern generators to initiate stepping during the swing phase when TS pulses were delivered. These findings were recently confirmed in three persons with chronic complete SCI when TS was combined with EAW for 12 weeks.[46] The authors noted an increase in the amplitude of the knee extensors after using TS with EAW compared with EAW only both at the stance and the swing phased of the gait cycle.[46] The amplitude of the extensor muscle was still enhanced even when lowering the assistance provided with EAW. Two of the three participants showed a considerable reduction in the robotic assistance needed during EAW with the use of TS.[46]

Similar to TS, the addition of ES to locomotor training alone has resulted in neuromodulation of the spinal cord circuitries in individuals with SCI.[61–64] These preliminary findings indicated successful overground stepping and walking in persons with complete SCI.[63,64] In a case report, Gorgey et al. found that using ES combined with EAW improved motor control during stepping in an individual with a complete SCI.[55] This participant underwent 24 sessions of EAW over 12 weeks. As EAW assistance decreased (100% to 35%), the ratio of walk time to stand time increased (0.77–0.86). Electromyography patterns revealed accompanying improvements in lower extremity motor function. Clearly, these results demonstrated improvements in motor control; however, these improvements only occurred while ES was on.[55]

A randomized clinical trial suggested that powered EAW may improve gait recovery by shaping the neuroplasticity of specific brain centers.[65] After enrolling 40 participants with stroke into either EAW plus overground training (n = 20) or only overground training (n = 20) for 8 weeks, individuals were evaluated on their gait performance (10-MWT), gait cycle, and muscle activation pattern using electromyography.[65] Neural connectivity was evaluated using transcranial magnetic pulses to evoke motor potentials at the relaxed abductor hallucis muscle, conditioning electrical stimulation of the big toe as well as high-input EEG unit. Both groups showed improvement in the10-MWT and the Rivermead Mobility Index as well as a reduced Timed Up and Go (TUG) Test; however, the overall improvement was greater in the EAW plus overground training group compared to the overground training only group.[65]

The use of EAW to enhance neuroplasticity and subsequently motor recovery has expanded to other clinical populations with different neuromuscular disorders. One study demonstrated that the use of the HAL exoskeleton in conjunction with treadmill training enhanced 10-MWT, 6-MWT, and TUG Test following 8 weeks in limb-girdle muscular dystrophy patients.[66] In two people with SCI with severe spasticity, peroneal nerve stimulation was used to stimulate flexor withdrawal reflex to suppress the extensor tone during swing phase with EAW. This facilitated hip flexion and knee flexion during the gait cycle.[67] The two subjects had difficulty performing toe-off during the swing phase prior to applications of peroneal nerve stimulation.[67] Hybrid technologies have been developed combining FES and exoskeleton (i.e., FEXO) to facilitate neurorehabilitation. However, the integration of these two different technologies is challenging as far as timing, and they require a closed-loop system (i.e., feedforward control of FES and feedback control of the exoskeleton) to ensure harmonic movements. This hybrid technology provides a successful marriage of FES and the exoskeleton to overcome several of the caveats of using each system separately. For example, FES results in excessive muscle fatigue and is unlikely to promote walking for a long distance in persons with SCI.[68] In healthy and paralyzed individuals, the integration of the FEXO Knee system was successful in enhancing the rhythmicity of central pattern generators and promoting torque production for effective movement. The use of the knee exoskeleton compensated for insufficient torque production and detected torque error during FES to induce leg flexion and extension.[67]

In summary, EAW shows promise to improve different activities, functions, and QOL for individuals living with SCI and other neurologic conditions. The addition of EAW to rehabilitation programs for individuals living with paralysis can translate to potential improvements in physical activity (i.e., locomotion), pulmonary function, lower extremity motor function, seated balance, spasticity, and bowel function. BWSTT provides similar benefits for individuals with neurologic conditions; however, it appears that the addition of a robotic exoskeleton to therapy sessions may be more feasible. Other neuromodulatory methods have also been used in addition to the robotic exoskeleton in both animal and human studies. The findings from these studies suggest that EAW is an effective task-specific modality for the enhancement of overground locomotion in persons with neurologic disabilities. Robotic exoskeletons offer a feasible platform to combine with other neuromodulatory approaches that may facilitate integration of spinal and supraspinal neural controls to enhance motor recovery following neurologic disorders. This combination offers a selection of multimodal rehabilitation interventions that promote neuroplasticity at different levels and ensures widespread, safe practice in clinical settings.

References

1. Leach JB, Achyuta AK, Murthy SK. Bridging the divide between neuroprosthetic design, tissue engineering and neurobiology. *Front Neuroeng*. 2010;2:18.
2. Lotter JK, Henderson CE, Plawecki A, et al. Task-specific versus impairment-based training on locomotor performance in individuals with chronic spinal cord injury: a randomized crossover study. Neurorehabil Neural Repair. 2020 Jul;34(7):627–639.
3. Tefertiller C, Rozwod M, Wojciehowski S, et al. A comparison of one year outcomes between standardized locomotor training and usual care after motor incomplete spinal cord injury: community participation, quality of life and re-hospitalization. *J Spinal Cord Med*. 2021 Oct 6;44:1–10.
4. Dobkin B, Apple D, Barbeau H, et al. Weight-supported treadmill vs over-ground training for walking after acute incomplete SCI. *Neurology*. 2006;66(4):484–493.
5. Behrman AL, Harkema SJ. Physical rehabilitation as an agent for recovery after spinal cord injury. *Phys Med Rehabil Clin N Am*. 2007;18(2):183–202, v.
6. Dolbow DR, Gorgey AS, Recio AC, et al. Activity-based restorative therapies after spinal cord injury: inter-institutional conceptions and perceptions. *Aging Dis*. 2015;6(4):254–261.

7. Gorgey AS, Poarch H, Miller J, Castillo T, Gater DR. Locomotor and resistance training restore walking in an elderly person with a chronic incomplete spinal cord injury. *NeuroRehabilitation*. 2010;26(2):127–133. https://doi.org/10.3233/NRE-2010-0544.
8. Gorgey AS, Poarch H, Harnish C, Miller JM, Dolbow D, Gater DR. Acute effects of locomotor training on neuromuscular and metabolic profile after incomplete spinal cord injury. *NeuroRehabilitation*. 2011;29(1):79–83.
9. Ryu HX, Kuo AD. An optimality principle for locomotor central pattern generators. *Sci Rep*. 2021;11(1):13140.
10. Lovely RG, Gregor RJ, Roy RR, Edgerton VR. Effects of training on the recovery of full-weight-bearing stepping in the adult spinal cat. *Exp Neurol*. 1986;92(2):421–435.
11. Lovely RG, Gregor RJ, Roy RR, Edgerton VR. Weight-bearing hindlimb stepping in treadmill-exercised adult spinal cats. *Brain Res*. 1990;514(2):206–218.
12. Winstein CJ, Stein J, Arena R, et al. Guidelines for adult stroke rehabilitation and recovery: a guideline for healthcare professionals from the American Heart Association/American Stroke Association. *Stroke*. 2016;47(6):e98–e169.
13. Picelli A, Munari D, Modenese A, et al. Robot-assisted arm training for treating adult patients with distal radius fracture: a proof-of-concept pilot study. *Eur J Phys Rehabil Med*. 2020;56(4):444–450. https://doi.org/10.23736/S1973-9087.20.06112-2.
14. Dickstein R. Rehabilitation of gait speed after stroke: a critical review of intervention approaches. *Neurorehabil Neural Repair*. 2008;22(6):649–660. https://doi.org/10.1177/1545968308315997.
15. Ada L, Dean CM, Vargas J, Ennis S. Mechanically assisted walking with body weight support results in more independent walking than assisted overground walking in non-ambulatory patients early after stroke: a systematic review. *J Physiother*. 2010;56(3):153–161. https://doi.org/10.1016/s1836-9553(10)70020-5.
16. English C, Hillier S. Circuit class therapy for improving mobility after stroke: a systematic review. *J Rehabil Med*. 2011;43(7):565–571. https://doi.org/10.2340/16501977-0824.
17. Mehrholz J, Elsner B, Werner C, Kugler J, Pohl M. Electromechanical-assisted training for walking after stroke: updated evidence. *Stroke*. 2013;44(10):e127–e128. https://doi.org/10.1161/strokeaha.113.003061.
18. Wagner TH, Lo AC, Peduzzi P, et al. An economic analysis of robot-assisted therapy for long-term upper-limb impairment after stroke. *Stroke*. 2011;42(9):2630–2632.
19. Gorgey A, Sumrell R, Goetz L. Exoskeletal assisted rehabilitation after spinal cord injury. Atlas of orthoses and assistive devices. 5th ed. Elsevier; 2018:440–447.
20. Kressler J, Thomas CK, Field-Fote EC, et al. Understanding therapeutic benefits of overground bionic ambulation: exploratory case series in persons with chronic, complete spinal cord injury. *Arch Phys Med Rehabil*. 2014;95:1878–1887.e4.
21. Bach Baunsgaard C, Vig Nissen U, Katrin Brust A, et al. Gait training after spinal cord injury: safety, feasibility and gait function following 8 weeks of training with the exoskeletons from Ekso Bionics. *Spinal Cord*. 2018;56:106–116.
22. Miller LE, Zimmermann AK, Herbert WG. Clinical effectiveness and safety of powered exoskeleton-assisted walking in patients with spinal cord injury: systematic review with meta-analysis. *Med Devices (Auckl)*. 2016;9:455–466.
23. Asselin P, Knezevic S, Kornfeld S, et al. Heart rate and oxygen demand of powered exoskeleton-assisted walking in persons with paraplegia. *J Rehabil Res Dev*. 2015;52:147–158.
24. Gorgey AS. Robotic exoskeletons: the current pros and cons. *World J Orthop*. 2018;9(9):112–119.
25. Gorgey AS, Wade R, Sumrell R, Villadelgado L, Khalil RE, Lavis T. Exoskeleton training may improve level of physical activity after spinal cord injury: a case series. *Top Spinal Cord Inj Rehabil*. 2017;23(3):245–255.
26. Gorgey AS, Holman ME. The future of SCI rehabilitation: understanding the impact of exoskeletons on gait mechanics. *J Spinal Cord Med*. 2018;41(5):544–546.
27. del-Ama AJ, Koutsou AD, Moreno JC, de-los-Reyes A, Gil-Agudo A, Pons JL. Review of hybrid exoskeletons to restore gait following spinal cord injury. *J Rehabil Res Dev*. 2012;49(4):497–514.
28. Esquenazi A, Talaty M, Packel A, Saulino M. The ReWalk powered exoskeleton to restore ambulatory function to individuals with thoracic-level motor-complete spinal cord injury. *Am J Phys Med Rehabil*. 2012;91(11):911–921.
29. Lester RM, Gorgey AS. Feasibility of robotic exoskeleton ambulation in a C4 person with incomplete spinal cord injury: a case report. *Spinal Cord Ser Cases*. 2018;4:36.

30. Hong E, Gorman PH, Forrest GF, et al. Mobility skills with exoskeletal-assisted walking in persons with SCI: results from a three center randomized clinical trial. *Front Robot AI.* 2020;7:93.
31. Xiang XN, Ding MF, Zong HY, et al. The safety and feasibility of a new rehabilitation robotic exoskeleton for assisting individuals with lower extremity motor complete lesions following spinal cord injury (SCI): an observational study. *Spinal Cord.* 2020;58(7):787–794. https://doi.org/10.1038/s41393-020-0423-9.
32. Spungen AM, Bauman WA, Biswas K, et al. The design of a randomized control trial of exoskeletal-assisted walking in the home and community on quality of life in persons with chronic spinal cord injury. *Contemp Clin Trials.* 2020;96:106102.
33. Knezevic S, Asselin PK, Cirnigliaro CM, Kornfeld S, Emmons RR, Spungen AM. Oxygen uptake during exoskeletal-assisted walking in persons with paraplegia. *Arch Phys Med Rehabil.* 2021;102(2):185–195.
34. Xiang XN, Zong HY, Ou Y, et al. Exoskeleton-assisted walking improves pulmonary function and walking parameters among individuals with spinal cord injury: a randomized controlled pilot study. *J Neuroeng Rehabil.* 2021;18(1):86. https://doi.org/10.1186/s12984-021-00880-w.
35. Tsai CY, Delgado AD, Weinrauch WJ, et al. Exoskeletal-assisted walking during acute inpatient rehabilitation leads to motor and functional improvement in persons with spinal cord injury: a pilot study. *Arch Phys Med Rehabil.* 2020;101(4):607–612.
36. Aach M, Cruciger O, Sczesny-Kaiser M, et al. Voluntary driven exoskeleton as a new tool for rehabilitation in chronic spinal cord injury: a pilot study. *Spine J.* 2014;14(12):2847–2853. https://doi.org/10.1016/j.spinee.2014.03.042.
37. Juszczak M, Gallo E, Bushnik T. Examining the effects of a powered exoskeleton on quality of life and secondary impairments in people living with spinal cord injury. *Top Spinal Cord Inj Rehabil.* 2018;24(4):336–342. https://doi.org/10.1310/sci17-00055.
38. Tsai CY, Asselin PK, Hong E, et al. Exoskeletal-assisted walking may improve seated balance in persons with chronic spinal cord injury: a pilot study. *Spinal Cord Ser Cases.* 2021;7(1):20. https://doi.org/10.1038/s41394-021-00384-8.
39. Chisholm AE, Alamro RA, Williams AM, Lam T. Overground vs. treadmill-based robotic gait training to improve seated balance in people with motor-complete spinal cord injury: a case report. *J Neuroeng Rehabil.* 2017;14(1):27. https://doi.org/10.1186/s12984-017-0236-z.
40. Stampacchia G, Rustici A, Bigazzi S, Gerini A, Tombini T, Mazzoleni S. Walking with a powered robotic exoskeleton: subjective experience, spasticity and pain in spinal cord injured persons. *NeuroRehabilitation.* 2016;39(2):277–283. https://doi.org/10.3233/NRE-161358.
41. Chun A, Asselin PK, Knezevic S, et al. Changes in bowel function following exoskeletal-assisted walking in persons with spinal cord injury: an observational pilot study. *Spinal Cord.* 2020;58(4):459–466.
42. Gorman PH, Forrest GF, Asselin PK, et al. The effect of exoskeletal-assisted walking on bowel and bladder function: results from a randomized trial. *International Symposium on Wearable Robotics.* Springer; 2020:209–214.
43. Raab K, Krakow K, Tripp F, Jung M. Effects of training with the ReWalk exoskeleton on quality of life in incomplete spinal cord injury: a single case study. *Spinal Cord Ser Cases.* 2016;2:15025. Erratum in. *Spinal Cord Ser Cases.* 2016;2:16019. https://doi.org/10.1038/scsandc.2015.25.
44. van Dijsseldonk RB, van Nes IJ, Geurts AC, Keijsers NL. Exoskeleton home and community use in people with complete spinal cord injury. *Sci Rep.* 2020;10(1):1–8.
45. Ramanujam A, Cirnigliaro CM, Garbarini E, Asselin P, Pilkar R, Forrest GF. Neuromechanical adaptations during a robotic powered exoskeleton assisted walking session. *J Spinal Cord Med.* 2018;41(5):518–528.
46. Sutor TW, Ghatas MP, Goetx LL, Lavis TD, Gorgey AS Exoskeleton Training and Trans-Spinal Stimulation for Physical Activity Enhancement After Spinal Cord Injury (EXTra-SCI): an exploratory study. Front Rehabil Sci. 2022;2:789422. https://doi.org/10.3389/fresc.2021.789422.
47. Jayaraman A, O'Brien MK, Madhavan S, et al. Stride management assist exoskeleton vs functional gait training in stroke: a randomized trial. *Neurology.* 2019;92(3):e263–e273.
48. Postol N, Grissell J, McHugh C, Bivard A, Spratt NJ, Marquez J. Effects of therapy with a free-standing robotic exoskeleton on motor function and other health indicators in people with severe mobility impairment due to chronic stroke: a quasi-controlled study. *J Rehabil Assist Technol Eng.* 2021;8 20556683211045837. https://doi.org/10.1177/20556683211045837.
49. Li J, Morrow C, Barnes S, et al. Gut microbiome composition and serum metabolome profile among individuals with spinal cord injury and normal glucose tolerance or prediabetes/type 2 diabetes. *Arch Phys Med Rehabil.* 2021;103(4):702–710. S0003-9993(21)00438-X.

50. Ivanenko Y, Ferris DP, Lee K, Sakurai Y, Beloozerova IN, Lebedev M. Editorial: Neural prostheses for locomotion. *Front Neurosci.* 2021;15:788021.
51. Florez JM, Shah M, Moraud EM, et al. Rehabilitative soft exoskeleton for rodents. *IEEE Trans Neural Syst Rehabil Eng.* 2017;25(2):107–118.
52. Wenger N, Moraud EM, Gandar J, et al. Spatiotemporal neuromodulation therapies engaging muscle synergies improve motor control after spinal cord injury. *Nat Med.* 2016;22(2):138–145.
53. van den Brand R, Heutschi J, Barraud Q, et al. Restoring voluntary control of locomotion after paralyzing spinal cord injury. *Science.* 2012;336(6085):1182–1185.
54. Gad P, Gerasimenko Y, Zdunowski S, et al. Weight bearing over-ground stepping in an exoskeleton with non-invasive spinal cord neuromodulation after motor complete paraplegia. *Front Neurosci.* 2017;11:333.
55. Gorgey AS, Gill S, Holman ME, et al. The feasibility of using exoskeletal-assisted walking with epidural stimulation: a case report study. *Ann Clin Transl Neurol.* 2020;7(2):259–265.
56. Dolbow DR, Gorgey AS, Sutor TW, Bochkezanian V, Musselman K. Invasive and non-invasive approaches of electrical stimulation to improve physical functioning after spinal cord injury. *J Clin Med.* 2021;10(22):5356.
57. Shapkova EY, Pismennaya EV, Emelyannikov DV, Ivanenko Y. Exoskeleton walk training in paralyzed individuals benefits from transcutaneous lumbar cord tonic electrical stimulation. *Front Neurosci.* 2020;14:416.
58. Murphy DP, Bai O, Gorgey AS, et al. Electroencephalogram-based brain-computer interface and lower-limb prosthesis control: a case study. *Front Neurol.* 2017;8:696.
59. Zhang D, Ren Y, Gui K, Jia J, Xu W. Cooperative control for a hybrid rehabilitation System combining functional electrical stimulation and robotic exoskeleton. *Front Neurosci.* 2017;11:725.
60. MacLean MK, Ferris DP. Energetics of walking with a robotic knee exoskeleton. *J Appl Biomech.* 2019;35(5):320–326.
61. Harkema S, Gerasimenko Y, Hodes J, et al. Effect of epidural stimulation of the lumbosacral spinal cord on voluntary movement, standing, and assisted stepping after motor complete paraplegia: a case study. *Lancet.* 2011;377(9781):1938–1947. https://doi.org/10.1016/S0140-6736(11)60547-3.
62. Angeli CA, Edgerton VR, Gerasimenko YP, Harkema SJ. Altering spinal cord excitability enables voluntary movements after chronic complete paralysis in humans. *Brain.* 2014 May;137(Pt 5):1394–1409. Erratum in: *Brain.* 2015;138(Pt 2):e330. https://doi.org/10.1093/brain/awu038.
63. Wagner FB, Mignardot JB, Le Goff-Mignardot CG, et al. Targeted neurotechnology restores walking in humans with spinal cord injury. *Nature.* 2018;563(7729):65–71.
64. Angeli CA, Boakye M, Morton RA, et al. Recovery of over-ground walking after chronic motor complete spinal cord injury. *N Engl J Med.* 2018;379(13):1244–1250.
65. Calabrò RS, Naro A, Russo M, et al. Shaping neuroplasticity by using powered exoskeletons in patients with stroke: a randomized clinical trial. *J Neuroeng Rehabil.* 2018;15(1):35.
66. Sczesny-Kaiser M, Kowalewski R, Schildhauer TA, et al. Treadmill training with HAL exoskeleton-a novel approach for symptomatic therapy in patients with limb-girdle muscular dystrophy-preliminary study. *Front Neurosci.* 2017;11:449.
67. Ekelem A, Goldfarb M. Supplemental stimulation improves swing phase kinematics during exoskeleton assisted gait of SCI subjects with severe muscle spasticity. *Front Neurosci.* 2018;12:374. https://doi.org/10.3389/fnins.2018.00374.
68. Gorgey AS, Black CD, Elder CP, Dudley GA. Effects of electrical stimulation parameters on fatigue in skeletal muscle. *J Orthop Sports Phys Ther.* 2009;39(9):684–692.

8

Robots on the Battlefield and for Space Travel

Douglas P. Murphy

KEY POINTS

- Robotic devices are providing first-line assessments and interventions on the battlefield to save the lives of the wounded and to protect medical personnel.
- Robotic devices can provide sophisticated medical care to soldiers in remote locations.
- Robots and artificial intelligence provide many advantages to astronauts to maintain their health in space.

Medical care on the battlefield has developed some interesting sophistications to ensure the optimal recovery and treatment of soldiers who have been injured in battle. A critical triage system exists to move soldiers to better equipped and better staffed locations. However, the circumstances of battle can make the recovery of wounded soldiers quite difficult as enemy fire can block the movement of medical personnel to the fallen individual. Clearly robotic systems can play a useful role in these situations. Unmanned robotic vehicles can be directed to help without putting medics and other soldiers in harm's way. These vehicles and devices can be directed from afar and can provide medical personnel with important information on the health status of the soldier to initiate treatment as quickly as possible in a situation where any delay can result in disastrous outcomes.

In this chapter some of the various devices that have been developed will be looked at in some detail to see how they work, how they help to provide safe and effective care, and how much they have influenced medical care on the battlefield. The companies that produce these devices are spread across the globe, and their approaches show similarities but also quite interesting variations.

Battlefield Extraction–Assist Robot

The Battlefield Extraction–Assist Robot, or BEAR[1], was designed by Vecna Technologies Inc. to operate in a variety of situations that could include rescue within buildings and areas of challenging terrain. The robot has the capability to lift 500 pounds and can be controlled either with a motion-capture glove or a M-4 rifle grip controller. It travels on a dual-track system that allows it to travel upstairs. It can stand upright. The device can be guided remotely to rescue and retrieve a wounded soldier particularly if under fire. Using karate chop movements of its arms and hands, it can break through doors within buildings. Development of the robot was assisted with funding from The US Army Medical Research and Materiel Command's Telemedicine & Advanced Technology Research Center (TATRC) and Defense Advanced Research Projects Agency (DARPA).

Vecna Technologies also has the QC Bot, which is a robotic truck-like device that has applications in hospitals for delivery of medicines and supplies. The machine has important safety features that allow it to stop if an individual comes in its path but also to strategize a way to keep moving without compromising anyone.

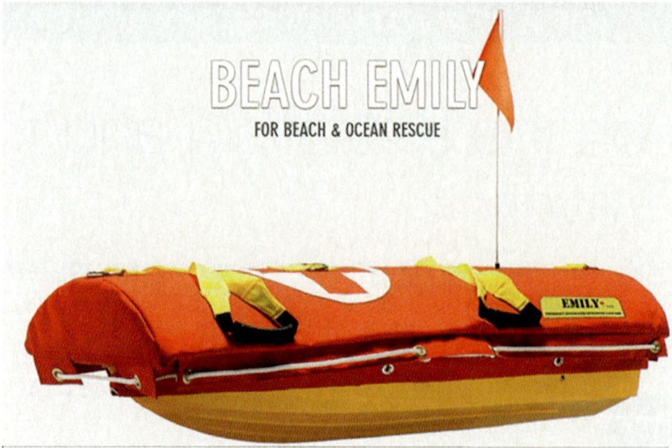

Fig. 8.1 Emily by Hydronalix—advanced small surface robotic systems. (From Hydronalix. https://www.hydronalix.com/Emily.)

Emergency Integrated Lifesaving Lanyard

EMILY is an acronym for Emergency Integrated Lifesaving Lanyard and is a device that can travel up to 25 mph[2] and can pound through surf to reach someone in distress in the water and provide a platform for rest until help can arrive (Fig. 8.1). It is 4 feet long and weighs 25 pounds and is available for use in Navies and Coast Guards around the world. It also has been used for civilian applications such as an assist for coast guards on beaches. The US Navy provided some funding for the development of this robotic device. Tony Mulligan is the inventor and chief executive officer and president of Arizona-based Hydronalix Inc., which also makes several other similar products such as NIX, AMY, and AMB that can serve a variety of purposes.

The company participates in advanced research and development programs for the Office of Naval Research, Naval Air Systems Command, Naval Sea Systems Command, Naval Surface Warfare Center, DARPA, Department of Homeland Security, Domestic Preparedness Support Initiative, National Oceanic Atmospheric Administration, Naval Information Warfare Center, and the National Science Foundation. The company also collaborates with many fire departments and has clients in many foreign countries.

Demining Robots

Although strictly speaking these robots are not directly for health care, brief mention is made here of the robots available to demine militarized zones. Since many soldier injuries are due to the explosion of mines such as improvised explosive devices, these robots serve an important role in the prevention of catastrophic injuries that would impose on soldiers a lifetime of severe disability. DOK-ING, a company headquartered in Zagreb, Croatia,[3] makes several robots of this category and these include its MV-2 Honey Badger (Fig. 8.2), MV-4 Scorpion, and MV-10 Bison. These are large autonomous vehicles that vary in their capacity to detect and destroy mines in a variety of terrains.

THE MISSION MASTER

The Rheinmetall Mission Master series[4] is a multifunctional group of unmanned ground vehicles (Fig. 8.3) whose purposes include the evacuation of injured personnel. The units consist of the Mission Master SP and the Mission Master XT. The first is the smaller of the units, and the

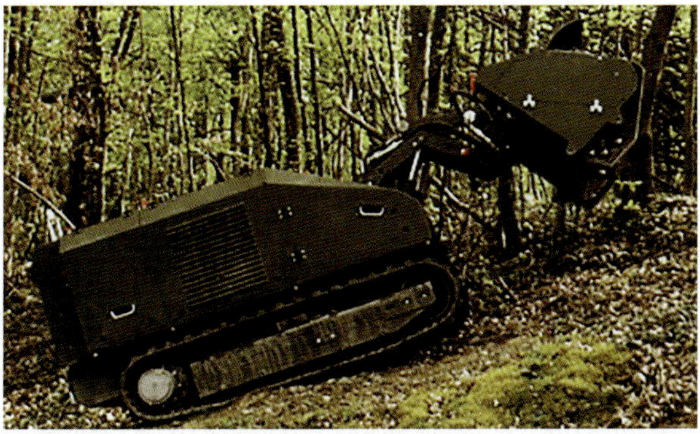

Fig. 8.2 MV-2 Honey Badger. (From DOK-ING. https://dok-ing.hr/defence-security/mv-2.)

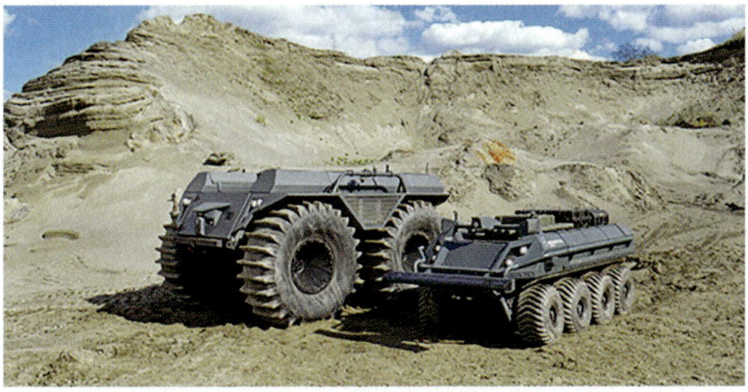

Fig. 8.3 Rheinmetall Mission Master A-UGVs. (From Robotics and Animation, "MOD Orders Surveillance UGVs," by Katie Searles, May 4, 2022. https://www.roboticsandinnovation.co.uk/news/defence/mod-orders-surveillance-ugvs.html. Rheinmetall https://www.rheinmetall-defence.com/en/rheinmetall_defence/systems_and_products/unbemannte_fahrzeuge/mission_master/index.php.)

larger one has amphibious capabilities as well. They are optionally manned. In addition to medical evacuation, they serve the purposes of reconnaissance, surveillance, tactical overwatch, and fire support. Autonomous driving and navigation functions are managed through the Rheinmetall PATH autonomy kit. Through controllers such as a tablet, smartwatch, soldier controller and single-hand controller, various modes can be implemented that include "follow me," convoy, and autonomous navigation. The artificial intelligence (AI) features are upgradable as advancements occur. Rheinmetall AG is a large, globally oriented corporation with products for the automotive industry as well as defense and security.

Bell APT 70

APT[5] is for "autonomous pod transport". This unmanned vehicle transports supplies that could include medical supplies in addition to others such as food or ammunition to soldiers on the battlefield. Since it is unmanned, there is no danger to personnel from antiaircraft defenses. Further protections include a neutral heat signature due to the electric engines and low radar visibility. It can carry payloads of up to 110 pounds. It measures 6 feet by 9 feet as it sits on the ground with a vertical height of 6 feet. It takes off vertically and then tilts forward to achieve speeds of 115 miles per hour with a range of 35 miles. It can travel from origin to destination without human interaction. The payload sits between the four booms for the rotors.[6]

ZIPLINE

These autonomous drones[7] can deliver medical supplies to remote or inaccessible locations quickly from a central staging area. The drones are propelled like small airplanes through an electric motor that propels them forward at about 100 km/h and a round trip range of 160 km. The drones have a modular design and prior to flight the package is stored, the wings applied, and the battery inserted. The GPS location is programmed into the system. The machine is sent rapidly into the air through a pulley system and electric motor that operate like a slingshot. This system accelerates the drone from a stationary position to its flight speed in 0.3 seconds. Once the drone reaches its destination, it drops its cargo, which falls to the ground through a small, disposable parachute, and then it turns around and goes home. Once back at its home station, a wire catches the drone on a hook on its fuselage. The drone communicates with the catching system and misses occur only 10% of the time. In this case the drone accelerates its engines and returns for another try.

ROBOTIC SURGERY IN THE BATTLEFIELD

Robotic surgery can enhance the timeliness and expertise of surgery needed for soldiers in the battlefield. Different options provide three different capabilities. The systems include supervisory-controlled, telesurgical, and shared-control options. In the first the surgeon loads a program suited to the required surgical needs of the patient. The surgical robot then performs the surgery independently. In the second method the surgeon operates the robot from a distance. In the last method, the robot assists the surgeon in various ways in the performance of the surgery such as steadying movements or increasing the precision of fine movements. Other considerations involve the portability of the robotic system as the larger more cumbersome units are not as suitable for transport into the battlefield. Downsides of these systems include a long and intensive training time for surgeons, the steep cost, and the increased time under anesthesia.

Trauma Pod[8]

DARPA has initiated the Trauma Pod project (Fig. 8.4)[8–10], which is a mobile, autonomous, robotic platform that can be deployed to the battlefield and serve injured soldiers without any immediate

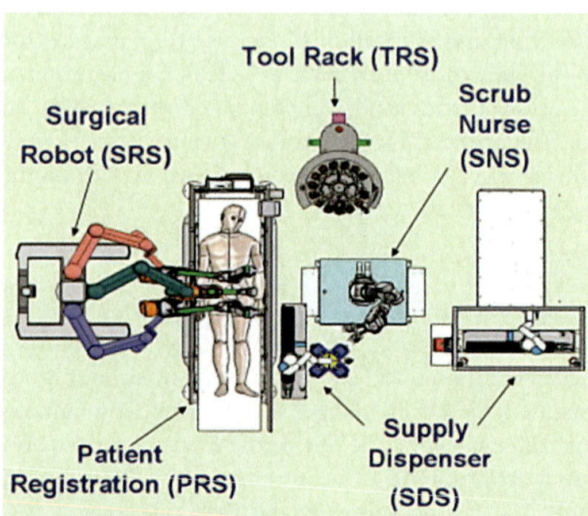

Fig. 8.4 Trauma Pod Layout.[8] (From Garcia P, Rosen J, Kapoor C, et al. Trauma Pod: a semi-automated telerobotic surgical system. Int J Med Robot. 2009;5(2):136–146.)

human intervention. Doctors and surgeons can remotely control the robotic surgical and assessment devices and thus through robotic avatars provide expert care. There are multiple subcontractors[11] that provide services such as the University of Maryland, the University of Washington, the University of Texas at Austin, Oak Ridge National Laboratory, General Dynamics, Intuitive Surgical, General Electric, and Integrated Medical Systems.

Raven

LSTAT, Life Support for Trauma and Transport System, is a snakelike robotic arm attached to a stretcher. A human operator monitors the patient through the robot's sensor and camera and manipulates the bot through a wireless system. The snakelike arm can be directed to any part of the body for assessment. The system contains the equivalent of a small-scale intensive care unit with a ventilator, defibrillator, pulse oximeter, and so on. Once the patient is moved to the stretcher the patient can be assessed, stabilized, and evacuated to more extensive medical systems.

In addition to using specific newly developed robots for targeted purposes, the military is attempting to organize a uniform system that employs robotics and AI[12] to address all the unique concerns that face the military when trying to provide medical care in a battlefield situation. An analogous civilian situation is a mass disaster, such as an earthquake or tsunami, in which there are mass casualties in a focused geographic region that require the efforts of many trauma-trained health-care workers and physicians, and yet the local systems have an inadequate supply of such personnel. The military, according to Dr. Cindy Crump of the Applied Physics Laboratory at Johns Hopkins University, faces a somewhat similar shortage and seeks to fill that gap at least partially through AI systems and robotics. An AI infrastructure would provide many advantages in that a lot of care could be automated from assessment to intervention and intervention could include as mentioned robotic surgeries. Challenges in this system exist. One is the cybersecurity of the devices used, because many commercial options do not provide sufficient cybersecurity to protect military personnel and the integrity of the military data systems. Another issue concerns device interoperability where different devices need to interface with each other.

The US Army Medical Research and Development Command has formed the Artificial Intelligence in Medical Sciences, or AIMS, task force to address such issues.[12] As part of its directives this task force identifies appropriate medical research for incorporation into ongoing programs, creates collaborative research efforts to generate information and technological developments that will support the care of warfighters, formulates partnerships with industry and academia, and assures that medical care is evidence based and that autonomous care such as from AI systems meets those standards as well. The model proposed is the AI Stack method of perceive, learn, decide, and act. This model would involve the appropriate AI computer software and hardware with a large, relevant data input and access to an immense database of reference and journal material. Although the AI systems would have some autonomy, the human interaction and modulation of such a system would be retained.

In a similar vein the Medical AI Autonomy Stack is also proposed. These layers consist of (1) sensors, medical devices, actuators, controls, and network connectivity; (2) data commons, open sources data base, repository, tools; (3) learn, replan, synchronize, prevent; (4) assess; (5) decide; (6) intervene. This stack is being approached through a collaboration between The Defense Health Agency and the US Army Medical Research and Development Command to establish MDIRA, or the medical device interoperability reference architecture.

A mixed collaboration between industry, academics, and various governmental groups has been assembled to tackle these objectives such as closed-loop control systems for medical care that is autonomous or semiautonomous and AI-assisted clinical support. Safe and secure systems are of course mandatory.

Efforts Outside the United States for Battlefield Robotics

Russia has made a commitment to develop robots for military medicine. Their areas of focus are much like those of other countries, and these include evacuation of injured soldiers on the battlefield and surgical robots for the battlefield. Their ministry of defense has planned a staged development program that would finish at the end of 2022, and they have allocated about 249,982,141 Rubles (US $3,617,241.58) to be portioned out in phases.[13] Some of the main challenges for the program involved the development of algorithms to rapidly diagnose injuries on the battlefield. Robots will rescue soldiers in combat situations, diagnose their injuries, and transport them to nearby centers where robotic surgical devices would perform the necessary surgeries. The entire flow of these events could be monitored remotely, and the use of robots would prevent human casualties in case of any mass attacks. The robots would be designed to operate effectively in conditions of extreme temperatures as well. This system would also find a place in the civilian setting and could replace paramedics. Through such programs fewer military personnel would be necessary, and one in four workers would no longer be necessary. The Russian surgical robot is lighter than the da Vinci system and has four arms, one of which is used for a video camera and the other three for surgical instruments. The Russian robotic system is designed to carry out procedures autonomously.

Pulki Gaur founded Gridbots in 2007 with a focus on AI and machine vision. Headquartered in Ahmedabad, Gridbots has clients such as the Ministry of Home Affairs in New Delhi, the National Institute of Design in Ahmedabad, the Indian Navy, Bhabha Atomic Research Center, Oil and Natural Gas Corporation (ONGC), TATA Power, Indian Space Research Organisation Physical Research Laboratory (ISRO PRL) and the Gujarat Police. The contribution of this company spread into many areas and include space robotics, defense, painting, welding, injection molding, nuclear robotics, power plants, and underwater robotics.

Robots and Artificial Intelligence in Space Programs

Travel into outer space and residence in a space station lend themselves naturally to the use of robotics and AI, both of which can enhance survival and the achievement of missions for astronauts who often function under arduous conditions.[14] Some of the traditional ways that these technologies can assist in the exploration of space consist of the following items. The most obvious would be for these to be assistants to the astronauts as they went about their duties. One example of this function is the AI assistant CIMON, which began its trial aboard the International Space Station (ISS) in December 2019. CIMON performs some of the duties that astronauts are required to perform. Another AI/robotic device is Robonaut, which will be able to off-load tasks and perform some of the riskier tasks aboard the ISS. The second area of use is mission design and planning. Daphne is an AI system that is used in the development of satellites. Travel to distant planets would be facilitated by such programs. Satellites pose significant challenges both for data that is produced and for issues related to their own healthy functioning. AI systems can be adapted for both these functions. With over 34,000 objects greater than 10 cm, outer space poses dangers due to the level of space debris floating around. The immense computational power of AI could help to track, monitor, and warn traveling astronauts of any such danger in their path. The final traditional purpose would be for navigational systems. One of the first such systems developed by researchers from National Aeronautics and Space Administration (NASA) in collaboration with technologists from Intel, utilized the multitude of images of our solar system to develop an AI method of navigation for exploring the planets. Clearly more such developments will accrue in the future.

Aside from these technical issues, the health and physiologic integrity of astronauts become major concerns particularly because space flight can create a host of medical issues. Astronauts often return with weakness. More prolonged stays can affect nearly all if not all physiological systems and organs. Examples of these include increased intracranial pressure, space flight–associated neuro-ocular syndrome, lunar dust pulmonary toxicity, alterations in gut microbiome, increased heart rate, decreased blood pressure, increased risk of cardiac dysrhythmias, kidney stones, anemia, loss of bone mineral content, immune deficiency, radiation-induced cancers, altered circadian rhythms, mood disturbances, among others. Many of these are worse with longer stays and can persist for long periods of time after the return to Earth. Ophthalmic symptoms fall into this category. In addition to space flight–associated neuro-ocular syndrome, globe flattening, optic nerve edema, retinal folds, refractive error shifts, and nerve fiber layer infarcts can occur. Cardiovascular issues can be quite concerning as dangerous dysrhythmias can occur. After even 6 months of being in space, changes occur in the structure and conduction paths of the heart. There are both immediate and chronic changes from microgravity as shifts in the distribution of blood occur as well as alterations in pumping capacity and changes in cardiac reflex activity. The risks of these changes once the astronaut returns to Earth at the present time are not known. Dust from the moon, Mars, and other planets has a known adverse effect on humans that is not limited to the pulmonary system, but which can also affect the neurologic and cardiovascular systems. Microgravity also exerts a negative effect on the musculoskeletal system, prompting loss of mineralization of bones and perhaps some loss of cartilage as well. Spinal pathologies can increase as a result. Diet and exercise can have some deterrent effect on these changes.

Consequently, the monitoring of the health and physiological systems of space travelers becomes of paramount importance. Several AI solutions have been proposed. These include wearable technology, biosensors, surveillance, diagnostic imaging, augmented and virtual reality, telemedicine, and telesurgery or robotic surgery. For AI to work, many factors must come into play. As noted previously in this book, deep learning systems function best when large amounts of data are fed into its processing systems for it to produce the most successful analyses. Due to the limited number of missions, optimal databases may not yet be available. Also, the AI systems need accurate and timely physiological data from the space travelers. There are multiple technologies that can be deployed to achieve these ends.

As mentioned previously, there are a host of wearables that can provide pertinent physiological information. Wrist-worn actigraphs[15,16] can provide rest data and already are in use. Important parameters to measure are bone density, cardiac output, energy expenditure, and muscle strength. Bone density of course provides an indication of whether an astronaut is at risk for fractures or approaching the risk for fractures and thus would allow preemptive action to prevent such decreases from occurring. A newer technological advance provides monitoring through electronic skin that can take different manifestations. The electronic nose can detect harmful substances while the electronic ear can pick up lung sounds for interpretation within an AI program. Such sensors could provide an early warning system for lunar dust (regolith). Other potential wearables could measure physical fatigue, mental decline, electroencephalographic data through caps or helmets. Wearables could be integrated into T-shirts or spacesuits. Prototypes for some of these options already exist such as the BRAINCARE, which can measure intracranial pressure.

Biosensors represent a useful tool to ensure the ongoing well-being of space travelers. Combined with AI,[17] they make a powerful system for health analysis and monitoring. This type of device can assess chemical factors in the blood and tissues and provide feedback about the effects of space travel on the physiology and metabolism of any given individual under these conditions. Any body fluid or tissue potentially could be analyzed such as blood, urine, feces, hair, muscle, and saliva. Panomics,[18] although generally requiring the use of bulky devices not suited for space flight, have the potential for being incorporated into space travel once the AI systems become miniaturized enough to bypass weight and space concerns. Under the umbrella of panomics resides genomic, transcriptomic, proteonic, and metabolomics.[18] Biosensors allowed the implementation of an interesting twin study where one twin spent a year on the ISS and other spent the same year on Earth. Multiple biological parameters were studied and compared. A vaccine study on the two did not show any difference in the immunologic system. However, there were significant differences in areas such as telomere length, epigenetics, gastrointestinal microbiome, inflammatory cytokines, ocular parameters, metabolites within the blood. Some of these normalized after return to Earth but others did not, and thus some systems appeared to be more adversely affected than others. Thus, the beginning of data sets for deep learning machines is accompanying the growth of technology to gather data.

Augmented and virtual reality will also find a place in these scenarios. A proposed aid to the psychological well-being of astronauts would be the enhanced visual and auditory input these systems would provide for relief of a somewhat monochromic space experience. Skin haptic systems would add the sensory input to the visual and auditory ones for a more comprehensive experience. This option has been discussed in relation to a proposed trip to Mars, which would take around 3 years with just a handful of astronauts in a confined space. Augmented and virtual reality would allow these astronauts some relief from the monotony and the stress of such an experience. Psychological well-being is not the only benefit or purpose being proposed. Maintaining cognitive and intellectual sharpness through stimulating and challenging games could also be a benefit as well.

Given that computed tomography and magnetic resonance imaging machines are far too bulky and heavy to hoist into space, medical care now relies on diagnostic ultrasound or teleultrasound to provide imaging guidance in the diagnosis of a variety of medical conditions. The ISS currently employs ultrasound for the residents there. Crew members of the ISS, for example, are trained in the focused assessment in sonographic technique to assist in the imaging. They perform the mechanics of moving the probe over the appropriate areas at the appropriate settings, and the images are then sent to Earth for analysis. Robot and AI assistance in this medical imaging technique is certainly anticipated. The members of the ISS can direct this technique toward critical intrabdominal, intrathoracic, and ocular issues. Studies have been done on the application of ultrasound to evaluation of the lumbar spine to better understand the development of back pain during these missions. Study and development of this modality has occurred through the program of NASA Extreme Environment Missions Operations in underwater conditions of a submarine. Robot assistance to the probe movements is sought as well. Physicians provide input remotely. Doppler ultrasound coupled with AI can do velocity comparisons of carotid versus femoral artery blood flow to assess the risk of cerebrovascular conditions.

So, although telemedicine for astronauts is now routinely employed, the difficulties with maintaining a continuous or real-time communication channel cause some obstacles to the delivery of care. Utilizing AI with the integration of data from wearables and biosensors and imaging can offset such difficulties and allows astronauts to receive a much higher level of care when not in communication with physicians located on Earth. One unique aspect of space medicine and research is that 3D printed tissue structures that would normally collapse under their own weight on Earth will sustain their shape in outer space in a microgravity environment (Fig. 8.5). Onboard AI can optimize imaging from ultrasound to enhance medical diagnosis and treatment. To increase the effectiveness of AI intervention, Astroskin[19–22] (Fig. 8.6) is used to monitor multiple biological parameters and uses the following: three-axis accelerometer, electrocardiogram (ECG)/heart rate, respiration rate and volume, oxygen saturation, systolic blood pressure, and skin temperature. Various trials have been performed to demonstrate its feasibility and usefulness. Prior to Astroskin, the method employed was the blood pressure/electrocardiogram kit which is capable of measuring ECG, heart rate, and blood pressure. Bulky and heavy, the kit also uses a lot of energy. One such test trial of Astroskin occurred at NASA's Human Exploration Research Analog, or HERA, within the Johnson Spaceflight Center. HERA allowed the simulation of isolation, remote conditions, and confinement associated with spaceflight. The Astroskin consisted of an upper-body garment and a headband, all of which contained sensors of the sort mentioned previously. In this study there were eight subjects, four women and four men. The study consisted

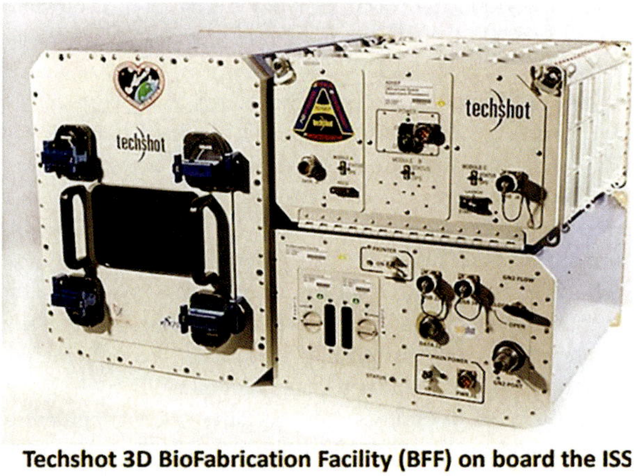

Fig. 8.5 Techshot 3D BioFabrication Facility on board the International Space Station.[23] (From NASA.gov. https://www.nasa.gov/mission_pages/station/research/experiments/explorer/Facility.html#id=7599.)

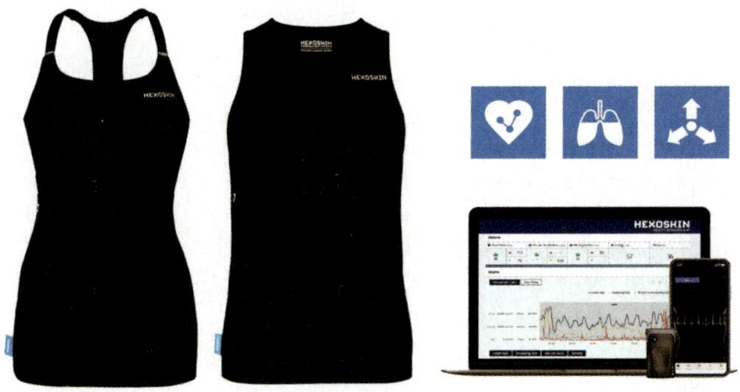

Fig. 8.6 Astroskin. (From Hexoskin. https://www.hexoskin.com/collections/all.)

of a permission baseline, 4 days of continuous monitoring during full workdays, and a postmission baseline. The results of the study indicated that the garment overall was user-friendly, was comfortable except for some issues with the headband, and could transmit reliably through Bluetooth technology good physiologic data. Sleep and fitness times were well monitored.

The health-care industry has branched into outer space where unique opportunities present themselves. NASA has identified two new imperatives for health care in outer space: (1) the health of astronauts to enable the completion of missions and (2) the health of civilian passengers to facilitate commerce in outer space. Radiation[24] in space poses hazards not encountered for humans living on the surface of Earth. For example, galactic cosmic rays and solar particle events both present risks such as damage to DNA and the development of cancer, as well as damage to other body systems such as the nervous and the cardiovascular systems. Several types of exposures comprise galactic cosmic rays such as high-charge and high-energy ions (HZEs), high-energy and secondary protons, neutrons and fragments produced through interactions with the shielding around spaceships and interactions with human tissue. The risks from solar particle events, on the other hand, come from low-energy to medium-energy protons. These exposures are different depending on whether they occur in a low Earth orbit or further out in space. With the former the geomagnetic field of the Earth provides some protective, modifying effect. HZEs cause greater damage to human tissue and DNA than the types of radiation normally encountered on the surface of the Earth. HZEs produce complex patterns of damage to DNA that are difficult to repair. Degenerative disorders can develop as a result of exposure to the radiation mentioned. These degenerative disorders can occur in the cardiovascular, neurologic, respiratory, immunologic, endocrine, and digestive systems. These exposures can increase the risk of cataracts, stroke, and myocardial infarctions. Risks can also be divided into acute and late ones. Neurocognitive dysfunction can occur during spaceflight, and later dementia and accelerated aging can occur. One study of mice who received varying levels of exposure showed measures of decreased dendritic sprouting for neurons proportional to the level of exposure. The NASA Human Research Program will seek to understand and mitigate all these risks through analysis of data collected from spaceflights, laboratory models, and computer modeling. A multidisciplinary approach is sought that covers a multitude of disciplines and specialists such as epidemiologists, physicians, clinicians, and computer modelers. Certainly, AI will play a role in such analyses. Robots also can serve to mitigate such risks because these can be deployed in riskier situations such as repairs outside the space capsule where exposures are more significant. Tools such as the Solar Energetic Particles (SEP) Acute Radiation Risk Tool will send radiation events[14] to the scientist on Earth in real time for biological predictions of the effects of any given event and for the quick implementation of counter measures. The tool was originally developed for Exploration Mission 1 where the Orion spacecraft looped around the moon.

Further protection of the health of astronauts comes using personal protective equipment such as the AstroRad vest[25,26] (Fig. 8.7), which can protect radiation-sensitive organs from predicted and unpredicted radiation events in space. Another study examines how the microgravity environment and the disruption of the 12-hour light-and-dark cycle affect the health and performance of certain organs, particularly those like the liver that are dependent on such cycles. A genetic link exists between the liver and genes associated with this 12-hour cycle.

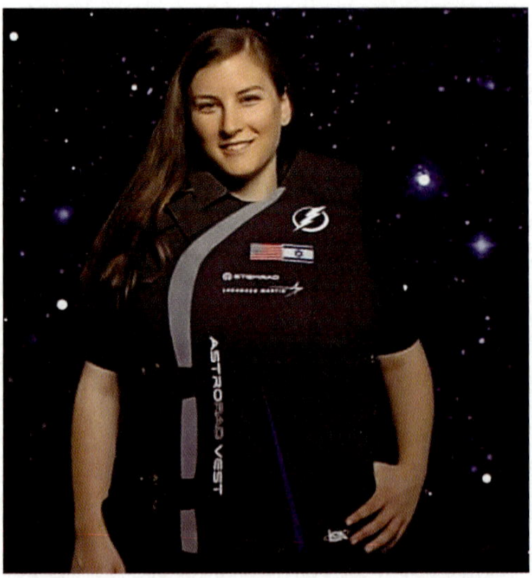

Fig. 8.7 AstroRad vest.[26] (StemRad Ltd.)

An interesting offshoot of such work occurred within a study at the Mayo Clinic. A convolutional neural network, or CNN, was trained through deep learning systems via data from 499,727 patients that consisted of ECG information. The purpose of the training was to see if the CNN could accurately predict a person's age based on a short time of interval of their ECG. Discrepancies potentially could be attributed to cardiac pathologies. Thus, potentially the CNN could be used to assess the cardiac health of individuals based on their ECG data. The AI system had a better accuracy if the individual had no history of cardiac issues and normal cardiac function as opposed to individuals with low ejection fractions, coronary artery disease, and other pathologies. When the latter occurred, the AI predicted an older age for the individual. Sex classification was achieved with a 90.47% accuracy.

Sensorimotor functions can deteriorate in microgravity conditions, and this deterioration can result in a decreased capability to control robots. To further study this phenomenon, NASA has created a system whereby astronauts in the ISS can practice controlling robots on Earth where their performances can be studied in parallel with their physiological functions.[23] This initiative is part of Analog-1 in which the European Space Agency is involved. Part of the purpose for this study is to elicit and resolve any difficulties prior to future missions on the moon and Mars, for example. The abilities of astronauts to navigate the lunar rover over varied terrain and courses and collect samples with a robotic arm come under scrutiny.

Another interesting project within NASA for the delivery of astronaut health-care concerns the construction of the Robonaut 2[27] (Fig. 8.8) that can combine nursing and physician skills. The robot has avatar capacities so that a remote physician could manipulate it from a distance. Sensors in its hand allow a gentle grabbing capacity, and it can lift items of moderate weight. The cameras can register the light spectrum that human eyes see and additionally can perceive the infrared range. The computing processing resides in its abdomen. Of course, not only remote individuals but the astronaut themselves can manipulate the robot in part to circumvent the delays in transmission from Earth. In addition to its medical and surgical duties, the robot should be able to perform maintenance tasks outside the space capsule or space station.

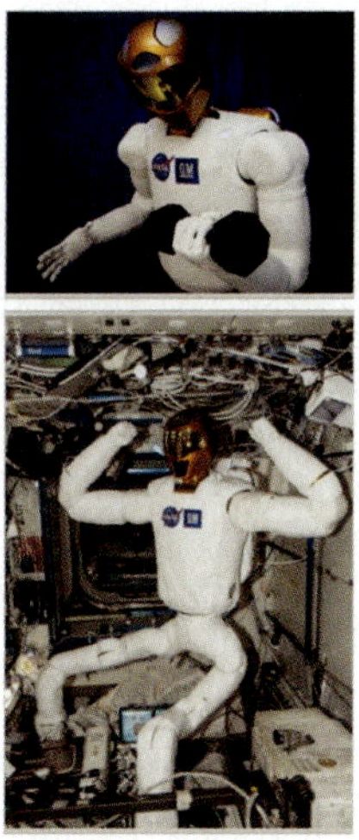

Fig. 8.8 National Aeronautics and Space Administration space robot Robonaut 2. (From Robonaut 2 (nasa.gov) National Aeronautics and Space Administration.)

References

1. Ruppert B. Robots to rescue wounded on battlefield. Published November 22, 2010. Accessed September 27, 2022. https://www.army.mil/article/48456/robots_to_rescue_wounded_on_battlefield
2. Advanced small surface robotic systems. Hydronallx (advanced, small, surface robotic systems). Accessed September 27, 2022. https://www.hydronalix.com/
3. About us. DOK-ING. Accessed September 27, 2022. https://dok-ing.hr/dok-ing-about-us/about-us/
4. The Rheinmetall Mission Master Family. Accessed September 27, 2022. https://rheinmetall-defence.com/en/rheinmetall_defence/systems_and_products/unbemannte_fahrzeuge/mission_master/index.php
5. Bell APT for Military. https://www.bellflight.com/products/bell-apt.
6. Tegler E. Bell learned that its APT 70 cargo drone can integrate with manned traffic during a demo flight. What did it learn about avoidance and 5G? Forbes. Published October 2, 2020. Accessed September 27, 2022. https://www.forbes.com/sites/erictegler/2020/10/02/bell-learned-that-its-apt-70-cargo-drone-can-integrate-with-manned-traffic-during-a-demo-flight-what-did-it-learn-about-avoidance-and-5g/?sh=5f7709692e1f
7. Zipline—vital on-demand delivery for the world. Zipline. https://www.flyzipline.com
8. Trauma Pod DARPA. Robot surgery—UMBC ebiquity. https://ebiquity.umbc.edu/project/html/id/63/Trauma-Pod
9. DARPA's Trauma Pod project. Published July 13, 2009. Accessed September 27, 2022. http://surgrob.blogspot.com/2009/07/darpas-traumapod-project.html
10. Martinic G. Glimpses of future battlefield medicine—the proliferation of robotic surgeons and unmanned vehicles and technologies. *J Mil Veteran Fam Health.* 2014;22(3). https://jmvh.org/article/glimpses-of-future-battlefield-medicine-the-proliferation-of-robotic-surgeons-and-unmanned-vehicles-and-technologies/
11. Garcia P, Rosen J, Kapoor C, et al. Trauma Pod: a semi-automated telerobotic surgical system. *Int J Med Robot.* 2009;5(2):136–146.
12. Crump C, Schlacta-Fairchild LM. Achieving a trusted, reliable, AI-ready infrastructure for military medicine and civilian care. Paper presented at the Proceedings SPIE 11413, Artificial Intelligence and Machine Learning for Multi-Domain Operations Applications II, 114130C; April 21, 2020. https://www.spiedigitallibrary.org/conference-proceedings-of-spie/11413/114130C/Achieving-a-trusted-reliable-AI-ready-infrastructure-for-military-medicine/10.1117/12.2557514.full
13. China developing medical military robots. Communal News: Online Business, Wholesale & B2B Marketplace News.
14. Five ways artificial intelligence can help space exploration. The Conversation. Published January 25, 2021. Accessed September 27, 2022. https://theconversation.com/five-ways-artificial-intelligence-can-help-space-exploration-153664
15. Rettner R. Sleepless in space: getting shut-eye is tough out there. NBC News. Published; August 8, 2014 Accessed September 27, 2022. nbcnews.com/id/wbna55821641.
16. Kawada T. Applicability of the actigraphy for astronauts in spaceflight. *Sleep Sci.* 2016;9(2):59.
17. Haney N, Urman A, Waseem T, Cagle Y, Morey J. AI's role in deep space. *J Med Artif Intell.* 2020;3:11.
18. Sandhu C, Qureshi A, Emili A. Panomics for precision medicine. *Trends Mol Med.* 2018;24(1):85–101.
19. DeLeon R., Cowings P., Toscano B. *Wearable biosensor monitor to support autonomous crew health and performance.* NASA Technical Reports Server (NTRS). Published; August 15, 2016 Accessed September 27, 2022. https://ntrs.nasa.gov/search?q=wearable%20biosensor%20monitor%20201
20. Kumar A, Levin E, Cowings P, Toscano WB.Evaluation of the accuracy of Astroskin as a behavioral health self-monitoring system for spaceflight. NASA Technical Reports Server (NTRS); August 22, 2015 Accessed September 27, 2022. https://ntrs.nasa.gov/search?q=evaluation%20of%20the%20accuracy%20of%20astroskin
21. Robillard C, et al. The Astroskin, a wearable body metrics garment to measure physiological parameters in non-clinical environments—health and spaceflight missions applications. Waterloo, Canada: 35th Annual International Gravitational Physiology Meeting; 2014.
22. Villa-Colin J, Shaw T, Toscano WB, Cowings P. Evaluation of Astroskin bio-monitor during high intensity physical activities. Memorias Del XLI Congreso Nacional De Ingeniera Biomedica. Sociedad Mexicana Ingeniera Biomedica. 2018. https://ntrs.nasa.gov/citations/20190000238

23. Space portal events. NASA. Accessed September 27, 2022. https://www.nasa.gov/ames/partnerships/spaceportal/news
24. Patel ZS, Brunstetter TJ, Tarver WJ, et al. Red risks for a journey to the red planet: the highest priority human health risks for a mission to Mars. *NPJ Microgravity*. 2020;6:33.
25. Cawdrey K. New technology could improve radiation risk warnings for future deep-space astronauts. August 20, 2018. Accessed September 27, 2022. https://phys.org/news/2018-08-technology-future-deep-space-astronauts.html#:~:text=New%20technology%20could%20improve%20radiation%20risk%20warnings%20for%20future%20deep%2Dspace%20astronauts,-by%20Kathryn%20Cawdrey&-text=New%20technology%20that%20detects%20radiation,according%20to%20a%20new%20study
26. Space Radiation Protection. AstroRad shield for astronauts and commercial spaceflight. StemRad. Accessed September 27, 2022. https://stemrad.com/astrorad-4/#:~:text=The%20AstroRad%20is%20personal%20protective,solar%20particle%20events%20(SPE).
27. Espiner T. Nasa's Robonaut 2 scrubs up for space surgery. BBC News. Published April 4, 2014. Accessed September 27, 2022. https://www.bbc.com/news/technology-26872884

9

The Economics of the Robotic Industry

Robert Trainer

KEY POINTS

- The robotics industry has grown rapidly both in production and in revenue and should continue to experience rapid growth in the coming years.
- The growth of this industry is changing the nature of health care in many ways.
- All aspects of robotic technology from artificial intelligence to humanoid robots are being brought into service in health-care settings.
- Profits from these technologies come from nay different sources.

Mention of robots brings to mind many different things for all of us, in large part based on how popular culture has shaped our individual understanding of what robots are and what they can and should do. In this chapter we discuss some of the economics behind the field of robotics in health care, an area that has been steadily growing boosted in large part because of the recent pandemic and stay-at-home orders issued in various parts of the world. As Brakman points out in an article by the same name, "robots do not get the coronavirus."[1] The response to the COVID-19 pandemic saw their use expand to reduce loneliness in nursing homes[2] and ramp up ventilator production[3] and many jobs in between. In China an entire hospital was "run" by robots,[4] reducing spread, repurposing staff roles, and maintaining morale.

For this discussion we define a robot as "a machine that resembles a living creature in being capable of moving independently (as by walking or rolling on wheels) and performing complex actions (such as grasping and moving objects)" (Merriam Webster). It is quite difficult as one can imagine to discuss robotics without mentioning artificial intelligence (AI) since the incredible data storage and "real-time" data usage obviates the need for fixed machines in some cases. We will at least try to exclude machine learning, virtual reality, and avatar technology, which represent another burgeoning area for growth and development. We will discuss the economics of surgical robots, rehabilitation robots, noninvasive radiosurgery robots, and hospital and pharmacy robots and discuss briefly robot process automation and implant technology. The introduction of robotics and AI can be lucrative to the manufacturer for a multitude of reasons. The robot unit itself will most likely require integration with hospital network systems, cloud-based storage, and software updates as well as disposables that are tailored to be specific to the hardware unit, thereby setting up a system built around the integration of the robot, which will setup for net increased annual profit indefinitely.

Scope of the Health-Care Robotics Market Report

The global health-care robotics market was valued at $7.7492 trillion in 2020 and will reach $16.830 trillion by the end of 2027, growing at a Compound Annual Growth Rate (CAGR) of 13.8%

from 2022 to 2027. The latest published report by 360 Research Reports, the global "Healthcare Robotics Market Segment Forecast, 2021–2027," key players/manufacturers identified are:

- Agilent Technologies
- Abbott Diagnostics
- CareFusion
- Accuray
- Roche Holding
- Siemens Healthcare
- Stryker
- Aurora Biomed
- Hansen Medical
- iRobot
- Kirby Lester
- Mazor Robotics
- Renishaw
- Baxter International
- Intuitive Surgical
- BioTek Instruments
- Aesynt
- Titan Medical
- ReWalk Robotics
- Hocoma

To answer the economic question how profits are realized, we might ask, "Why is Elon Musk the richest man in the world?" A quick analysis of TSLA financial statement shows a market cap of $1.04 trillion with a price-to-earnings ratio of 329 as of this writing. (This is evidence that the stock is priced to reflect the fact that he is believed to be an innovator. Alphabet's [GOOGL] price-to-earnings ratio by comparison is 30, and Intuitive Surgical [ISRG], the maker of the da Vinci robot, which has dominated the hospital surgical market for 15 years, is 75.) Clearly then stock price is an incomplete measure but illustrates the *belief* of production to some degree. It is not an empty vessel, however, because with more cash on hand there is more room for innovation, further research and development, and more patents that can be achieved. Tesla has over 3200 patents, iRobot has 1500, and Intuitive Surgical has 600. That is most impressive since the car company in this example is relatively young. Being in a fast-changing field can be an advantage as a true innovator can and must change quickly. Imagine Ford founded in 1903 changing 60+ features in next year's model. For Mr. Musk, use of government facilities including the National Aeronautics and Space Administration's space launch pad does not hurt his side business either.

The typical funding source for *new* robotics companies is most often venture capitalist spending. As a sign that the field of robotics is gaining ground, according to Forbes, Venture Capitalists poured $6.3 billion during the pandemic (March 2019 to March 2020), up 50% from $4.3 billion the year before. In 2015 the total was $1 billion. The number of startups receiving funding is also up from 48 to 68.[5] Approximately one-third of this is industrial, which as we will see is often a testing ground for military and health-care applications. When TechCrunch asked 13 robotics-centered VCs for comment on the direction of the industry, the overwhelming reply that the previous mantra "hardware is hard" is being replaced by "RaaS" (robot as a service), reflecting the increase in the desire to enhance not replace human capability, which will fit into health care quite seamlessly.[6]

If we discuss where you might encounter robots in health care, I think the easiest way to illustrate this is take a *behind the scenes tour* in the hospital as a patient having surgery. Imagine two of the most common operations performed in the United States today, a surgery to remove an enlarged or cancerous prostate and a total hip replacement.

On your initial visit, the receptionist might check you in, alerting others logged into the electronic health record (EHR) of your presence (of course, after your copay and insurance information is confirmed and reconfirmed). A medical assistant will again add medical history, chief complaint, and vital signs to the EHR. Your preoperative laboratory values, imaging, and other scanned documents will already be in the chart from an outside laboratory of your primary care physician's office. So how does the EHR integrate the information into the online record? Complete with reminders: here AI provides various prompts based on comorbidities, age, and yes, insurance carrier. What happens to these data afterward is not completely clear. Data are used to keep the EHR working better. By using conglomerated patient data sets, predictive analytics can help build robotics (think IBM Watson) directly or be sold to other companies and health-care conglomerates interested in such data.

Take Inovalon, a data analytics company. Available data pertaining to a specified patient are aggregated from massive longitudinally linked data sets, connected partners, decision support platforms, EHRs, Health Information exchanges (HIEs), and a myriad of other platforms to improve economics across the health-care ecosystem.

The top 10 clients accounted for approximately 29% of revenues for the year ended December 31, 2020. The Inovalon and Humana engagement dates back to early 2019 which had expanded the relationship later in 2019 to include Inovalon's ScriptMed Cloud offering. Inovalon as a relatively new entity processes data pertaining to more than 1 million physicians, 574,000 clinical facilities, 332 million Americans, and nearly 61 billion medical events. This helped them add adaptive machine learning capabilities along with data on billions of known medical events to transform unstructured clinical data into highly valuable, structured data, which are then analyzed at massive scale in fractions of a second. So the technology builds newer technology all using data from patients, the ownership of which is unknown.

If after this visit you are deemed to be a good candidate, you will have a preoperative evaluation by an anesthesiologist. In the wake of COVID-19 and for convenience if you meet the criteria, you might be offered a telehealth visit—using a patient-facing secure platform for direct communication where you meet your doctor in a virtual room to discuss anesthesia risks, ask questions, and attempt to optimize solutions to any medical problems before surgery. For objective physical examination tests, a physical robot (where data would be uploaded for storage and retrieved later) might not be necessary if it can be replaced with directly communicated data. For example, to listen to your heart and lungs, remote devices with AI algorithms trained by over 12,000 auscultation sounds can be obtained and analyzed. If you participated in remote patient monitoring, metadata from a wearable device including a month's worth of pulse oximetry, heart rate, and any aberrant heart rhythm will be summarized and added to the chart.

On the day of surgery after you receive anesthesia clearance, drugs are drawn from one of many "omnicells" located throughout the hospital. Total stock of each medicine operates as part of a pharmacy tracking program. This essential piece engages in the provision of medication management automation solutions. It includes a platform and interoperability, central pharmacy dispensing, medication adherence, and point of care automation. An autonomous mobile robot will deliver the intravenous fluid, medications for pain, nausea prevention, hemodynamic control, and so on. That is not all; the same robot will likely be used for linens and medical waste encompassing food service and laboratory, environmental, nursing, and pharmacy roles at all points. The delivery system also ensures hospital employee ID scan-tracked handoff replacing prior tube systems without positive control of all of the above. At a hospital system such as University of California San Francisco, this robot can cover 115 miles in 24 hours. This same hospital system uses robots not only to dispense medications but also to prepare and track medications in an outfit that looks much like Amazon's warehouse. Is this profitable for the developer? Aethon is a Pittsburg-based firm that developed the TUG in 2004. The autonomous robot now carries 1400 pounds and navigates around people and the corridors of client facilities. When Aethon was acquired in 2017 to Singapore Technologies (ST) Engineering, it received $37 million and continued to operate as a subsidiary of ST Robotics. ST Engineering is traded on the Singapore stock exchange and is 1 of 82 robotics companies in the newly formed ROBO Global Robotics & Automation ETF (ROBO). The technology used is a simpler version of the laser guidance used to control missiles developed by the military and used most commonly in many of today's cars (Light detection and ranging or Lidar).

On to the operating room . . . The first documented use of a robot-assisted surgical procedure occurred in 1985 when the PUMA 560 robotic surgical arm was used in a neurosurgical biopsy. This led to its more common use in laparoscopic surgeries (Fig. 9.1), in which flexible fiberoptic cameras are utilized. More and more commonly, prostate removal is performed by a robot-assisted technology. The most common surgical setup is the da Vinci surgery apparatus (approved by the Food and Drug Administration in 2000) and disposables by intuitive surgical. The reason: after insufflation, approximately three to six 1- to 2-cm incisions are made for the robotic hands. Each one has seven axes of movement compared with the four of a human hand. Combined with scaled and filtered hand movements and high-definition, 3D, 12× magnified vision, the surgery is becoming the standard for reducing complications and speeding recover. With many centers purchasing two and three bases at approximately $1 million each, combining the fact that each surgery requires the separate purchase of disposables, that can be in excess of $30,000 per operation—it is easy to see profits rise. The company Intuitive Surgical has a market cap of $125 billion with a 360% rise in the last 5 years. Intuitive Surgical has dominated the robotic surgery industry for 15 years, and the company offers robotic surgery options for thoracic surgery, gynecologic surgery, and many more.

Ion's fully articulating catheter and flexible needle enable accurate biopsy, even in difficult-to-reach nodules outside airways. The catheter moves 180 degrees in all directions and enables fine adjustment for precise biopsy. The custom-designed needle can pass through tight-radius bends to

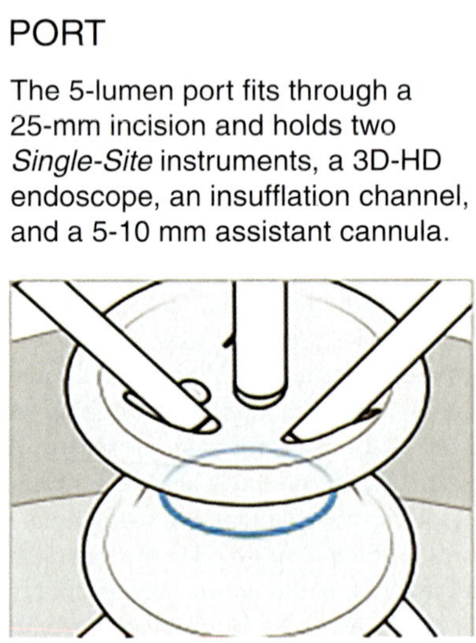

Fig. 9.1 Port adapter for the da Vinci robotic surgery system. HD, high-definition. (From Intuitive Surgical, da Vinci Robotic Surgery.)

perform transbronchial needle biopsies. Ion's ultra-thin robotic catheter and advanced maneuverability allow navigation far into the peripheral lung with robotic control of the catheter's position throughout the entire navigation and biopsy process.

And it all comes with a service: Excel with Genesis is an add-on service that helps hospitals and networks maximize efficiency, uncover cost saving opportunities, increase utilization and more. It comes with an annual contract, for a price.

Building on this robotic biopsy setup, as reported in nature,[7] development of AI into an existing system dubbed Smart Tissue Autonomous Robot (STAR) with a force sensor allows a robot arm to perform 20 sutures exactly the same by tracking the tissue when it moves and adjusting every stitch in an intestinal anastomosis. The same hardware is being trialed for heart valves and brain tumors.[8]

Say instead of minimally invasive surgery, you are having that joint replacement. Almost *1 million* hip and knee replacements are done in the United States every year. Becoming more precise and less invasive offers faster recovery, lower complications, and enhancing prosthetic life span. For this reason both surgeries are more often aided by a robot-assisted device with a recent study on hip replacement showing 5× better leg length matching and 2× the angle accuracy with use of a robot-assisted technique.[9]

The familiar uses of robots in surgery might be just that familiar. A human places and guides the arms and is in the room for the entire procedure. *In 2001*, surgeons in New York removed the gallbladder of a patient in France utilizing a remote-controlled robotic system. That same year cardiologist Tejas Patel performed five remote coronary procedures with the same device.[10] Now, 20 years later, there is renewed hope that the 5 G network enhancements may make a tele-hub-and-spoke surgery model more of a reality. Use of microbots is yet another area of rapid development as it combines remote control and miniaturization, allowing surgeons and medical doctors to render treatment in previously unreachable areas, which is discussed elsewhere. Cybersecurity concerns are also a factor with more devices coming online the susceptibility to cyberattack is heightened.

Robots in Rehabilitation

Imagine you have a complication from any of the above procedures, which causes a stroke or spinal cord injury. What would your tour of the rehabilitation unit look like now?

As discussed by Van der Loos et al,[11] Ekso Bionics, is one company who has paired with Project Walk to help spinal cord injury recovery using intelligent exoskeletons for paralyzed patients to gain function and independence. The company founded in 2005 as Berkely Bionics has been a pioneer in exoskeletons that have now become a common fixture in major rehabilitation facilities.

The global rehabilitation robot market is also anticipated to gain momentum from a rise in the geriatric population across the globe as the role of assistance.

Key players are involved in mergers and acquisition to strengthen their market position. Owing to increasing competition, frequent innovations are taking place in the market. Some of the companies operating the industry are:

- Cyberdyne Inc.
- Bionik
- Hocoma
- Rex Bionics Ltd.
- BioXtreme
- Ekso Bionics
- Corindus, Inc.
- ReWalk Robotics

One of the most common uses of exoskeletons in health care is probably poststroke rehabilitation.[12,13] Strong evidence is provided for inpatient improvement in muscle mass, density, and mitochondrial activity oxygen consumption.[14] There is also a role for its use post–spinal cord injury with and without implanted spinal cord stimulation devices. This *dual technology* takes advantage of targeted motor stimulation of the spinal cord below the level of a lesion with the proprioception gained by having a robotic assistance. Spinal Cord Stimulation (SCS) was approved by the US Food and Drug Administration in 1989 for the treatment of chronic intractable pain of the trunk or limbs and has become the most common of all neuromodulation therapies.

SCS has been applied off-label in many other disabling conditions, including motor disorders. It began with the serendipitous observation made in a patient with multiple sclerosis being treated for intractable back pain who regained considerable voluntary motor control with SCS. Subsequent studies described improved bladder function, reduced spasticity, and a feeling of lightness of the legs during movement as the primary benefits, along with increased endurance during ambulation and the recovery of some voluntary motor function with SCS. Is this a robot? If not, it is at least a human augmentation in line with the RaaS (robot as a service) concept much like a robotic arm. A recent case series of 13 patients with spinal cord injury with a complaint of diffuse, ongoing dysesthesias of a burning quality below the level of the lesion were implanted with SCS leads (16 contact placed at L1–S1). All received significant benefits in motor function and pain control.[15,16] It has been long believed that SCS (Figs. 9.2, 9.3) may augment rehabilitative science in treating SCI; if the technology can be made smaller, requiring less support, it might have utility in an outpatient basis. It is paired with the exoskeleton for optimal function.

Rehabilitation exoskeletons have begun to serve a dual purpose since many can imagine the industrial use of a device that can augment strength up to 20× with battery power, preventing injuries before they ever occur. Enter the Guardian XO: a complex humanoid robot that is not setting out to replace humans but instead to amplify their strength as they perform physically demanding (and often repetitive) tasks.

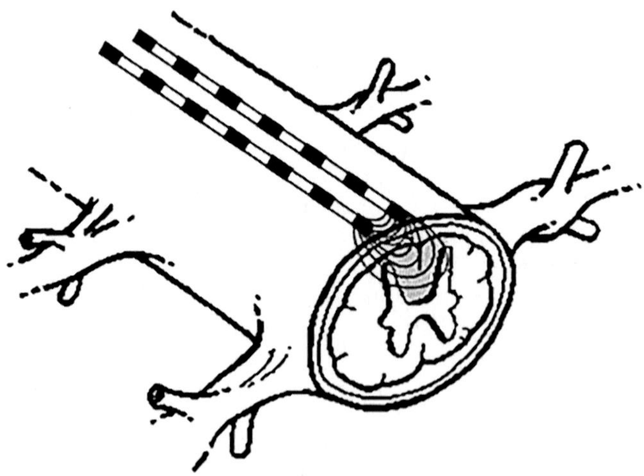

Fig. 9.2 Schematic of two scs leads driving energy to the dorsal columns. (From Dr. Robert Trainer.)

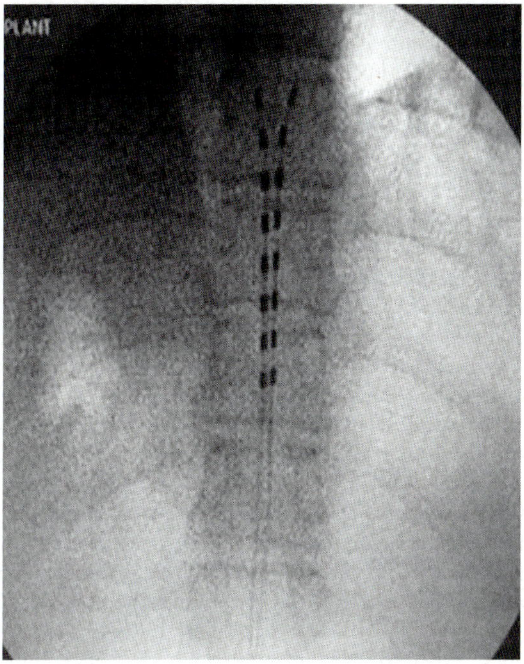

Fig. 9.3 Two eight-contact spinal cord stimulator leads placed in the thoracic spine. (From Dr. Robert Trainer.)

Government Funding Sources

We discussed earlier how the federal government can be a source of guaranteed income for companies with working products; it can also be an area where grant funding can help a newer or seasoned company in developing a product.

FedBizOpps (now SAM.gov) is a publicly available database of open projects—a search for "robot" yields 67 unique listings. Limiting it to health care does not change it drastically. The Veterans Affairs is the third largest budget at $269 billion, and there are 152 facilities nationwide with many having a community support facility. The national Institute of Health is a large drawer of contracts and grants for cutting-edge research. A few of the open contracts include Aethon's TUG pharmacy robot system repair contract, a robotic stereotactic system for neurosurgical application, the da Vinci surgical robot repair maintenance contract, robotic hand technology. There is also a call for using a robot system not just for well plating but to integrate entire laboratory systems in the National Institutes of Health.

The Department of Commerce's new budget provides $718 million for the National Institute of Standards and Technology to advance US innovation and technological development, as part of an all-of-government approach to ensure that the United States leads the world in the areas of AI, quantum information science, advanced manufacturing, and next-generation communications technologies such as 5G. The budget doubles National Institute of Standards and Technology's AI funding to accelerate the development and adoption of AI technologies and help ensure AI-enabled systems are interoperable.[17]

Future

Robot-assisted minimally invasive surgical techniques offer improved instrument precision and dexterity and reduced patient trauma and risk and promise to lessen the skill gap among surgeons.

These approaches are common in general surgery, urology, and gynecology. However, minimally invasive surgical techniques remain largely absent for surgical applications within narrow, confined workspaces, such as neuroendoscopy. The limitation stems from a lack of small yet dexterous robotic tools. In a newer technology using magnetically actuated forceps, the robot performance had an error rate of 11.2% compared with 14.9% without its use on a pineal gland tumor in a silicone phantom brain.[18]

A newer surgical technique, that of using robotic natural orifice transluminal endoscopic surgery (NOTES) as a scarless and gasless procedure has the potential to revolutionize minimally invasive surgery and allow alternate uses of robotics technology. Evangelisti et al. report[19] robotic NOTES hysterectomy is a feasible and safe. Other uses include transgastric, transcolonic, transanal approaches[20] for nephrectomy, appendectomy, among other uses.[21,22] This technology was essentially built on the endoscopy camera pill.[23] Video capsule endoscopy, an important innovation in diagnostic endoscopy, was approved in 2001 and is now widely available. In this system, the patient swallows a miniature high-resolution camera that is propelled by peristalsis through the gastrointestinal tract. It is particularly useful in examining the small intestine, which is difficult to visualize by conventional endoscopic techniques.[24] An update upon this would involve a "controllable" small device through a natural orifice or a surgically created entrance. Microbots have been increasingly more useful as some think the best way to deal with problems in the human body is to inject patients with tiny intelligent entities that can swim, crawl, and otherwise navigate through the body doing whatever is required of them. With that in mind, adaptable microrobots have been developed that are able to change shape to get around. The hope is that these origami-inspired shape-shifting robots could one day be used for performing surgery or delivering drugs wherever required. Microbots[25] have also been used for intracellular delivery of biomolecules[26] controlled by nanomagnets,[27] taking a note out of the playbook of the classic 1966 science-fiction movie *Fantastic Voyage*. Developments needed are still better imaging and control.[28]

When talking about innovators with high market caps, the names Google, Tesla, and Amazon come to mind for most people. Google just announced that it is spinning out its robotics division into a new company, called Intrinsic. For some background, Intrinsic was developed within Google's Alphabet X program, that is, its moonshot division. It incubates new businesses on the bleeding edge of technology. Intrinsic was developed for about 5.5 years within Alphabet X. It got a boost from Google's acquisition of Boston Dynamics back in 2013. As a reminder, Boston Dynamics developed the robot "dog" Spot.[29] But then, Google sold Boston Dynamics to SoftBank for a profit in 2017. The industry thought this was a sign that Google was getting out of the robotics business. Clearly that was not the case, as it seems that Google simply used Boston Dynamics to accelerate its own robotics technology. And now Intrinsic is ready to stand alone. It is not clear what Google's strategy is, but with the self-driving division Waymo, Google may be well placed to improve on some health-care adoptions we discussed earlier. Tesla is being secretive about their own Tesla Bot, a 5-foot, 8-inch 125 pound humanoid robot that runs on the same AI used by Tesla's fleet of autonomous vehicles. Its head will be kitted out with the autopilot cameras used by Tesla's vehicles to sense the environment and will contain a screen to display information. Internally, it will be operating via Tesla's Full Self-Driving computer. They may adapt it to fit the home health-care market, which is expected to grow at a compound annual growth rate of 12.5% by 2025 according to researchandmarkets.com.[30] When you consider that the number of people >65 years old will make up 16% of the world's population by 2050, it seems like a safe play. Amazon's answer is the "Astro" robot which although less functional overall has mentioned you might call your parent who owns an Astro, and it will go find them to deliver the call. In fact, if you're doing a video call, Astro will move with you around the house.

Maybe one of the more obvious uses for robots is the robot factory recently opened in Shanghai. ABB has two other such factories in the United States and Sweden. The company has an Market cap of $66.63 billion with expected Earnings before interest and taxes (EBIT) margins increase by 300-plus basis points over the medium term. They expect to benefit from a demand tailwind for grid-management and energy-saving products. At the moment they are heavily exposed to demand for robotic arms for heavier industrial applications, and putting more of their products online for remote monitoring could expose them to cyberattacks.

Concluding Thoughts

In this short section, we discussed some of the nuances of a multibillion-dollar industry that is expected to grow by $1.5 trillion per year for the next 6 years. As you can discern, the introduction of robots into the health-care sector mandates entire health-care systems be retrofit to meet the new capabilities (i.e., increased cybersecurity, cloud storage, maintenance, purchase of disposables, AI software for updates, and other implications). We also saw how robotics can work together for increased capabilities as in the example of SCS and exoskeleton training for spinal cord injury. Similarly, improvements in surgical approach through natural orifices (NOTES) led to better cameras and finally "controllable" cameras with robotic capabilities. Development of robotics for health care can have utilization opportunities for industrial, military, and home use as a few examples, and the reverse is certainly true. Lastly, implementation of robotics in health care requires a system-wide change in infrastructure, purchase of specific disposables, maintenance agreements, and AI capabilities to manage the large amounts of data, much of which can be managed by the robotic manufacturer themselves, thus guaranteeing ongoing income. In the 20 years since the first robotic surgical system has been adopted and 15 years after autonomous service robots have become commonplace, and considering the pace of advancement for robot implementation and infrastructure, AI, and cloud development built around the greater demand for the physical presence of human performance-enhancing and intelligent robots, the current numbers probably underestimate just how much of our individualized care will be performed by their increased presence.

References

1. Brakman S, Garretsen H, van Witteloostuijn A. Robots do not get the coronavirus: the COVID-19 pandemic and the international division of labor. *J Int Bus Stud.* 2021;52:1215–1224. https://doi.org/10.1057/s41267-021-00410-9.
2. Follmann A, Schollemann F, Arnolds A, et al. Reducing loneliness in stationary geriatric care with robots and virtual encounters-a contribution to the COVID-19 pandemic. *Int J Environ Res Public Health.* 2021;18(9):4846–4847.
3. Malik AA, Masood T, Kousar R. Reconfiguring and ramping-up ventilator production in the face of COVID-19: can robots help? *J Manuf Syst.* 2021;60:864–875.
4. R LB, Keri VC, Sinha TP, Bhoi S. Re-purposing humanoid robots for patient care in COVID-19 pandemic. *Int J Health Plann Manage.* 2020;35(6):1629–1631.
5. Feldman A. Robotics Firms Garnered $6.3 Billion in venture funding during the pandemic year. March; 12:2021. https://www.forbes.com/sites/amyfeldman/2021/03/12/robotics-firms-garnered-63-billion-in-venture-funding-during-the-pandemic-year/?sh=6b74f58a3c1a.
6. TechCrunch "Leading robotics VCs talk about where they're investing" November 26, 2019.
7. Svoboda E. Your robot surgeon will see you now. Nature. 2019;573:S110–S111.
8. Saeidi H, Opfermann JD, Kam M, Raghunathan S, Leonard S, Krieger A. A confidence-based shared control strategy for the Smart Tissue Autonomous Robot (STAR). *Rep U S.* 2018;2018:1268–1275.
9. Taha TA, Bejcek C. Robotic arm-assisted total hip arthroplasty to correct leg length discrepancy in a patient with spinopelvic obliquity. *Arthroplast Today.* 2020;6(4):784–791.
10. Grochola LF, Soll C, Zehnder A, Wyss R, Herzog P, Breitenstein S. Robot-assisted single-site compared with laparoscopic single-incision cholecystectomy for benign gallbladder disease: protocol for a randomized controlled trial. *BMC Surg.* 2017;17(1):13.

11. Van der Loos HM, Reinkensmeyer DJ, Guglielmelli E Rehabilitation and health care robotics. In: Siciliano B, Khatib O, eds. Springer Handbook of Robotics. Springer, Cham: Springer Handbooks; 2016. https://doi.org/10.1007/978-3-319-32552-1_64.
12. Bhagat NA, Yozbatiran N, Sullivan JL, et al. Neural activity modulations and motor recovery following brain-exoskeleton interface mediated stroke rehabilitation. *Neuroimage Clin*. 2020;28:102502.
13. Caliandro P, Molteni F, Simbolotti C, et al. Exoskeleton-assisted gait in chronic stroke: an EMG and functional near-infrared spectroscopy study of muscle activation patterns and prefrontal cortex activity. *Clin Neurophysiol*. 2020;131(8):1775–1781.
14. Louie DR, Mortenson WB, Durocher M, Teasell R, Yao J, Eng JJ. Exoskeleton for post-stroke recovery of ambulation (ExStRA): study protocol for a mixed-methods study investigating the efficacy and acceptance of an exoskeleton-based physical therapy program during stroke inpatient rehabilitation. *BMC Neurol*. 2020;20(1):35.
15. Edgerton VR, Harkema S. Epidural stimulation of the spinal cord in spinal cord injury: current status and future challenges. *Expert Rev Neurother*. 2011;11(10):1351–1353.
16. Angeli CA, Boakye M, Morton RA, et al. Recovery of over-ground walking after chronic motor complete spinal cord injury. *N Engl J Med*. 2018;379(13):1244–1250.
17. Office of Management and Budget. A budget for America's future. https://www.govinfo.gov/content/pkg/BUDGET-2021-BUD/pdf/BUDGET-2021-BUD.pdf
18. Lim A, Schonewille A, Forbrigger C, Looi T, Drake J, Diller E. Design and comparison of magnetically-actuated dexterous forceps instruments for neuroendoscopy. *IEEE Trans Biomed Eng*. 2021;68(3):846–856.
19. Evangelisti G, Barra F, Centurioni MG, D'Alessandro G, Alessandri F, Ferrero S. Vaginal natural orifice transluminal endoscopic surgery (NOTES) for treating benign adnexal diseases: past results and future developments. *J Invest Surg*. 2020;35(2):1–3.
20. Chen T, Xu A, Lian J, Chu Y, Zhang H, Xu M. Transcolonic endoscopic appendectomy: a novel natural orifice transluminal endoscopic surgery (NOTES) technique for the sessile serrated lesions involving the appendiceal orifice. *Gut*. 2021;70(10):1812–1814.
21. Wang S, Guan F, Wang F, Wen P. Transgastric natural orifice transluminal endoscopic surgery (NOTES) to remove a foreign body from the abdominal cavity of a 12-year old boy. *Endoscopy*. 2021.
22. Arezzo A, Zornig C, Mofid H, et al. The EURO-NOTES clinical registry for natural orifice transluminal endoscopic surgery: a 2-year activity report. *Surg Endosc*. 2013;27(9):3073–3084.
23. Kovac C. "Video pill" may supplement standard endoscopy. *BMJ*. 2001;323(7309):358.
24. Panescu D. Emerging technologies. An imaging pill for gastrointestinal endoscopy. *IEEE Eng Med Biol Mag*. 2005;24(4):12–14.
25. Vilela D, Stanton MM, Parmar J, Sanchez S. Microbots decorated with silver nanoparticles kill bacteria in aqueous media. *ACS Appl Mater Interfaces*. 2017;9(27):22093–22100.
26. Latiyan S, Suneet K, Jain S. Magneto-conducting multifunctional Janus microbots for intracellular delivery of biomolecules. *J Tissue Eng Regen Med*. 2021;15(7):625–633.
27. Zhao X, Kim Y. Soft microbots programmed by nanomagnets. *Nature*. 2019;575(7781):58–59.
28. Medina-Sanchez M, Schmidt OG. Medical microbots need better imaging and control. *Nature*. 2017;545(7655):406–408.
29. Brown J. Amazon is designing new chips for data centers. Brownstone Research. Published April 12, 2021. Accessed September 27, 2022. https://www.brownstoneresearch.com/bleeding-edge/amazon-is-designing-new-chips-for-data-centers/
30. Home Healthcare Market - Growth, Trends, COVID-19 Impact, and Forecasts (2022 - 2027) (researchandmarkets.com) January, 2022, ID: 5529469. https://www.researchandmarkets.com/reports/5529469/home-healthcare-market-growth-trends-covid#product--toc

10

Brain-Controlled Assistive Robotics and Prosthetics

Kavya Pramod Puthuveetil ■ Dean J. Krusienski

KEY POINTS

- Brain-computer interfaces use electrical activity recorded from electrodes on the scalp or surgically implanted in the brain.
- Brain-computer interfaces for rehabilitation and assistive devices strive to replace, supplement, or restore lost function.
- Significant challenges remain for brain-computer interfaces to achieve their full potential and practicality.

This chapter provides an overview of prior and prospective work related to the control of assistive robotics and prostheses via direct measurements of brain activity. Specifically, this chapter focuses on brain-controlled robotic devices that *replace*, *supplement*, or *restore* lost motor function.[1] The chapter does not include brain-controlled robotic devices that have been developed for rehabilitation or therapeutic applications, which are included in Chapter 6. The present chapter introduces noninvasive and invasive brain signal–recording modalities, common brain-actuated control signals, and a survey of applications in assistive robotics and prosthetics. The chapter concludes with a discussion of current challenges and future prospects of these technologies.

Brain-Computer/Brain-Machine Interfaces

A brain-computer interface (BCI) is a system that directly translates neuronal signals into actionable inputs for an external device, as shown in Fig. 10.1. The term "brain-computer interface" is generally synonymous with brain-machine interface, with the terms emerging from the noninvasive and invasive research communities, respectively. This general field of research originated as a means to help severely disabled individuals (e.g., suffering from late-stage amyotrophic lateral sclerosis [ALS] or brain stem stroke) communicate and perform tasks of daily living.[2] Although the field has since evolved to include other nonmedical applications, there is still significant focus on medical applications of BCI.

Because the original impetus for BCIs was to restore, replace, or supplement lost function, much of the early work was focused on controlling motor prostheses, orthotics, and assistive devices.[3] Ideally, the ultimate objective is to completely restore natural motor function that has been lost by the user. However, approaching such naturalistic and transparent control in practice requires precise measurement of large-scale neural activity that can currently only be achieved via invasive measurements of brain activity (e.g., surgical implantation of high-density electrodes into the brain).

Due to the inherent risks of surgical implants, much of the research has been conducted in animal models (primarily nonhuman primates[4–7]) and, in special cases, on humans undergoing

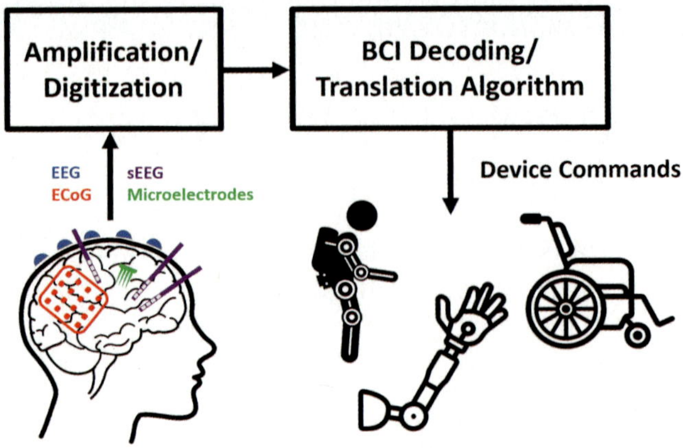

Fig. 10.1 Block diagram of a brain-computer interface (BCI). ECoG, Electrocorticography; EEG, electroencephalogram; sEEG, stereotactic electroencephalography.

surgical procedures for intractable epilepsy and glioma removal.[8,9] Additionally, there have been a limited number of long-term human implants exclusively for BCI research.[10–14] In contrast, current modalities for noninvasive measurement of brain activity cannot provide sufficient fidelity to achieve natural, refined control of a motor prosthetic. Nevertheless, the ability to control assistive devices with as few as 2 to 3 degrees of freedom (DoFs) (e.g., wrist rotation and hand grasp) has the potential to greatly improve the user's performance on activities of daily living.[15]

Broadly, there are two classes of brain activity measurements that are relevant for such applications: (1) electrophysiologic and (2) hemodynamic. Hemodynamic activity can be measured with functional magnetic resonance imaging, positron emission tomography, and functional near-infrared imaging. Because of the comparatively slow hemodynamic response on the order of 1 to 2 seconds and the impractical size and cost of the devices for independent daily use (in the case of functional magnetic resonance imaging and positron emission tomography), these modalities are generally not well suited for real-time robotic control applications.

Conversely, electrophysiologic measurements of brain activity provide response times on the order of milliseconds and can be designed to be portable or fully implantable, making them suitable for real-time control and independent daily use. The established modalities for invasively and noninvasively acquiring electrical brain activity for BCI applications are described next.

INVASIVE RECORDINGS

There are three general categories of implanted electrodes, characterized by the method of implantation, depth of penetration, and size of the recording contacts. The most commonly used types of implanted electrodes are shown in Fig. 10.2A–C.

Microelectrodes

Microelectrodes are penetrating electrodes designed to record from individual neurons, commonly referred to as *single units*. Most modern microelectrodes are configured as arrays of needlelike probes with electrodes along the shafts of each probe.[16] The electrodes generally have surface areas and spacings on the order of 1 to 10 μm and are fabricated using silicon substrates. Individual microelectrode arrays are typically designed for sampling tens of hundreds,[17,18] and potentially thousands,[19,20] of neurons simultaneously.

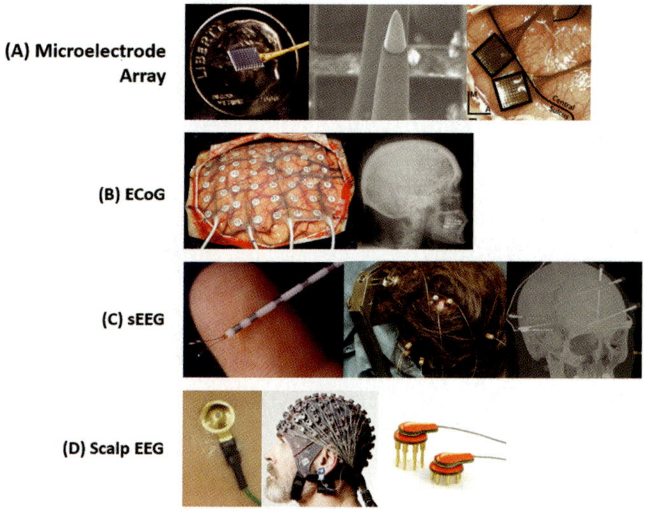

Fig. 10.2 Types of invasive/noninvasive electrodes. (A) Microelectrode array; individual electrode tip; implanted electrode. (B) Electrocorticography (ECoG) grid during craniotomy; postoperative computed tomography. (C) Stereotactic electroencephalography (sEEG) electrode with microwires at tip; view of scalp after implantation; postoperative computed tomography. (D) Wet electroencephalogram (EEG) electrode; EEG electrode cap; dry EEG electrode.

Ideally, each microelectrode contact will measure action potentials from a single neuron. In practice, only a subset of contacts will yield clean recordings of action potentials from individual neurons. Otherwise, contacts can also measure local field potentials, representing a superposition of electrical activity from surrounding neurons.

The acquisition of action potentials from a population of neurons in the motor cortex can precisely determine movement intentions based on a phenomenon known as *population coding*.[21] Put simply, individual neurons in the motor cortex have been shown to have firing rates that follow a cosine tuning curve, in which the firing rate of each neuron maximally corresponds to a preferred direction of movement and minimally corresponds to movements in the opposite direction (i.e., 180 degrees), with intermediate directions following a cosine curve (as shown in Fig. 10.3A–B). By sampling a sufficient number of neurons in the motor cortex, shown to be as few as 10 to 100,[22] continuous motor movements can be accurately reconstructed by taking the vector sum of the predicted movement directions for each neuron in the population as prescribed by the predetermined tuning curves (Fig. 10.3C). Because the resulting control signal represents a fairly direct mapping of the measured neuronal function, this approach yields naturalistic control of motor prostheses.[10]

Electrocorticography and Stereotactic Electroencephalography

Electrocorticography (ECoG) uses comparatively larger disk electrodes in rectangular arrays or strips placed on the cortical surface via a craniotomy.[9] The standard clinical electrodes are 5 mm in diameter with 1 cm spacing between contacts, although micro-ECoG arrays also have been used with diameters and spacings on the order of tens of microns.[23] Although ECoG does not penetrate the brain or record single unit activity, it can provide detailed information for decoding sensory, motor, and cognitive processes for a BCI. ECoG recording provide signals that are morphologically similar to local field potentials with spectral bandwidth of roughly 0 to 250 Hz. ECoG is used clinically for localizing and mapping as part of surgical planning for intractable epilepsy and intraoperatively for glioma removal. To minimize the extent of the required

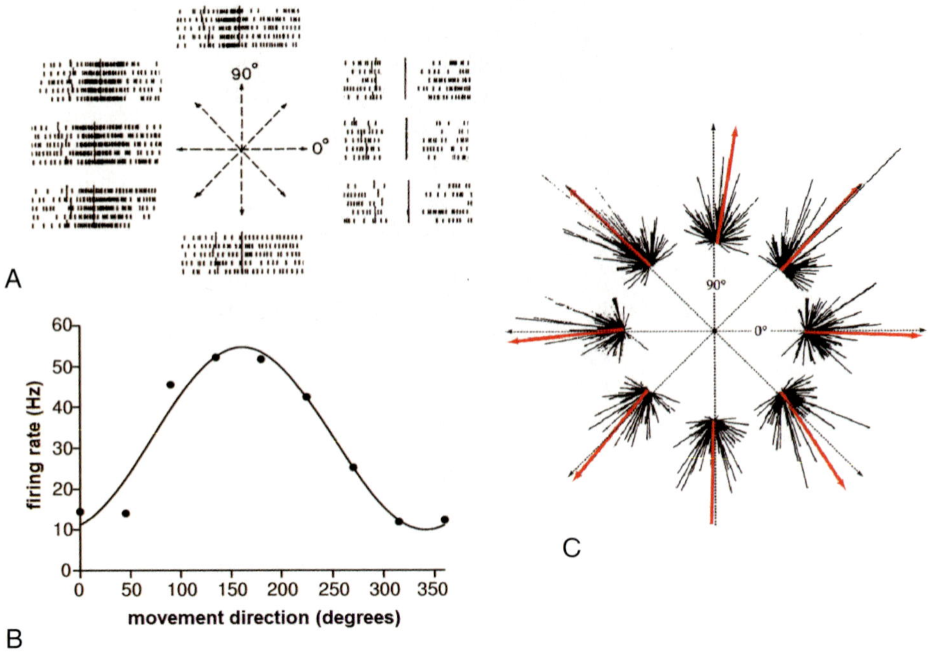

Fig. 10.3 Population coding of cortical motor neurons. (A) Hand reaching directions and associated spike raster plots from a single neuron. (B) Corresponding cosine tuning curve for the neuron. (C) Predicted direction vectors (red) based on the individual tuning curves of a population of neurons. (Modified from Georgopoulos AP, Schwartz A, Kettner R. Neuronal population coding of movement direction. *Science*. 1986;233(4771):1416–1419.[21])

craniotomy, ECoG grid placement is typically localized to particular cortical areas associated with the patient's pathology, typically on a single hemisphere. For clinical purposes, the number of implanted ECoG electrodes typically ranges from 16 to 128, depending on the nature and location of the pathology.

A related technology employed for epileptic seizure localization is stereotactic electroencephalography (sEEG).[8] sEEG electrodes are positioned along a cylindrical shaft (~1 mm in diameter), which is inserted deeper into the brain through small burr holes in the skull using stereotactic guidance. The surface area, number of electrodes implanted, and nature of the measured signals of sEEG for clinical purposes are roughly comparable to ECoG, although higher-density contacts and microwires can be used. Although, in contrast to ECoG, sEEG electrodes penetrate brain tissue, there is evidence that the procedures are as effective as ECoG and have improved surgical recovery outcomes compared with the craniotomy required for ECoG. Also, unlike the single, localized craniotomy for ECoG, the comparatively minute burr holes for sEEG electrodes allows for a broader but sparse sampling of both superficial and deeper brain structures. This creates a trade-off for investigating and utilizing specific brain regions and networks compared with the generally superior local cortical resolution provided by ECoG.

Although the traditional lower-frequency rhythms can be observed in intracranial recordings, one unique and commonly used feature of ECoG/sEEG signals for BCI control is broadband gamma activity.[24] This activity manifests as roughly uniform fluctuations in the signal spectrum over the approximate range of 70 to 250 Hz, which resembles a broadband noise process and is not practically observable in scalp EEG, as illustrated in Fig. 10.4.[25] This activity has been shown to be

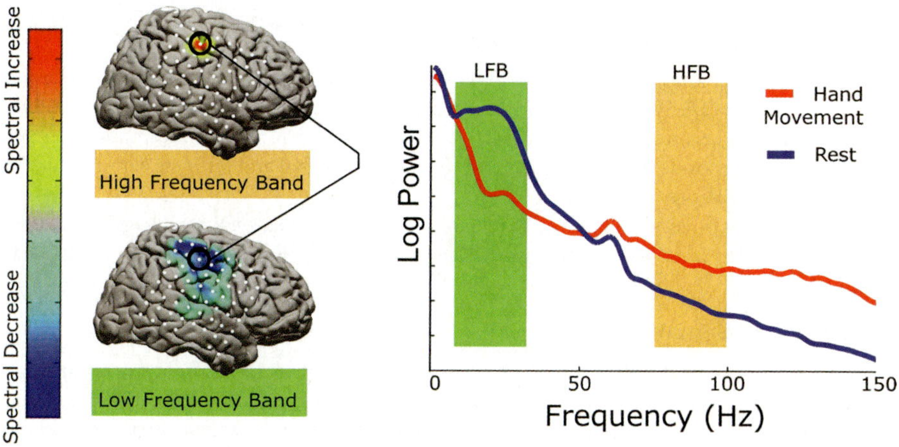

Fig. 10.4 Electroencephalogram power spectral bands for hand movement versus rest.[25] LFB, Low frequency band; HFB, high frequency band. (Modified from Miller KJ, Sorensen LB, Ojemann JG, Nijs M. Power-law scaling in the brain surface electric potential. *PLoS Comput Biol*. 2009;5.[25])

highly correlated with a wide variety of cognitive and behavioral function. It is important to note that although high-frequency oscillations exist, broadband gamma is generally not considered a brain oscillation akin to lower-frequency gamma (~40–70 Hz) or the traditional lower-frequency EEG bands below 40 Hz (i.e., delta, theta, alpha, beta).[26]

Other Implanted Electrodes

One of the earliest demonstrations of invasive BCI control in humans was using neurotrophic electrodes.[13] Neurotrophic electrodes consist of a 1- to 2-mm hollow glass cone attached to several gold conductive wires. The electrode is filled with trophic factors to encourage the growth of axons and dendrites into the cone.[27] Unique features of neurotrophic electrodes are their ability to isolate and record from single or small groups of neurons and their biocompatibility for long-term implantation.[28] However, compared with modern microelectrode arrays, neurotrophic electrodes have not been designed to conveniently sample larger numbers of neurons and have therefore not been widely adopted for BCI research.

More recently, an endovascular thin-film stent-electrode array was implanted in the superior sagittal sinus adjacent to the primary motor cortex of two participants with ALS.[29] This sensor array, known as a *stentrode*, consists of 17 circumferential sensors on an 8 mm × 40 mm monolithic, self-expanding nitinol scaffold designed for minimally invasive intracranial delivery using catheter venography. The array is connected to a 50-cm flexible transvascular lead and inserted into an inductively powered wireless telemetry unit. For this feasibility study, the participants were able to successfully perform a typing task using attempted movements in combination with an eye tracker for cursor navigation.[29]

NONINVASIVE RECORDINGS

The primary modality for noninvasive electrophysiologic recordings of the brain is the scalp electroencephalogram (EEG). EEG is acquired via metallic electrodes placed directly on the scalp. EEG electrode diameters are generally on the order of centimeters, and the number of electrodes used can be anywhere from 2, giving a single bipolar channel, to 256 or even more for detecting subcortical activity and source localization.[30] To provide conductivity through hair, the electrodes are either filled with electrolytic gel (i.e., wet electrodes) or have barbs designed to pass through hair (i.e., dry electrodes), as shown in Fig. 10.2D.

Due to the signal attenuation caused by the skull and scalp layers, noninvasive recordings are lower in amplitude (10–100 μV) and are more prone to movement and muscle artifacts compared with invasive recordings. The use of active electrodes, which contain preamplifier circuitry embedded in the electrode housing, can effectively boost the signal and mitigate certain noise and artifacts in the recordings.

EEG signals for direct BCI control can broadly be categorized as *active* or *reactive*,[31] depending on whether the brain activity is primarily modulated by endogenous or exogenous means, respectively.

Active Control Signals

The most commonly used active control signals for robotic control applications are event-related desynchronization/synchronization (ERD/ERS)[32] and sensorimotor rhythms (SMRs).[33] These are more naturalistic control signals since they are generated from the motor cortex during actual and imagined movements.

SMRs are idling rhythms occurring in the alpha band of the motor cortex during rest, which can be observed in an estimated 80% of the population.[33] To distinguish from unrelated alpha-band activity, these are often referred to as mu rhythms.[34] A defining characteristic of these rhythms is that the amplitude is attenuated over the corresponding area of the motor cortex during continued actual or imagined movements.[35] Related modulations can also be observed in the beta and gamma bands, although it is not clear whether these are contributed by distinct neural processes or are simply, in part, a by-product of the unique temporal morphology of mu rhythms.[36] Users can learn to modulate SMR amplitudes continuously to achieve continuous, dimensional BCI control (e.g., imagine right-hand movement to move a cursor to the right).[37] The temporal, spatial, and spectral characteristics and how they can be mapped to dimensional BCI control are illustrated in Fig. 10.5A.

ERD refers to the transient decrease in alpha-band power over the motor cortex associated with the onset of isolated movement or imagery, followed by the transient ERS increase as the motor activity returns to the resting state, as shown in Fig. 10.5B. Thus, this transient activity can be used as a discrete switch, for instance to activate/deactivate a hand grasp orthotic.[38]

Other active control signals exist, such as alpha-band modulation during cognitive processes such as mental math or object rotation.[39,40] However, although these modulations can be reliably detected in the EEG, they require the user to perform a mental task that is not directly related to the primary robotic control task. This can be unnatural, unintuitive, and distracting and is ultimately not an ideal control signal for a practical assistive device.

Although ERD/ERS and SMR represent the most natural and intuitive scalp EEG activity for dimensional control of robotic or assistive devices, these signals tend to be nonstationary, and significant task training may be required for users to reliably modulate these signals to achieve practical device control.[41]

Reactive Control Signals

Reactive control signals result from predictable changes in brain activity generated from the user's attention to specific sensory stimuli that are mapped to aspects of the control task.[42] These predictable changes in brain activity are known as stimulus evoked potentials (SEPs). SEPs can either be transient, which are generally time-locked with the sensory stimulus and resolve on the order of a second, or steady state, which continue as long as attention to the stimulus is maintained.

One of the earliest scalp EEG BCIs is the P300 speller.[43] It operates based on the brain's response to a rare or novel sensory stimulus. This brain response is known as an event-related potential (ERP), which is a specific type of SEP that includes a cognitive component (opposed to

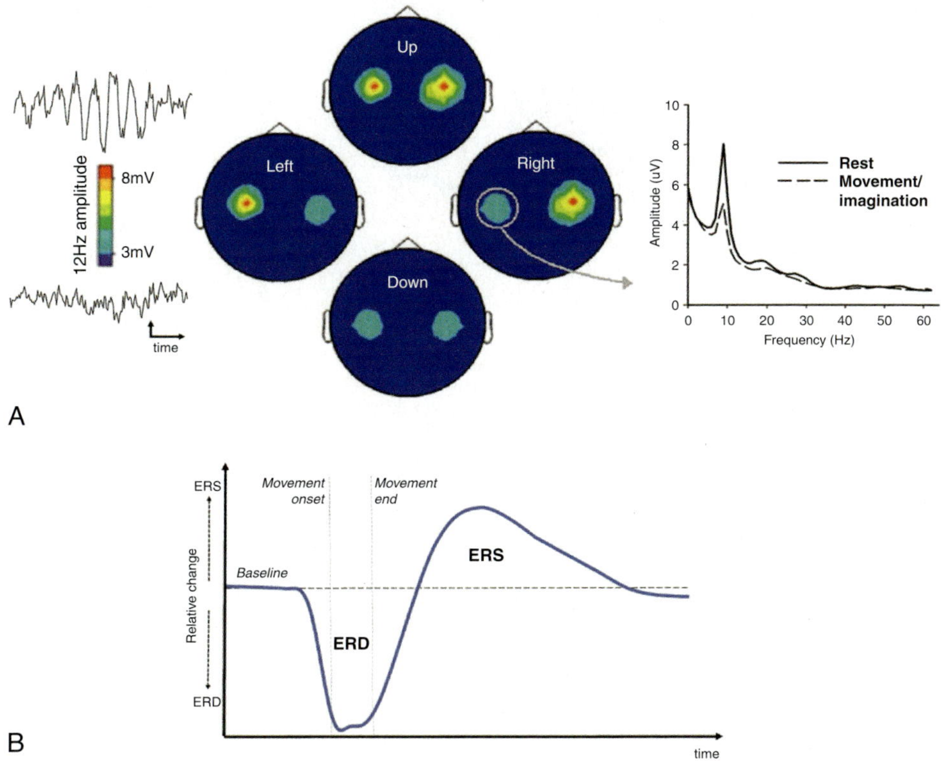

Fig. 10.5 Active control signals. (A) Topographical and spectral representations of sensorimotor rhythms for dimensional control using left- and right-hand movement/imagery. (B) ERS/ERD of the alpha band corresponding to an isolated movement/imagery. ERD, Event-related desynchronization; ERS, event-related synchronization.

a purely sensory reflex). In this case, the cognitive component is the recognition that the stimulus is rare or novel.

In a simple P300 speller paradigm, the user is presented with a matrix of flashing symbols on a computer monitor, for instance, similar to a visual keyboard. The user attends to the desired symbol as each symbol is flashed in a random sequence. The general concept is illustrated in Fig. 10.6. Because the user does not know when the desired symbol will be flashed, an ERP is generated when the symbol is flashed while the user maintains fixed attention. Multiple ERPs must be accumulated over multiple stimulus sequences to reliably represent the characteristic brain response and determine the desired symbol. This process can be made more efficient via row/column flashing[43] or a variety of other enhancements to the original paradigm.[44,45] Although the original P300 speller paradigm was based on visual attention, auditory[46] or tactile[47] attention can also be utilized with decreased performance compared with visual paradigms.

Effectively, such paradigms provide discrete command selection, equivalent to a computer keyboard—albeit at a much slower rate (~4–5 symbols per minute).[45] These commands can be mapped to achieve discrete dimensional[48] or goal-oriented[49] control of a robot, for example.

To achieve continuous dimensional control, steady-state sensory evoked potentials can be used, the most practical being the steady-state visual evoked potential (SSVEP).[50] Unlike transient evoked potentials resulting from a single stimulus event, the steady-state evoked potentials result from a repeating stimulus pattern, such as a blinking light. As such, rather than generating a

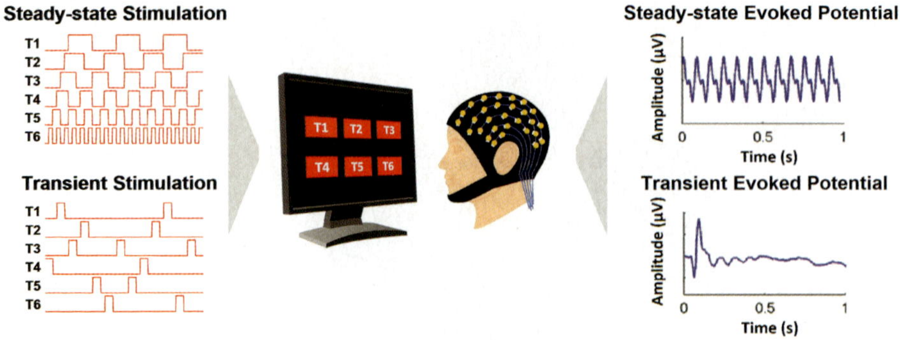

Fig. 10.6 Reactive control signals for a visual paradigm. Six targets presented on a computer monitor flash independently according to (1) a steady-state pattern with a unique stimulus frequency for each target or (2) transient pulses with a unique stimulus onsets for each target. The user focuses visual attention on a single target and (1) the electroencephalogram (EEG) over the occipital cortex oscillates at the target stimulus frequency (plus harmonics) for the steady-state stimulus scenario or (2) an EEG-evoked potential can be detected over the visual cortex (and potentially other areas) with respect to the stimulus onset for the transient stimulus scenario.

transient EEG response, predictable, continuous repeating EEG patterns over the occipital cortex are generated with attention to the repeating stimulus patterns. These EEG patterns manifest as distinct spectral peaks in the frequency domain that can be reliably identified and tracked, in contrast to the time-domain techniques used to identify transient evoked potentials.

A typical SSVEP interface consists of a spatial array of individual lights or symbols on a screen, each concurrently repeating with a unique temporal flashing pattern and mapped to a control command, as shown in Fig. 10.6. When the user focuses attention to a specific light/symbol, the brain activity unique to that symbol is detected and the associated command is executed. In contrast to transient evoked potentials, the command can be maintained with continued attention to the stimulus and can be readily changed by shifting attention to a different stimulus to execute the associated control command in a continuous fashion. This can enable joystick-like dimensional control of a robotic device with latency on the order of 0.5 to 1 seconds.[51] It is also possible to achieve high communication rates with discrete selection via keyboard-like interfaces using SSVEP and related variants.[52,53] As with transient responses, BCIs that utilize steady-state auditory[54] and tactile (somatosensory)[55] potentials, have also been developed.

Control paradigms that rely on visual evoked potentials have several limitations. Foremost, performance can drastically decrease with inability to control eye movements,[56,57] which is the case for many patients with locked-in syndrome. Also, these interfaces often create a visual cacophony, can be unnatural and fatiguing, and can be distracting from the primary control task,[58] which can make them inconvenient and impractical for long-term use.

Applications to Assistive Robotics and Prosthetics

UPPER-LIMB PROSTHETICS

Foundational work exploring the application of BCI for control of robotic arms was first performed in animal models. In 1999, Chapin et al. showed how rats could position a single-DoF robotic arm in real time using a BCI driven by neuronal population activity in the primary motor cortex and ventrolateral thalamus.[5] Just a year later, Wessberg et al. demonstrated an open-loop BCI for real-time control of 3-DoF robotic arms, which better represent the complex arm movements needed to accomplish a reach-and-grasp task.[7] In their approach, cortical neural ensemble activity, recorded from owl monkeys who received no feedback while completing the reach-and-grasp tasks, was used to predict 3D hand trajectories that controlled robotic movement. Further work succeeded in closing the loop for continuous neuronal control of robotic prostheses by nonhuman primates by introducing visual feedback, which resulted in stabilization of performance and more effective learning of neuromodulation.[4,6]

Velliste et al. demonstrated embodied control, involving real-time interaction with the physical environment, of a 4-DoF prosthetic arm using cortical signals in a closed-loop system.[59] Modulation of cortical signals represented not only the velocity of the end effector in Cartesian space, but also the aperture velocity of the gripper's fingers. This BCI enabled monkeys to continuously control the prosthetic device to reach to a food target, grasp the food, and then feed themselves. Physical interaction with the environment using the robotic arm enabled displays of embodiment unseen in previous virtual cursor control experiements via behaviors inessential to task completion. For example, the monkey treated the prosthetic arm as if it was its own by moving the gripper to its mouth to lick it instead of only reaching to grasp the food target.

Initial results for BCI control of prosthetic devices by humans was demonstrated by Hochberg et al. in their report describing the first participant in a trial for BrainGate, a neuromotor prosthetic system consisting of a single cortically implanted, 96-channel sensor and external signal processors.[22] In this work, a patient with tetraplegia was enabled to grasp and move objects using a robotic arm controlled via neuronal ensemble spiking activity.

A follow-up clinical trial of the BrainGate system, dubbed BrainGate2, showed how participants from the original BrainGate trial were able to use continuous neuronal ensemble control to operate a robotic arm for 3D reach-and-grasp movements.[60] Using the BCI system, one participant with tetraplegia was able to manipulate and drink from a bottle without assistance for the first time in 14 years. The results from this work were achieved in participants whose intracortical arrays were implanted more than 5 years prior, which is promising evidence that the development of neural interfaces using chronically implanted intracortical sensors may be feasible.

Independent of the BrainGate trials, Collinger et al. demonstrated how a human with tetraplegia could control a 7-DoF prosthetic arm using an intracortical activity recorded from two 96-channel arrays implanted in the motor cortex.[10] Continuous control was achieved by relating neural firing rates and movement velocity in each control dimension (3D translation, 3D orientation, 1D grasp) using a linear model, as previously demonstrated in nonhuman primate studies.[59] The participant was able to achieve clinically significant improvements of function, as well as complex, coordinated movements, on par with that of able-bodied people, sustained over several weeks of testing. Fig. 10.7 shows the participant feeding herself using the robotic arm.

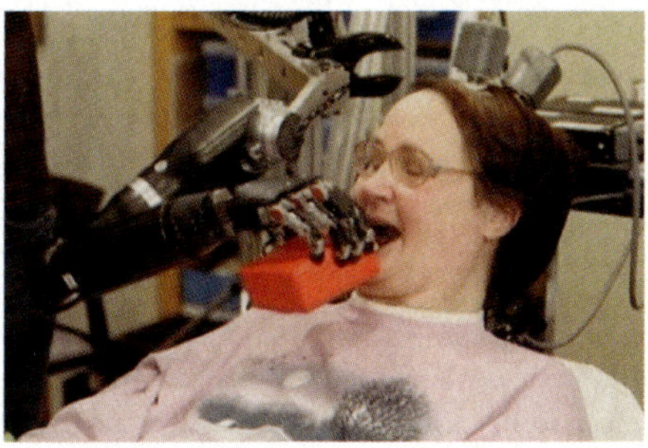

Fig. 10.7 Real-time brain-machine interface prosthetic arm control using microelectrode arrays implanted in the motor cortex. University of Pittsburgh. (Reprinted with permission from Elsevier (The Lancet, Volume 381, Issue 9866, 16–22 February 2013, Pages 557-564).)

In follow-up work with the same patient, Wodlinger et al. expanded the one-dimensional grasp, which simply allowed binary open/close, to now include four dimensions to control hand shape, which introduced a new emphasis on object-interaction behavior.[61] The study demonstrated that object interaction when calibrating neural activity to intended control behaviors was important to achieve 10-dimensional operation of a prosthetic arm using the previously demonstrated linear model for neural decoding.[10]

More recent work has considered the role of bidirectional BCIs, which integrate both sensory and motor modalities for robust restoration of function,[62] for the control of robotic arms.[11,63,64] Flesher et al. builds on previous demonstrations of high-dimensional continuous control of robotic arms using cortical activity and visual feedback alone[10,61] by introducing tactile feedback.[11] Tactile percepts were evoked by intracortical microstimulation of the somatosensory cortex based on contact-and-grasp forces measured via sensors in the robotic arm, resulting in perceived tactile sensations at the palm and fingers. A participant with tetraplegia achieved higher performance when performing grasp-and-reach tasks, namely through reduction of grasp attempt time, with the systems with tactile sensation than with BCI systems with only visual feedback.

ORTHOTICS AND EXOSKELETONS

The application of BCI for the control of orthotics and exoskeletons has also been explored, often in the context of rehabilitation.[65] We restrict the scope of this chapter to focus only on the control of orthotics or exoskeletons using BCIs, not on the use and assessment of these systems for neurologic rehabilitation.

One of the earliest demonstrations of BCI control of orthoses was by Pfurtscheller et al.[66] Using an EEG-based BCI, a patient with tetraplegia was able to operate a hand orthosis. The participant was trained to modulate mu oscillations via a motor imagery approach, allowing users to close or open the orthosis by imagining movement of their feet or hands, respectively. More recently, P300-based BCI systems for hand-orthosis control have also been demonstrated.[67,68] Delijorge et al.[69] introduced a P300-based BCI to allow patients with ALS to control a robotic hand orthosis. Compared with previous work that only allows binary opening/closing of the hand,[66,67] this system enabled patients to control the movement of individual fingers.

EEG-based BCIs have also been demonstrated to control lower-limb exoskeletons. Kwak et al.[70,71] presented an asynchronous SSVEP-based BCI system that controlled a leg exoskeleton to provide healthy participants with support while walking forward, turning, sitting, and standing. The oscillatory nature of SSVEPs makes them a reasonable candidate to decode user intention for exoskeleton control despite the poor signal-to-noise ratio in the EEG signal, caused by the introduction of additional artifacts while walking or broadband distortion by the exoskeleton. SSVEP-based control of lower-limb prostheses has been replicated by Wang et al.[72] In the same study, motor imagery-based control was also demonstrated and high-accuracy performance was achieved by both approaches. In an approach that can be directly applied to knee orthoses, Murphy et al. presented ERD-based control to lock and unlock a prosthetic knee for the swing phase of gait or for sitting.[73]

In an initial clinical proof-of-concept, Benabid et al.[74] showed how an individual with tetraplegia could control a four-limb, 14-DoF exoskeleton using an ECoG-based BCI. This exoskeleton is depicted in Fig. 10.8. ECoG signals were recorded from the upper-limb sensorimotor areas of the brain using two epidural recorders implanted bilaterally. The number of DOFs the patient was able to control increased gradually with training over a period of 20 months, culminating in the ability to perform multilimb action to complete eight-dimensional, bimanual tasks. Over the total 24-month study, recalibration of the BCI was only required after considerably long intervals of time—more than 1.5 months. The results of this study suggest that ECoG may be a promising modality to enable higher-dimensional control of exoskeletons by individuals with tetraplegia.

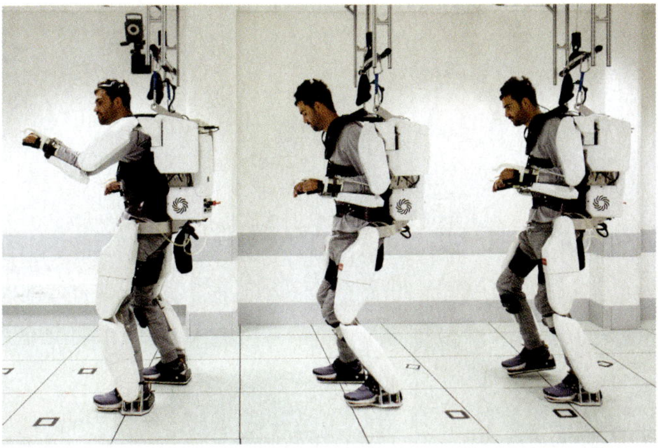

Fig. 10.8 BCI-controlled exoskeleton. Quadriplegic individual moves with the assistance of robotic arms and legs controlled by decoding motor cortex activity in real time. The brain signals are recorded with two 64-electrode electrocorticography implants.[74] (Reprinted with permission from Elsevier (The Lancet Neurology, 2019, Volume 18, Issue 12, Pages 1112-1122).)

WHEELCHAIRS, TELEPRESENCE, AND ASSISTIVE ROBOTS

BCI-controlled wheelchairs have the potential to improve the mobility of individuals with disabilities or movement disorders. Previously demonstrated BCI wheelchairs have largely been noninvasive, including P300-based,[75,76] motor imagery–based,[77,78] or ERD/ERS[79]-based paradigms. In the motor imagery approach developed by Carlson and Millán,[77] the user was able to provide turning commands via the BCI system to a forward moving a wheelchair equipped with automatic obstacle avoidance.

Waytowich and Krusienski[51] introduced an SSVEP-based BCI, utilizing signals recorded from five-channel dry-electrode EEG, for continuous control of a motorized wheelchair. Stimuli were superimposed over a live video feed of the environment, presented on an Android phone mounted in front of the user's face, and were placed on the peripheral edges of the screen, as shown in Fig. 10.9A. This approach allows users to observe both the control stimuli and the environment in front of them with latencies on the order of 0.5 to 1 second.

Although control of prosthetic or assistive robots generally focuses on allowing users to interact with their local environment, telepresence BCI systems can enable users to interact with their global environment through a remotely controlled robotic device. Noninvasive telepresence BCI systems have been demonstrated to control a variety of devices including quadcopters,[81] wheelchairs[51] (Fig. 10.9B), robotic arms,[7] humanoid robots,[82] and mobile robots,[83–85] among others. Millán et al.[85] showed how a mobile robot could be controlled using an asynchronous EEG-based BCI system to move between rooms of a simulated house. To achieve precise control despite the low bit rate of the EEG-based BCI, the user's brain activity was associated with high-level commands executed autonomously by the robot based on a behavior-based controller. BCI control of the mobile robot achieved similar task performance to manual control.

In this section, we distinguish BCI control of robotic arms as upper-arm prosthetics from their usage as assistive robots. As previously described, the former aims to achieve high-dimensional, continuous control that mimics natural function, typically using invasive BCI systems that decode cortical activity to control joint velocities. On the other hand, the latter consists of noninvasive BCI systems for goal-oriented or partially automated control.[49,80,86] For example, Johnson et al. achieved high-level control of a 6-DoF robotic arm using an adapted P300 speller interface,[49] as shown in

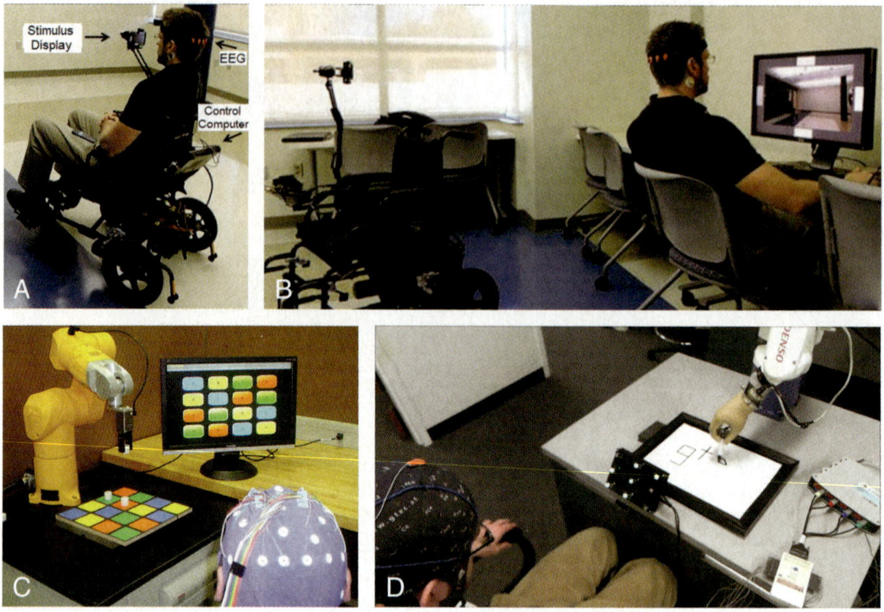

Fig. 10.9 Electroencephalogram (EEG)-based robotics control. (A) Continuous, real-time control of a motorized wheelchair via a steady-state visual evoked potential (SSVEP) paradigm displayed on a handheld device including pass-through camera view.[51] (B) Continuous, real-time control of a telepresence robot (remotely operated wheelchair with streaming camera view) via a remote SSVEP paradigm.[51] (C) Goal-oriented control of a pick-and-place robotic arm via a P300 paradigm.[49] (D) Continuous, real-time control of a robotic arm for writing via an SSVEP paradigm.[80]

Fig. 10.9C. This goal-oriented approach leverages the discrete selection capabilities of P300 spellers, allowing users to select a target for the robot's end effector to move toward in its workspace, represented as a 4 × 4 grid. Similar to Waytowich and Krusienski,[51] an SSVEP approach was applied for continuous control of a robotic arm for a real-time writing application[80] (Fig. 10.9D).

Some research has considered how near-continuous high-dimensional control of robotic arms can be achieved using noninvasive BCI systems. Meng et al. demonstrated a noninvasive ERD/ERS-based approach to control a robotic arm to complete 3D reach-and-grasp tasks.[87] High-accuracy, continuous control of a device in 3D space requires the user to have three independent pairs of motor strategies, which has not been robustly demonstrated using noninvasive EEG-based BCI alone, although some previous work used 3D gaze tracking in combination with SMR-based BCI to achieve such control.[88] This study achieved manipulation outcomes equivalent to fluid, 3D control by executing two low-dimensional control commands sequentially. In this approach, the user first continuously controls the end effector within a 2D plane to hover above some target object. Then, the 2D end-effector position is held constant by the system while the user controls the end effector in the third dimension to complete the grasp. This two-step approach, although more time-consuming than 3D fluid control, is able to achieve 3D reach-and-grasp tasks while reducing the number of DoFs the noninvasive BCI needs to simultaneously interpret.

Artificial Intelligence and Shared Control

Artificial intelligence employs sensors and processing algorithms to make decisions in response to environmental variables, often being implemented to adapt and learn new behaviors. Due to a variety of factors, such as limitations of brain activity–sensing technologies, the current state of

BCI control generally does not allow for perfectly precise and reliable execution of device commands. In particular, as the primary input for direct device control, current scalp-based EEG BCIs are generally slower and less reliable than using any residual volitional muscle movement as a simple binary control switch, for instance, especially for safety-critical applications. Thus, scalp-based BCIs are generally only practical for individuals that are in or nearing a locked-in state without volitional muscle control, such as those suffering from late-stage ALS or brain stem stroke.[2] Furthermore, for individuals in this state, the practical applications of robotic control become significantly more limited and specialized in terms of meeting their immediate basic needs.

To help mitigate the limitations of BCI as the primary controller, artificial intelligence can be employed to achieve shared control, in which some aspects of the robotic control are learned and automated by the machine, such as obstacle avoidance, trajectory planning, object interactions, balancing, and so on, and other aspects such as navigation or goal-oriented commands, for instance, remain under the user's direct control. This can provide interactions that are more functional, natural, convenient, and/or less demanding for the user. In this context, the degree of shared control can range from full user (BCI) control to full autonomous (artificial intelligence) control, with the relative proportion of user control depending on the nature and constraints of the application. Additionally, it is possible to dynamically vary the degree of user control depending on task demands and user workload, for example.

Depending on the application, artificial intelligence implementations can use a variety of sensing modalities mounted on or in proximity to the robot to acquire data for building a model of the environment. Such sensors may include cameras, optical sensors, accelerometers, ultrasonic sensors, and pressure sensors, for example.

Artificial intelligence is generally achieved via machine learning algorithms that implement supervised, unsupervised, or reinforcement learning strategies.[89] Supervised learning is when the system is trained using labeled data that correspond to predefined states, actions, goals, and so on. Unsupervised learning is when the data are not labeled, either because labels are not available or do not exist. Thus, unsupervised learning must find consistent patterns in the data to create or infer labels. Reinforcement learning can be applied when there are multiple approaches for achieving the same end goal. Here, specific actions are associated with a reward or penalty and, based on accumulated experience, the system learns appropriate sequences of actions to achieve the desired outcome by maximizing rewards and/or minimizing penalties.

Intelligent shared control has been implemented using a variety of strategies. For example, error-related potentials, ERPs that occur in response to observed errors,[90] have been introduced as a feedback signal to train intelligent controllers to achieve optimal behaviors for a given task. Interactive reinforcement learning using error-related potentials as implicit feedback has been shown for human-robot interaction (HRI),[91] including for coadaptation in HRI.[92] Error-related potentials have also been used to teach neuroprostheses optimal control policies for goal-directed movement, allowing users to give high-level commands that the trained policy develops low-level plans to execute.[93]

Computer vision–based strategies for shared control have also been demonstrated.[94,95] Muelling et al.[96] introduced a shared-control framework that combines computer vision, intent prediction, and human-robot control arbitration to reduce perceived difficulty when using BCI to control a 7-DoF robotic arm. Vision-based target-pose estimation can enable the robot to autonomously grasp targets once a person has moved its end effector close to the target via BCI control.[95] Applying target prediction in tandem with target-pose estimation allowed a shared controller to infer user intent and dynamically optimize user control commands to provide corrections while reaching or to autonomously grasp or place an object.[97]

In the context of wheelchair control and mobile manipulators, shared controllers are often used to autonomously move to a user-defined location in space,[75] to assist with obstacle avoidance during user control,[77] or some combination of these two approaches.[98–100] More recent approaches have considered how to dynamically modify when, or to what extent, wheelchair behavior is commanded by the human user or by a robot controller. Deng et al. showed how a Bayesian shared

BCI system for wheelchair control can intelligently arbitrate human and robot control commands generated via kinematic modeling and vision-based path planning.[98] Building off of this work, Deng et al.[99] propose a self-adaptive self-control system that evaluates subject's control ability from single trial SSVEP to modify the level of assistance provided by the robot for wheelchair control.

Current Challenges and Future Prospects

The aim of restoring natural function via a neuroprosthetic device (i.e., high DoF, continuous control), which will generally require invasive recordings from a large number of individual neurons, faces existing challenges that are distinctly different compared with that of a low-DoF assistive device that can be achieved via noninvasive means. For the former, population coding has proven to very reliably decode movement trajectories for motor prosthetics.

However, there are still open questions regarding the practicality and long-term viability of current approaches,[101] particularly with respect to the surgical risks. Furthermore, to move toward a fully transparent motor prosthetic, information from an increasing number of neurons must be incorporated. Significant efforts are going into the development of high-density recording devices,[19,20] including practical implantation and long-term stability considerations. Access to larger numbers of neurons requires new and improved large-scale decoding algorithms, which will, in turn, require additional behavioral data for training. Furthermore, to better model natural neuroplasticity in the brain, such models would likely need to be capable of adaptation, requiring data from appropriately designed closed-loop experiments. Because the user must also adapt to the model feedback, a precarious coadaptation scenario is created for which closed-loop experiments would need to carefully examine the nature, timing, dynamics, and accuracy of the feedback.[102]

Another critical consideration for developing fully natural motor prosthetics is the integration of sensory feedback, including tactile, visual, proprioceptive, and so on.[11] This requires a bidirectional BCI capable of providing coordinated and localized brain stimulation, which further complicates the aforementioned issues of electrode densities, locations, adaptive model development, and closed-loop experiments.

For lower-DoF assistive noninvasive devices, as mentioned in the "Artificial Intelligence and Shared Control" section, the primary limitation lies with the practicality and fidelity of noninvasive recordings—particularly if the user has any residual volitional muscle control. Thus, such BCIs are generally only practical for locked-in users, and the development of improved goal-oriented and shared-control methods holds the most promise until significant advances are made in noninvasive recording technologies. However, it must also be recognized that as the BCI moves further toward goal-oriented or shared control, users may lose a sense of agency relative to when they have truly continuous control. Otherwise, noninvasive BCIs do hold promise for motor rehabilitation,[65] as well as potential integration of passive cognitive-state estimates such as cognitive workload, attention, affect, and so on into the BCI feedback control loop.[103]

Overall, the BCI field is rapidly advancing and is beginning to receive serious commercial and investor interest, which is further accelerating the advances. With the recent developments in large-scale neural recording modalities and machine learning methods to handle the resulting "big data," practical BCI-controlled motor prosthetics, exoskeletons, and assistive robotics for disabled end users will become an eventual reality.

References

1. Wolpaw J, Wolpaw E. Brain–Computer Interfaces: Principles and Practice (2012; online edn, Oxford Academic, 24 May 2012). https://doi.org/10.1093/acprof:oso/9780195388855.001.0001. Accessed 2 Mar 2023.
2. Wolpaw J, Birbaumer N, McFarland D, Pfurtscheller G, Vaughan T. Brain–computer interfaces for communication and control. *Clin Neurophysiol.* 2002;113:767–791.

3. Shih J, Krusienski D, Wolpaw J. Brain-computer interfaces in medicine. *Mayo Clin Proc.* 2012;87(3):268–279.
4. Carmena JM, Lebedev MA, Crist RE, O'Doherty JE, Santucci DM, et al. Learning to Control a Brain–Machine Interface for Reaching and Grasping by Primates. *PLOS Biology.* 2003;1(2):e42. https://doi.org/10.1371/journal.pbio.0000042.
5. Chapin JK, Moxon KA, Markowitz RS, Nicolelis MAL. Real-time control of a robot arm using simultaneously recorded neurons in the motor cortex. *Nat Neurosci.* 1999;2:664–670.
6. Lebedev MA, Carmena JM, O'Doherty JE, Zacksenhouse M, Henriquez CS, Príncipe JC, Nicolelis MA. Cortical Ensemble Adaptation to Represent Velocity of an Artificial Actuator Controlled by a Brain-Machine Interface. *The Journal of Neuroscience.* 2005;25:4681–4693.
7. Wessberg J, Stambaugh CR, Kralik JD, et al. Real-time prediction of hand trajectory by ensembles of cortical neurons in primates. *Nature.* 2000;408:361–365.
8. Herff C, Krusienski DJ, Kubben P. The Potential of Stereotactic-EEG for Brain-Computer Interfaces: Current Progress and Future Directions. *Front Neurosci.* 2020 Feb 27;14:123. https://doi.org/10.3389/fnins.2020.00123. PMID: 32174810; PMCID: PMC7056827.
9. Schalk G, Leuthardt E. Brain-computer interfaces using electrocorticographic signals. *IEEE Rev Biomed Eng.* 2011;4:140–154.
10. Collinger J, Wodlinger B, Downey J, et al. High-performance neuroprosthetic control by an individual with tetraplegia. *Lancet.* 2013;381:557–564.
11. Flesher SN, Downey J, Weiss J, et al. A brain-computer interface that evokes tactile sensations improves robotic arm control. *Science.* 2021;372:831–836.
12. Gilja V, Pandarinath C, Blabe CH, et al. Clinical translation of a high-performance neural prosthesis. *Nat Med.* 2015;21:1142–1145.
13. Kennedy P, Bakay R, Moore M, Adams K, Goldwaithe J. Direct control of a computer from the human central nervous system. *IEEE Trans Rehab Eng.* 2000;8(2):198–202.
14. Willett F, Avansino DT, Hochberg L, Henderson J, Shenoy K. High performance brain-to-text communication via handwriting. *Nature.* 2021;593(7858):249–254.
15. Gull MA, Bai S, Bak T. A review on design of upper limb exoskeletons. *Robotics.* 2020;9:16.
16. Chen R, Canales A, Anikeeva P. Neural Recording and Modulation Technologies. *Nat Rev Mater.* 2017 Feb;2(2):16093. https://doi.org/10.1038/natrevmats.2016.93. Epub 2017 Jan 4. PMID: 31448131; PMCID: PMC6707077.
17. Maynard EM, Nordhausen CT, Normann RA. The Utah intracortical electrode array: a recording structure for potential brain-computer interfaces. *Electroencephalogr Clin Neurophysiol.* 1997;102(3):228–239.
18. Vetter RJ, Williams JC, Hetke JF, Nunamaker EA, Kipke DR. Chronic neural recording using silicon-substrate microelectrode arrays implanted in cerebral cortex. *IEEE Trans Biomed Eng.* 2004;51:896–904.
19. Jun J, Steinmetz NA, Siegle JH, et al. Fully integrated silicon probes for high-density recording of neural activity. *Nature.* 2017;551:232–236.
20. Musk E, Neuralink. An Integrated Brain-Machine Interface Platform With Thousands of Channels. *J Med Internet Res.* 2019 Oct 31;21(10):e16194. http://doi.org/10.2196/16194. PMID: 31642810; PMCID: PMC6914248.
21. Georgopoulos AP, Schwartz A, Kettner R. Neuronal population coding of movement direction. *Science.* 1986;233(4771):1416–1419.
22. Hochberg L, Serruya M, Friehs G, et al. Neuronal ensemble control of prosthetic devices by a human with tetraplegia. *Nature.* 2006;442:164–171.
23. Kellis SS, House P, Thomson K, Brown R, Greger B. Human neocortical electrical activity recorded on nonpenetrating microwire arrays: applicability for neuroprostheses. *Neurosurg Focus.* 2009;27(1):E9.
24. Miller K, Honey C, Hermes D, et al. Broadband changes in the cortical surface potential track activation of functionally diverse neuronal populations. *Neuroimage.* 2014;85:711–720.
25. Miller KJ, Sorensen LB, Ojemann JG, den Nijs M. Power-law scaling in the brain surface electric potential. *PLoS Comput Biol.* 2009 Dec;5(12):e1000609. https://doi.org/10.1371/journal.pcbi.1000609. Epub 2009 Dec 18. PMID: 20019800; PMCID: PMC2787015.
26. Kennedy P. The cone electrode: a long-term electrode that records from neurites grown onto its recording surface. *J Neurosci Methods.* 1989;29:181–193.
27. Miller K, Leuthardt E, Schalk G, et al. Spectral changes in cortical surface potentials during motor movement. *J Neurosci.* 2007;27:2424–2432.

28. Gearing M, Kennedy P. Histological Confirmation of Myelinated Neural Filaments Within the Tip of the Neurotrophic Electrode After a Decade of Neural Recordings. *Front Hum Neurosci.* 2020 Apr 21;14:111. https://doi.org/10.3389/fnhum.2020.00111. PMID: 32372930; PMCID: PMC7187752.
29. Oxley T, Yoo P, Rind G, et al. Motor neuroprosthesis implanted with neurointerventional surgery improves capacity for activities of daily living tasks in severe paralysis: first in-human experience. *J Neurointerv Surg.* 2020;13:102–108.
30. Seeber M, Cantonas LM, Hoevels M, Sesia T, Visser-Vandewalle V, Michel CM. Subcortical electrophysiological activity is detectable with high-density EEG source imaging. *Nat Commun.* 2019 Feb 14;10(1):753. https://doi.org/10.1038/s41467-019-08725-w. PMID: 30765707; PMCID: PMC6376013.
31. Zander T, Kothe C. Towards passive brain-computer interfaces: applying brain-computer interface technology to human-machine systems in general. *J Neural Eng.* 2011;8(2):025005.
32. Pfurtscheller G, Silva FLD. Event-related EEG/MEG synchronization and desynchronization: basic principles. *Clin Neurophysiol.* 1999;110:1842–1857.
33. Schomer D, Silva FLD. Niedermeyer's electroencephalography: basic principles, clinical applications, and related fields, 7 edn (New York, 2017; online edn, Oxford Academic, 1 Nov. 2017). https://doi.org/10.1093/med/9780190228484.001.0001, accessed 22 Feb. 2023.
34. Arroyo S, Lesser R, Gordon B, Uematsu S, Jackson D, Webber R. Functional significance of the mu rhythm of human cortex: an electrophysiologic study with subdural electrodes. *Electroencephalogr Clin Neurophysiol.* 1993;87(3):76–87.
35. Pfurtscheller G, Neuper C, Flotzinger D, Pregenzer M. EEG-based discrimination between imagination of right and left hand movement. *Electroencephalogr Clin Neurophysiol.* 1997;103(6):642–651.
36. McFarland DJ, Miner LA, Vaughan TM, Wolpaw JR. Mu and beta rhythm topographies during motor imagery and actual movements. *Brain Topogr.* 2004;12:177–186.
37. Wolpaw J, McFarland D. Control of a two-dimensional movement signal by a noninvasive brain-computer interface in humans. *Proc Natl Acad Sci U S A.* 2004;101(51):17849–17854.
38. Pfurtscheller G, Solis-Escalante T, Ortner R, Linortner P, Muller-Putz G. Self-paced operation of an SSVEP-based orthosis with and without an imagery-based "brain switch": a feasibility study towards a hybrid BCI. *IEEE Trans Neural Syst Rehabil Eng.* 2010;18:409–414.
39. Jeunet C, N'Kaoua B, Subramanian S, Hachet M, Lotte F. Predicting Mental Imagery-Based BCI Performance from Personality, Cognitive Profile and Neurophysiological Patterns. *PLoS One.* 2015 Dec 1;10(12):e0143962. https://doi.org/10.1371/journal.pone.0143962. Erratum in: PLoS One. 2023 Feb 23;18(2):e0282281. PMID: 26625261; PMCID: PMC4666487.
40. Wang Q, Sourina O. Real-time mental arithmetic task recognition from EEG signals. *IEEE Trans Neural Syst Rehabil Eng.* 2013;21:225–232.
41. McFarland DJ, Wolpaw JR. Brain-computer interface use is a skill that user and system acquire together. *PLoS Biol.* 2018 Jul 2;16(7):e2006719. https://doi.org/10.1371/journal.pbio.2006719. PMID: 29965965; PMCID: PMC6044535.
42. Misulis K, Fakhoury T. Spehlmann's evoked potential primer. Boston : ButterworthHeinemann; 2001.
43. Farwell L, Donchin E. Talking off the top of your head: toward a mental prosthesis utilizing event-related brain potentials. *Electroencephalogr Clin Neurophysiol.* 1988;70(6):510–523.
44. Kaufmann T, Schulz S, Grünzinger C, Kübler A. Flashing characters with famous faces improves ERP-based brain-computer interface performance. *J Neural Eng.* 2011;8(5):056016.
45. Townsend G, LaPallo BK, Boulay C, et al. A novel P300-based brain–computer interface stimulus presentation paradigm: moving beyond rows and columns. *Clin Neurophysiol.* 2010;121:1109–1120.
46. Furdea A, Halder S, Krusienski DJ, et al. An auditory oddball (p300) spelling system for brain-computer interfaces. *Psychophysiology.* 2009;46(3):617–625.
47. Zhao J, Li W, Li M. Comparative Study of SSVEP- and P300-Based Models for the Telepresence Control of Humanoid Robots. *PLoS One.* 2015 Nov 12;10(11):e0142168. https://doi.org/10.1371/journal.pone.0142168. PMID: 26562524; PMCID: PMC4642929.
48. Zhao J, Li W, Li M. Comparative study of ssvep- and p300-based models for the telepresence control of humanoid robots. *PLoS One.* 2015;10.
49. Johnson GD, Waytowich NR, Cox D, Krusienski DJ. Extending the discrete selection capabilities of the P300 speller to goal-oriented robotic arm control. Proceedings of the 2010 *3rd IEEE RAS & EMBS International Conference on Biomedical Robotics and Biomechatronics.* The University of Tokyo, Tokyo, Japan, IEEE. September 26-29, 2010.

50. Middendorf M, McMillan G, Calhoun G, Jones KS. Brain-computer interfaces based on the steady-state visual-evoked response. *IEEE Trans Rehab Eng*. 2000;8(2):211–214.
51. Waytowich NR, Krusienski D. Development of an extensible SSVEP-BCI software platform and application to wheelchair control. *2017 8th International IEEE/EMBS Conference on Neural Engineering (NER)*. IEEE. 2017:259–532. ieee.org.
52. Bin, Guangyu & Gao, Xiaorong & Wang, Yijun & Hong, Bo & Gao, Shangkai VEP-based brain-computer interfaces: Time, frequency, and code modulations [Research Frontier]. *IEEE Comp. Int. Mag*. 2009;4:22–26. https://doi.org/10.1109/MCI.2009.934562.
53. Chen X, Wang Y, Nakanishi M, Gao X, Jung T, Gao S. High-speed spelling with a noninvasive brain–computer interface. *Proc Natl Acad Sci U S A*. 2015;112:E6058–E6067.
54. Higashi H, Rutkowski TM, Washizawa Y, Cichocki A, Tanaka T. EEG auditory steady state responses classification for the novel BCI. *2011 Annual International Conference of the IEEE Engineering in Medicine and Biology Society*. IEEE. 2011:4576–4579. ieee.org.
55. Ahn S, Kim K, Jun SC. Steady-State Somatosensory Evoked Potential for Brain-Computer Interface-Present and Future. *Front Hum Neurosci*. 2016 Jan 14;9:716. https://doi.org/10.3389/fnhum.2015.00716. PMID: 26834611; PMCID: PMC4712271.
56. Brunner P, Joshi S, Briskin S, Wolpaw J, Bischof H, Schalk G. Does the "P300" speller depend on eye gaze? *J Neural Eng*. 2010;7(5):056013.
57. Treder M, Blankertz B. Covert attention and visual speller design in an ERP based brain-computer interface. *Behav Brain Funct*. 2010;6. Published 2010 May 28. https://doi.org/10.1186/1744-9081-6-28.
58. Waytowich NR, Krusienski D. Spatial decoupling of targets and flashing stimuli for visual brain-computer interfaces. *J Neural Eng*. 2015;12(3):036006.
59. Velliste M, Perel S, Chance Spalding M, Whitford AS, Schwartz AB. Cortical control of a prosthetic arm for self-feeding. *Nature*. 2008;453:1098–1101.
60. Hochberg LR, Bacher D, Jarosiewicz B, et al. Reach and grasp by people with tetraplegia using a neurally controlled robotic arm. *Nature*. 2012;485:372–375.
61. Wodlinger B, Downey JE, Tyler-Kabara EC, Schwartz AB, Boninger ML, Collinger JL. Ten-dimensional anthropomorphic arm control in a human brain machine interface: difficulties, solutions, and limitations. *J Neural Eng*. 2015;12(1):016011.
62. Hughes CL, Herrera AJ, Gaunt RA, Collinger JL. Bidirectional brain computer interfaces. *Handb Clin Neurol*. 2020;168:163–181.
63. Quick KM, Weiss JM, Clemente F, Gaunt RA, Collinger JL Intracortical microstimulation feedback improves grasp force accuracy in a human using a brain-computer interface. *Annu Int Conf IEEE Eng Med Biol Soc*. 2020;2020:3355–3358. https://doi.org/10.1109/EMBC44109.2020.9175926.
64. Wendelken S, Page DM, Davis T, Wark HAC, Kluger DT, Duncan C, Warren DJ, Hutchinson DT, Clark GA. Restoration of motor control and proprioceptive and cutaneous sensation in humans with prior upper-limb amputation via multiple Utah Slanted Electrode Arrays (USEAs) implanted in residual peripheral arm nerves. *J Neuroeng Rehabil*. 2017 Nov 25;14(1):121. https://doi.org/10.1186/s12984-017-0320-4. PMID: 29178940; PMCID: PMC5702130.
65. Mane R, Chouhan T, Guan C. BCI for stroke rehabilitation: motor and beyond. *J Neural Eng*. 2020 Aug 17;17(4):041001. https://doi.org/10.1088/1741-2552/aba162. PMID: 32613947.
66. Pfurtscheller G, Guger C, Müller GR, Krausz G, Neuper C. Brain oscillations control hand orthosis in a tetraplegic. *Neurosci Lett*. 2000;292:211–214.
67. Stan A, Irimia D, Botezatu N, Lupu R. Controlling a hand orthosis by means of P300-based brain computer interface. *2015 E-Health and Bioengineering Conference (EHB)*. 2015:1–4.
68. Syrov N, Novichikhina KA, Kir'yanov DA, Gordleeva SY, Kaplan AY. The changes of corticospinal excitability during the control of artificial hand through the brain–computer interface based on the P300 component of visual evoked potential. *Hum Physiol*. 2019;45:152–157.
69. Delijorge J, Mendoza-Montoya O, Gordillo JL, Caraza R, Martinez HR, Antelis JM. Evaluation of a P300-Based Brain-Machine Interface for a Robotic Hand-Orthosis Control. *Front Neurosci*. 2020 Nov 27;14:589659. https://doi.org/10.3389/fnins.2020.589659. PMID: 33328860; PMCID: PMC7729175.
70. Kwak NS, Müller KR, Lee SW. A lower limb exoskeleton control system based on steady state visual evoked potentials. *J Neural Eng*. 2015;12(5):056009.
71. Gui K, Liu H, Zhang D. Toward multimodal human-robot interaction to enhance active participation of users in gait rehabilitation. *IEEE Trans Neural Syst Rehabil Eng*. 2017;25(11):2054–2066. https://doi.org/10.1109/TNSRE.2017.2703586.

72. Wang C, Wu X, Wang Z, Ma Y. Implementation of a brain-computer interface on a lower-limb exoskeleton. *IEEE Access*. 2018;6:38524–38534.
73. Murphy DP, Bai O, Gorgey AS, Fox J, Lovegreen WT, Burkhardt BW, Atri R, Marquez JS, Li Q, Fei DY. Electroencephalogram-Based Brain-Computer Interface and Lower-Limb Prosthesis Control: A Case Study. *Front Neurol*. 2017 Dec 15;8:696. https://doi.org/10.3389/fneur.2017.00696. PMID: 29326653; PMCID: PMC5736540.
74. Benabid A, Costecalde T, Eliseyev A, et al. An exoskeleton controlled by an epidural wireless brain–machine interface in a tetraplegic patient: a proof-of-concept demonstration. *Lancet Neurol*. 2019;18:1112–1122.
75. Iturrate I, Antelis JM, Kübler A, Minguez J. A noninvasive brain-actuated wheelchair based on a P300 neurophysiological protocol and automated navigation. *IEEE Trans Robot*. 2009;25:614–627.
76. Rebsamen B, Burdet E, Guan C, Zhang H, et al. A brain-controlled wheelchair based on P300 and path guidance. *The First IEEE/RAS-EMBS International Conference on Biomedical Robotics and Biomechatronics, 2006. BioRob 2006*. IEEE. 2006:1101–1106. ieee.org.
77. Carlson T, Millán JR. Brain-controlled wheelchairs: a robotic architecture. *IEEE Robot Autom Mag*. 2013;20:65–73.
78. Tanaka K, Matsunaga K, Wang HO. Electroencephalogram-based control of an electric wheelchair. *IEEE Trans Robot*. 2015;21:762–766.
79. Huang D, Qian K, Fei DY, Jia W, Chen X, Bai O. Electroencephalography (EEG)-based brain–computer interface (BCI): a 2-d virtual wheelchair control based on event-related desynchronization/synchronization and state control. *IEEE Trans Neural Syst Rehabil Eng*. 2012;20:379–388.
80. gtec medical engineering. *SSVEP Control of a Robotic Arm. Published*. July 2011. https://www.youtube.com/watch?v=8eOSlzDdOpg.
81. Lafleur K, Cassady K, Doud A, Shades K, Rogin E, He B. Quadcopter control in three-dimensional space using a noninvasive motor imagery-based brain-computer interface. *J Neural Eng*. 2013;10(4):046003.
82. Bell CJ, Shenoy P, Chalodhorn R, Rao RPN. Control of a humanoid robot by a noninvasive brain-computer interface in humans. *J Neural Eng*. 2008;5(2):214–220.
83. Carlson T, Tonin L, Perdikis S, Leeb R, Millán JR. A hybrid BCI for enhanced control of a telepresence robot. *2013 35th Annual International Conference of the IEEE Engineering in Medicine and Biology Society (EMBC)*. IEEE. 2013:3097–3100. ieee.org.
84. Leeb R, Tonin L, Rohm M, Ferro Desideri L, Carlson T, Millán JR. Towards independence: a BCI telepresence robot for people with severe motor disabilities. *Proc IEEE Inst Electr Electron Eng*. 2015;103:969–982.
85. Millán JR, Renkens F, Mouriño J, Gerstner W. Noninvasive brain-actuated control of a mobile robot by human EEG. *IEEE Trans Biomed Eng*. 2004;51(6):1026–1033. https://doi.org/10.1109/TBME.2004.827086.
86. McFarland D, Wolpaw J. Brain-Computer Interface Operation of Robotic and Prosthetic Devices. *Computer*. Oct. 2008;41(10):52–56. https://doi.org/10.1109/MC.2008.409.
87. Meng J, Zhang S, Bekyo A, Olsoe J, Baxter B, He B. Noninvasive Electroencephalogram Based Control of a Robotic Arm for Reach and Grasp Tasks. *Sci Rep*. 2016 Dec 14;6:38565. https://doi.org/10.1038/srep38565. Erratum in: Sci Rep. 2020 Apr 15;10(1):6627. PMID: 27966546; PMCID: PMC5155290.
88. Onose G, Grozea C, Anghelescu A, et al. On the feasibility of using motor imagery EEG-based brain–computer interface in chronic tetraplegics for assistive robotic arm control: a clinical test and long-term post-trial follow-up. *Spinal Cord*. 2012;50:599–608.
89. Kroemer O, Niekum S, Konidaris GD. A review of robot learning for manipulation: challenges, representations, and algorithms. *J Mach Learn Res*. 2021;22:1–82.
90. Kumar A, Gao L, Pirogova E, Fang Q. A review of error-related potential-based brain–computer interfaces for motor impaired people. *IEEE Access*. 2019;7:142451–142466.
91. Kim SK, Kirchner EA, Stefes A, Kirchner F. Intrinsic interactive reinforcement learning - Using error-related potentials for real world human-robot interaction. *Sci Rep*. 2017 Dec 14;7(1):17562. https://doi.org/10.1038/s41598-017-17682-7. PMID: 29242555; PMCID: PMC5730605.
92. Ehrlich SK, Cheng G. Human-agent co-adaptation using error-related potentials. *J Neural Eng*. 2018;15(6):066014.

93. Iturrate I, Chavarriaga R, Montesano L, Minguez J, Millán Jdel R. Teaching brain-machine interfaces as an alternative paradigm to neuroprosthetics control. *Sci Rep*. 2015 Sep 10;5:13893. https://doi.org/10.1038/srep13893. PMID: 26354145; PMCID: PMC4564803.
94. Tang J, Zhou Z. A shared-control based BCI system: for a robotic arm control. *2017 First International Conference on Electronics Instrumentation & Information Systems (EIIS)*, IEEE: Harbin, China. 2017:1–5. https://doi.org/10.1109/EIIS.2017.8298767.
95. Xu Y, Zhang H, Cao L, Shu X, Zhang D. A Shared Control Strategy for Reach and Grasp of Multiple Objects Using Robot Vision and Noninvasive Brain–Computer Interface. *IEEE Transactions on Automation Science and Engineering*. Jan. 2022;19(1):360–372. https://doi.org/10.1109/TASE.2020.3034826.
96. Muelling K, Venkatraman A, Valois JA, et al. Autonomy infused teleoperation with application to brain computer interface controlled manipulation. *Auton Robots*. 2017;41:1401–1422.
97. Cao L, Li G, Xu Y, Zhang H, Shu X, Zhang D. A brain-actuated robotic arm system using non-invasive hybrid brain-computer interface and shared control strategy. *J Neural Eng*. 2021 May 5;18(4): https://doi.org/10.1088/1741-2552/abf8cb. PMID: 33862607.
98. Deng X, Yu ZL, Lin C, Gu Z, Li Y. A bayesian shared control approach for wheelchair robot with brain machine interface. *IEEE Trans Neural Syst Rehabil Eng*. 2020;28:328–338.
99. Deng X, Liang Yu Z, Lin C, Gu Z, Li Y. Self-adaptive shared control with brain state evaluation network for human-wheelchair cooperation. *J Neural Eng*. 2020 Jul 13;17(4):045005. https://doi.org/10.1088/1741-2552/ab937e. PMID: 32413885.
100. Han X, Lin K, Gao S, Gao X. A novel system of SSVEP-based human-robot coordination. *J Neural Eng*. 2019;16(1):016006.
101. Polikov VS, Tresco PA, Reichert WM. Response of brain tissue to chronically implanted neural electrodes. *J Neurosci Methods*. 148:1–18, 2005.
102. Cheng G, Ehrlich SK, Lebedev M, Nicolelis MAL. Neuroengineering challenges of fusing robotics and neuroscience. *Sci Robot*. 2020 Dec 9;5(49):eabd1911. https://doi.org/10.1126/scirobotics.abd1911. PMID: 33298517.
103. Alimardani M, Hiraki K. Passive Brain-Computer Interfaces for Enhanced Human-Robot Interaction. *Front Robot AI*. 2020 Oct 2;7:125. https://doi.org/10.3389/frobt.2020.00125. PMID: 33501291; PMCID: PMC7805996.

11

Artificial Intelligence in Radiology

M. Rehan Khan

KEY POINTS

- The convergence of artificial intelligence and radiology was a natural development as these two fields evolved technologically.
- Different types of artificial intelligence such as supervised learning and deep learning have their applications to radiology.
- Machines can interpret radiologic images through multiple techniques and can provide speed and accuracy.
- The ability to process large numbers of images rapidly offers the radiologist some relief for the increasing demands of this specialty.
- The future role of AI in radiology is evolving with pitfalls and promises, and radiologists should have a strong role in its development.

Background

RADIOLOGY

Radiology as a discipline has been on the forefront of advances in medicine and always been one of the early adopters of computing revolutionary technologies. Since 1895, when Wilhelm Rontgen took the first x-ray of his wife's hand, there have been significant developments in this field.

DIGITAL RADIOLOGY

The use of digital technology in radiology started in 1967 with the advent of CT (computed tomography) scanners.[1] Next, a major shift happened with the advent of MRI (magnetic resonance imaging) in the 1980s. Since then, various more technologies like single-photon emission CT, positron emission CT, multidetector CT, dual-energy CT scanners, and positron emission tomography with MRI, with significantly higher level of computing sophistications evolved. As development continued, the concept of imaging networks evolved mainly for the purpose of image storage and distribution, called PACS (picture archiving and communication systems), and is now widely used throughout small and large medical enterprises.

ARTIFICIAL INTELLIGENCE

The term "artificial intelligence" (AI) was introduced for the first time by John McCarthy of Dartmouth college in the summer of 1956 at a conference, and he defined AI as "the science and engineering of making intelligent machines."[2]

COMPUTERIZED DECISION-MAKING TOOL

These early intelligent machines started to get utilized in different fields of life, and in 1972 one of the earliest computerized clinical decision tools in medicine was developed in the United Kingdom. This clinical decision system was called AA Phelp, and it helped in diagnosing the cause of abdominal pain based on clinical symptoms. This computer system was more accurate than the diagnosis made by senior physicians (91% vs. 79%); however, the problem back then was that computers took a few hours to make the diagnosis.[3]

COMPUTER VISION AND IMAGE RECOGNITION

Even with so much success made by intelligent machines, the progress in the field of image recognition or analysis was relatively slow. Things changed in 2009, when researchers from Princeton University, under the leadership of Li Fei-Fei, developed a new database for computer vision and pattern recognition. They built this new database using 3.2 million images and named that database ImageNet.[4]

After 2009, this revolutionary ImageNet database was used by multiple groups to improve computer vision and pattern recognition, who presented their results at annual ILSVRC (ImageNet Large Scale Visual Recognition Challenge). In 2012, a group took significant leap when graphics processing unit (GPU) was used for the first time in convolutional neural network (CNN) named AlexNet, which performed significantly better at the annual ILSVRC.

In 2015, a team of computer scientist introduced new type of CNN called ResNet (residual neural network), which won the first prize at the annual ILSVRC and for the first time outperformed human vision for certain tasks. This neural network is fundamentally different from other CNNs, in which not all the layers are connected to each other, so it is more time-efficient and accurate.[5]

Technical Knowledge

CENTRAL PROCESSING UNIT VERSUS GRAPHICS PROCESSING UNIT

GPU is a special processor different from the regular central processing unit (CPU) microprocessor as shown in Fig. 11.1 and has thousands of small cores that can handle multiple computation in parallel. Originally it was used in video games and was optimized in such a way that each pixel value can be processed by each core. More hardware is allocated to computations and less to fast cache memory in GPU, the opposite of CPU, where memory is much more important. CPU is good in performing serial tasks that take a lot of memory versus GPU, which performs a lot of parallel computations.[6]

COMPUTER LANGUAGES

Python and R are the two most used programming languages for data science in deep learning and AI.

ARTIFICIAL INTELLIGENCE

AI is any computer algorithm that can perform a task at human level. AI includes all type of machine learning (ML). ML includes all types of deep learning and deep learning includes all types of CNNs (Fig. 11.2).[7,8]

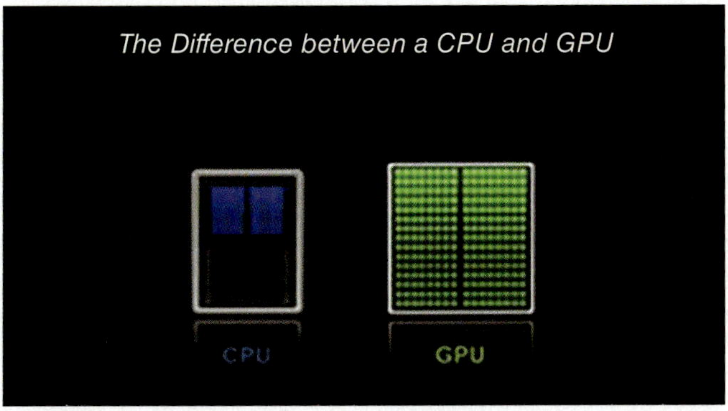

Fig. 11.1 Architectural difference between central a processing unit (CPU) and a graphics processing unit (GPU), which has multiple microprocessors versus two or three in a CPU. (Modified from https://blogs.nvidia.com/blog/2009/12/16/whats-the-difference-between-a-cpu-and-a-gpu/.)

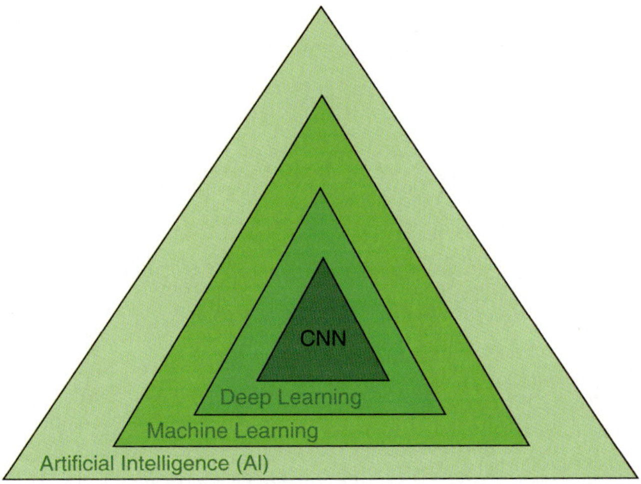

Fig. 11.2 All types of convolutional neural network (CNN) are subset of deep learning, all forms of deep learning are subset of machine learning, and all machine learning is a subset of artificial intelligence.

MACHINE LEARNING

- ML is defined by computer scientist Tom Mitchel as "the study of computer algorithms that improve automatically through experience." ML is when data train the computer to perform tasks, instead of programming the computer. ML can be supervised by humans, if needed.
- In supervised ML (Fig. 11.3), the data are labeled, which means that some data already know the right answer. Regression and classification are two types of supervised learning based on output variables. When the output is a real number, it is called regression, like height, weight, or size. Classification is the other type, when the output variable is in the form of category or class, like choosing between different colors (e.g., red or blue) (Fig. 11.4).
- In unsupervised ML, the input data are not labeled, and developers let the machine discover answers on its own. Unsupervised learning can be of two types: clustering and association.

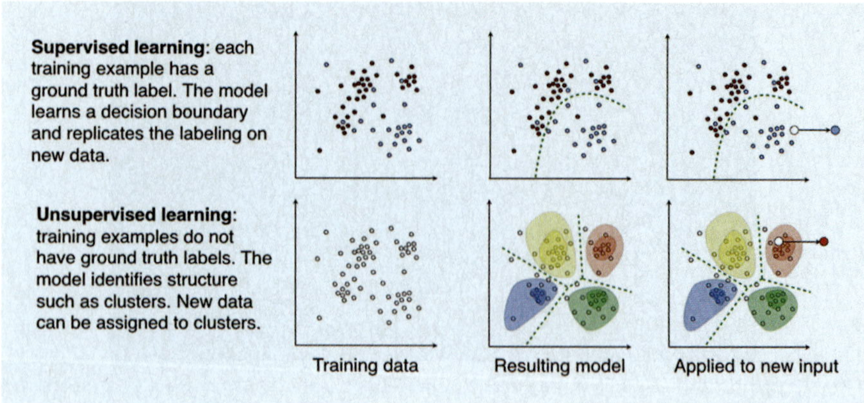

Fig. 11.3 Difference in training and resulting model and how it is applied to new input between supervised and unsupervised learning.

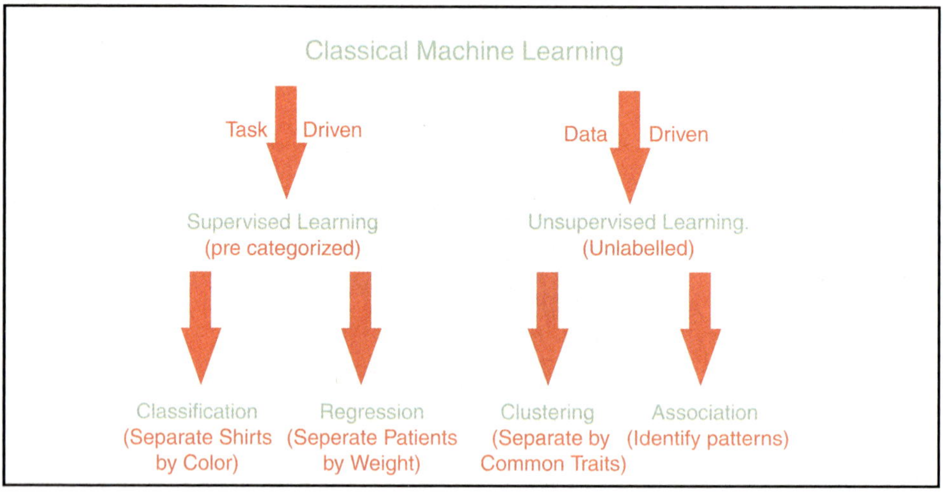

Fig. 11.4 Types of classical machine learning.

Clustering is applied by developers when they like to identify structure or pattern in uncategorized data; for example, uncategorized data of thyroid nodules can be categorized based on shape, size, and calcifications. Association, on the other hand, is when developers need to recognize associations between different data objects while evaluating large databases (Fig. 11.5).[9]

COMPUTER-AIDED DIAGNOSIS

Computer-aided diagnosis is a type of supervised ML. The earliest use of computer-aided diagnosis was in 1963 by Lodwick to evaluate chest x-rays. Current computers are 30 million times faster than what was used in 1963.[10–12]

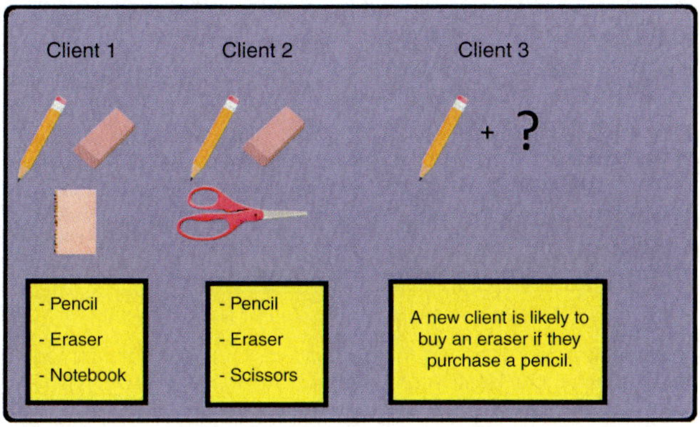

Fig. 11.5 Example of association type of unsupervised learning explains how computers recognize association between two data objects.

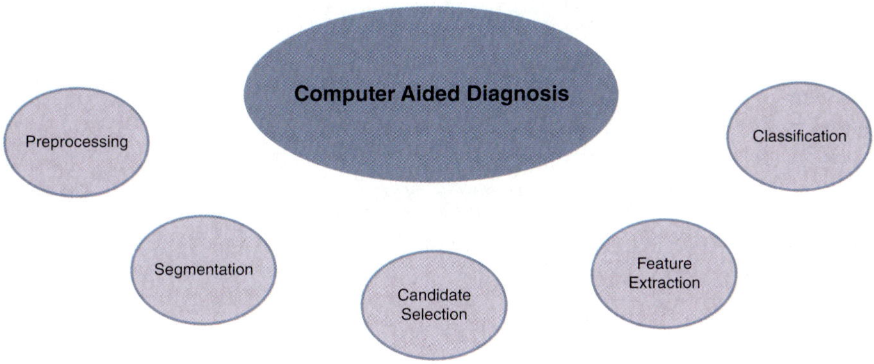

Fig. 11.6 Steps of computer-aided diagnosis.

In computer-aided diagnosis, images go through multiple steps (Figs. 11.6 and 11.7) like preprocessing, segmentation, candidate detection, feature extraction, and classification.[13]

1. Preprocessing means radiology images go through recalibration and noise removal.
2. Segmentation is the separation of image data, based on anatomy. It is considered one of the most interesting and studied areas in medical imaging.[14]
3. During candidate selection, areas that need more attention get identified (for example, density or calcification).
4. In the fourth step, the selected candidate's feature extraction is performed. This step requires vector space paradigm, which means each candidate is represented by a vector, which is a row of numbers and each number represents each feature of the candidate. Several features define the dimension of feature space and help with pattern classification also known as ML.
5. The last step is classification, in which normal and abnormal features are classified by trainers.

DEEP LEARNING

Deep learning is a type of ML (Fig. 11.8) where data trains multilayered network or deep neural networks and extract higher-level features. Deep neural networks are not the only way to perform deep learning, but they are the most used method.[15]

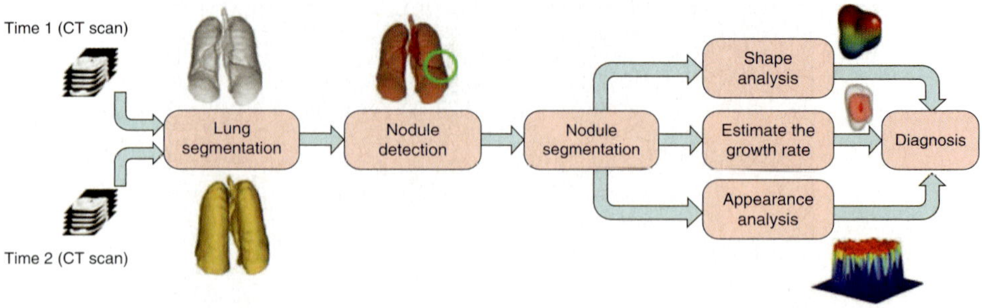

Fig. 11.7 Steps of computer aided diagnosis for lung nodule. CT, Computed tomography. (Modified from https://www.researchgate.net/figure/Typical-computer-aided-diagnosis-CAD-system-for-lung-cancer-The-input-of-a-CAD-system_fig1_235691825.)

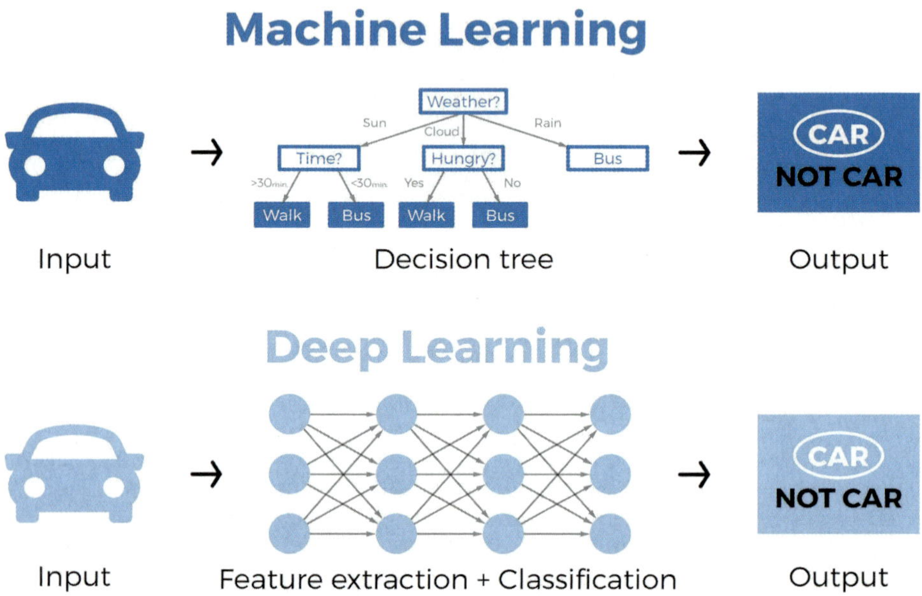

Fig. 11.8 Diagrammatic representation of differences in machine learning and deep learning (which is also a type of machine learning). (Modified from https://blog.bismart.com/en/difference-between-machine-learning-deep-learning.)

Neural networks are many interconnected processing elements that change their dynamic internal state due to external inputs/data.[16]

These concepts were first conceived in 1943.[8] In the 1990s neural networks were shallow and consisted primarily of only three layers: an input layer, a hidden layer, and an output layer. Each neuron in these layers receives input data, performs operation, and exports the results to the next layer. Deep neural networks have more than two hidden layers present, but very commonly, they can have 30 to 40 hidden layers.[7]

CNN

CNN is a type of artificial neural network that differs from others due to the convolutional layer. Convolutional in mathematics refers to producing a third function by combining two functions. Neural network convolution can be when a kernel (filter) is used with input data to create a feature map. In radiology, filters are commonly used to create edge sharpening and blurring and other appearances of images. The next step is pooling, which could be averaging the values or maximizing the values in the target area. In the fully connected layers, features extracted from convolutional and pooling layers get mapped into the final outputs of the model. Activation is one of the most integral components of CNN and transforms linear operations output (convolutions) into nonlinear, making them learn and perform complex tasks.

CNN is most widely used deep learning model in imaging due to following reasons:

1. Unlike other fully connected neural networks where every single neuron has to be connected to every single neuron of the next layer, in CNN only some of the neurons will be connected to some of the neurons of the next layer through a kernel or filter. It reduces the time it takes to train; for example, if there is an input layer of 64 × 64 and an output layer of 64 × 64, a total of 16,777,216 parameters needs to be trained versus if there is a kernel/filter of 3 × 3 used between 2 layers, then only 9 parameters needs to be trained.
2. The features that are relevant can be learned from the images. Most of the filters we use on regular photos are predefined, although in CNN filters they are not predefined but they learn to perform certain tasks from raw image data. Then these trained kernels are applied to the input images, which results in different feature maps.
3. It is very efficient for new tasks, as existing trained CNN can train itself for new tasks by transfer learning.
4. CNN has outperformed other algorithms on image analysis.

RESIDUAL NETWORK

Evidence suggest depth of the network is very important, and adding more layers increases the error rate.[17,18] Therefore, in ResNet (residual network) weightage is assigned to each stacked layer as well to allow some features to skip the layers so that the error rate, which was high with conventional plain multilayer system, can be reduced. In summary, adding layers are important but these can increase errors, which can be corrected by adding weightage and skipping the layers.

Convolutional Neural Network–Recurrent Neural Network

A CNN–recurrent neural network is a type of CNN that is good at processing *sequential* information like speech and language. It can be used to evaluate medical records or radiology reports. In one study, recurrent neural network–based natural language processing (NLP) was performed of the musculoskeletal imaging reports for fracture versus no fracture. Interestingly this project was not done based on vocabulary, grammar, or dictionary; instead, it generated annotation by output characters (which are not words) so in this study these 11 characters were used: f, r, a, c, t, u, e, n, o, -, EOS (end of sentence symbol). For example, the study was labeled fracture from the sentences like ("s/p intramedullary nailing in the femoral shaft" or "increased callus formation").[19,20]

Convolutional Neural Network–Generative Adversarial Network. In a CNN-generative adversarial network, two (generator and discriminator) networks work with and against each other. In radiology it can help to augment synthetic data to create realistic-appearing medical images. In a 2018 publication, artificial brain images were created (from very preliminary raw data) that could not be identified as artificial, even by a well-trained neuroradiologist. The generative adversarial network–based model can be very helpful in a scenario with difficult and sick patients and only have 5 to 10 minutes to obtain all relevant images instead of 20 to 30 minutes for brain MRI.[21,22]

TRANSFER LEARNING

It this process, a preexisting trained model gets retrained with the new data. This will significantly reduce the data demands for CNN model development and can have a significant role in radiology as abnormal medical images are very limited.

TRAINING A CNN MODEL

Although a child can recognize a cat from the dog, describing the exact features that help distinguish between them is difficult. Both animals have teeth, ears, eyes, and tongue. Similarly, CNN can reliably identify lesions without needing specific morphologic parameters; instead, they need lot of images labeled "fracture" or "no fracture." Images to train CNN do not typically require preprocessing, segmentation, or feature extraction. CNN models are typically described as a "black box" that extracts differentiating features and arrives at weighted probabilities for specific question. It is important to understand that CNN needs lot of images to train the system. If a CNN model is built on insufficient number of images, it will suffer from overfitting, which means it will not be applicable generally to other clinical images outside the training set. After the CNN model is trained on sufficient images, the model can be tested on a separate validation data set. Finally, the model can be tested on testing data set, which ideally should be different from training and validation data sets.[23]

RADIOMICS

Radiographic image data along with the clinical outcomes have led to the expansion of the field of radiomics. Radiomics is relatively a new field in radiology and deals with the extraction of a large number of features such as size, shape, texture analysis, image intensity histograms, and image voxel relationships from radiology images. These features include spatial information on pixel or voxel distribution and patterns and help in the diagnosis of diseases of the bone, muscle, and other organs, which can lead to precise treatment. AI with radiomics provides a smarter capability of managing enormous data sets efficiently than the traditional systems.[24–26]

ML techniques have led to expansion of the potential of radiomics to impact clinical care. One recent study applied ML-enhanced radiomics to differentiate sacral chordomas from sacral giant cell tumors on 3D CT.[27] The researchers found that contrast-enhanced CT characteristics were more useful than those from unenhanced imaging for differentiation of these two tumor types when comparing different feature selection and classification methods. In guiding more precise evaluations and treatments, there is potential for ML-enhanced radiomics in evaluating other Musculoskeletal (MSK) and non-MSK tumors as well.

DICE SIMILARITY COEFFICIENT

It is a measure of similarity between two samples. Dice similarity coefficient is commonly used to measure accuracy of image segmentation algorithms. It is important to know when reading radiology literature especially with AI.

Applications of Artificial Intelligence in Radiology

AI is considered one of the most disruptive and transformative technology of the present time, and its use in radiology is already felt to be groundbreaking. In the last 5 years alone, there have been more than 6000 citations in PubMed related to AI and radiology.

There is a strong argument that AI in medicine will be led by specialties like radiology because they generate multibillion images every year. Images in radiology are all digital and are stored and distributed via powerful network of computers like PACS (picture archiving and storage systems).[28]

The number of images provided to radiologist for review for each patient have increased multiple times over the last few decades. Average number of images radiologists review while reading a CT scan have increased by approximately 10 times from 82 images in 1999 to 679 images in 2010. For MRI, the average number of images increased from 164 images to 570 images, respectively.[29] The total number of radiologists needed is a lot more than the available workforce around the world. In the United States, the percentage of radiologists as a share of overall physician workforce has decreased from 8.8% in 1995 to 4.0 % in 2011.[30] In Japan, there is only 1 radiologist per 40,000 patient population compared with 1 regular physician per 500 patient population.[31] Overall accuracy in interpreting images is also decreasing as medical error rates are increasing. Radiologist error rates are as high as 30%[32] due to the large number of images, search patterns, and also the complexity of the examinations—for example, people who read three to five MRI liver examinations a day versus people who read three to five cases a week.[33] Per year, 40,000 to 80,000 deaths are related to diagnostic errors.[34] Economic cost associated with their diagnostic errors are more than $38 to $50 billion dollars.[32,35]

Use of AI can hopefully help improve much needed efficiency and efficacy in the field of radiology.[36]

In the next few sections, some of the direct roles of a radiologist and how AI can assist will be discussed. Some of the other potential roles of AI in advanced radiology department will also be discussed.

Pathology Detection

One of the primary roles of a radiologist is to evaluate and interpret images. There are multiple pathologies in which AI can help the radiologist, but the next few paragraphs will address more of musculoskeletal pathologies.

FRACTURE DETECTION

There are multiple published studies showing that fractures can be detected using deep learning. Some limitations of all these studies are that to train CNNs, thousands of images are needed for the same body part, images need labeling, and the ability to recognize fracture does not cross over to other body parts very easily (unlike humans who can transfer that knowledge). In addition, the results are binary, such as presence of a fracture or no fracture. Description or type of fractures present is currently not available.

In 2017, a group from Stanford introduced MURA (musculoskeletal radiograph), a large data set of musculoskeletal X-rays containing 40,561 images from 14,863 examinations, with each examination labeled manually by radiologists as normal or abnormal. They trained a 169-layer DenseNet baseline model to detect and localize abnormalities. Their model achieved an area under the receiver operating characteristic curve (ROC) of 0.929, with 0.815 sensitivity and 0.887 specificity. Model performance was comparable to the best radiologist performance in detecting abnormalities on finger and wrist studies. However, model performance was lower than best radiologist performance in detecting abnormalities on elbow, forearm, hand, humerus, and shoulder examinations.[37,38]

Since the time of publication, Stanford's large MURA data set was made public to encourage other groups to compete for fracture-detection algorithms. The performance of some of the models exceeded the original model and as of August 3, 2021, the top eight models have k values ranging 0.843 to 0.795, which is better than the best of the three radiologists in the original study (0.778).[23]

Compression fractures can be subtle, and differences in bone density in the spines can be very difficult to evaluate. A well-researched article was published in *Radiology* in 2017 in which an automated computer system was developed to detect, localize, and classify compression fractures and to measure bone density on spine CT scans. Sensitivity for detection or localization of compression fractures was 95.7%. Accuracy for classification by Genant type (anterior, middle, or posterior height loss) was 0.95. Accuracy for categorization by Genant height loss grade was 0.68. The average bone attenuation for T12–L4 vertebrae was 146 Hounsfield units (HU) ± 29 (standard deviation) in case patients and 173 HU ± 42 in control patients; this difference was statistically significant.[39]

In 2017 a Swedish study was published, in which 256,000 wrist, hand, and ankle x-rays were classified for fracture, laterality, body part, and view. Researchers used five openly available deep learning neural networks, and the results demonstrate that all five networks perform at 90% accuracy for laterality, body part, and examination view. Accuracy for recognizing fractures was 83% for the best performing deep learning neural network. These results were comparable to senior orthopedic surgeons evaluating images for fractures.[40]

In 2019, a study was performed on more than 20,000 images to detect hip fractures. Results were compared between orthopedic surgeons and deep CNN, and accuracy was 92% and 95%, sensitivity was 88% and 94%, and specificity was 97% and 97%, respectively. The performance of deep CNN outperformed the orthopedic surgeons. This could develop into very important application, which can help us detect hip fracture early and accurately, because missed hip fractures are associated with long-term pain and disability.[41]

CARTILAGE ABNORMALITY DETECTION

Cartilage abnormality detection is lot more difficult and different than fracture detection. It is usually done on MRIs. Cartilage first needs to be accurately segmented and then the segmented cartilage is divided into small patches/sections for abnormality detection. Other issue with cartilage is that it is inherently usually small or thin.

A study published in 2018, performed on knee MRI images to look for cartilage abnormality. In this study knee images had to go through two separate CNNs, one for the segmentations and other one for the characterization (detection) (Fig. 11.9). After segmentation, each knee cartilage surface area was divided into small patches. Each patch was evaluated separately, so total of 17,395 small patches from 175 patients were evaluated twice. Results show sensitivity of 84% and specificity of 85% for evaluation 1 and 80% and 88% for evaluation 2. AUC was 0.917 and 0.914 for evaluation 1 and 2. There was good interobserver agreement between two evaluations with a k of 0.76.

MENISCAL OR LIGAMENTOUS TEAR DETECTION

More work is getting done to detect abnormalities involving ligaments and menisci. Bien et al. from Stanford reported an AUC of 0.847 for detecting meniscal tears with their CNN model (MRNet; 1130 training and 120 validation examinations). The network was also trained to recognize anterior cruciate ligament tears and achieved an AUC of 0.937 on the internal validation set. When tested on an external validation set of 183 examinations obtained from a public data set of 917 examinations from Croatia, AUC was slightly lower (0.824) for the detection of anterior cruciate ligament tears. However, when MRNet was trained on the external data set, AUC improved to 0.911 on the external validation set.[43]

Segmentation

Drawing boundaries around normal anatomical structures or pathological findings for the purpose of quantification (volumes) is segmentation. It is extremely time-consuming with a high level

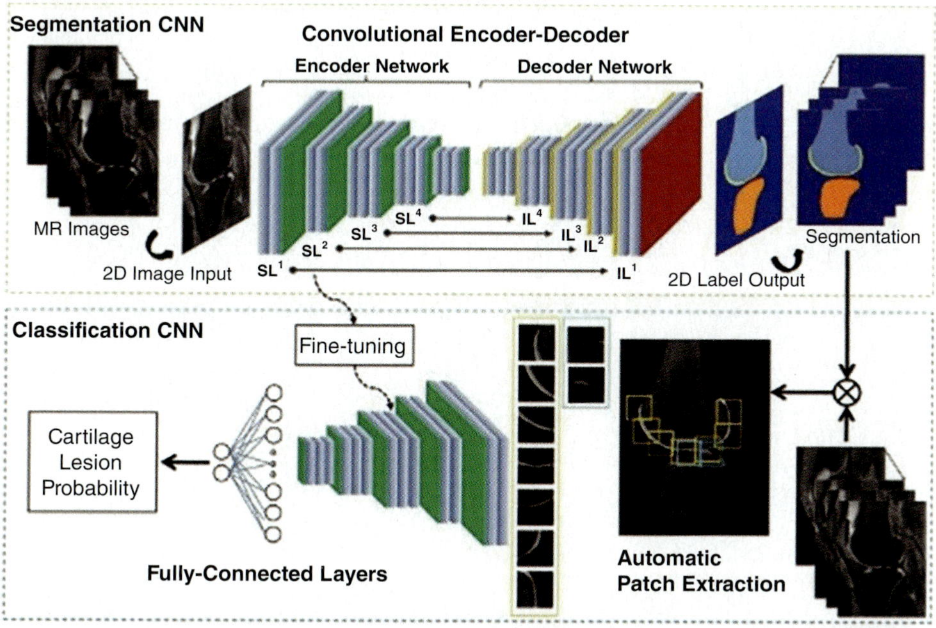

Fig. 11.9 Two separate convoluted neural networks (CNNs) used for the cartilage lesion detection, one for the segmentation *(top)* and one for the classification *(bottom)*.[42] (From Liu F, Zhou Z, Samsonov A, et al. Deep learning approach for evaluating knee MR images: achieving high diagnostic performance for cartilage lesion detection. *Radiology*. 2018;2891:160–169. doi:10.1148/radiol.2018172986.)

of variations and inaccuracies, which can have very important clinical ramifications, especially if long-term changes need to be tracked. Use of AI for autosegmentation will reduce the variability, and more accurate 3D volumes can be measured.[44]

MUSCLE SEGMENTATION

Most radiologists do not quantify a lot of information available on radiologic images, because it is extremely time-consuming and inaccurate. A good example of these is generalized muscle atrophy or decrease bone density. A study by Lee et al. tried to quantify muscle on CT scan and their best model achieved 0.93 Dice similarity coefficient.[45]

CARTILAGE SEGMENTATION

Osteoarthritis is one of leading causes of pain and disability, so early detection and quantification of cartilage loss can be helpful. Manual cartilage segmentation can be extremely time-consuming. One of the main hurdles in automated cartilage assessments tools is to clearly identify the cartilage; since the cartilage is most easily recognized in the knee, most of the AI work is performed on knee MRIs (Fig. 11.10). In a study published in 2019 by Gaj et al.,[46] a developed model was trained and tested on knee MRI images from the Osteoarthritis Initiative data set. The model provided excellent segmentation performance for cartilages with Dice coefficients ranging from 0.84 to 0.91. For meniscus segmentation, the model achieves 0.87 to 0.89 Dice coefficients.

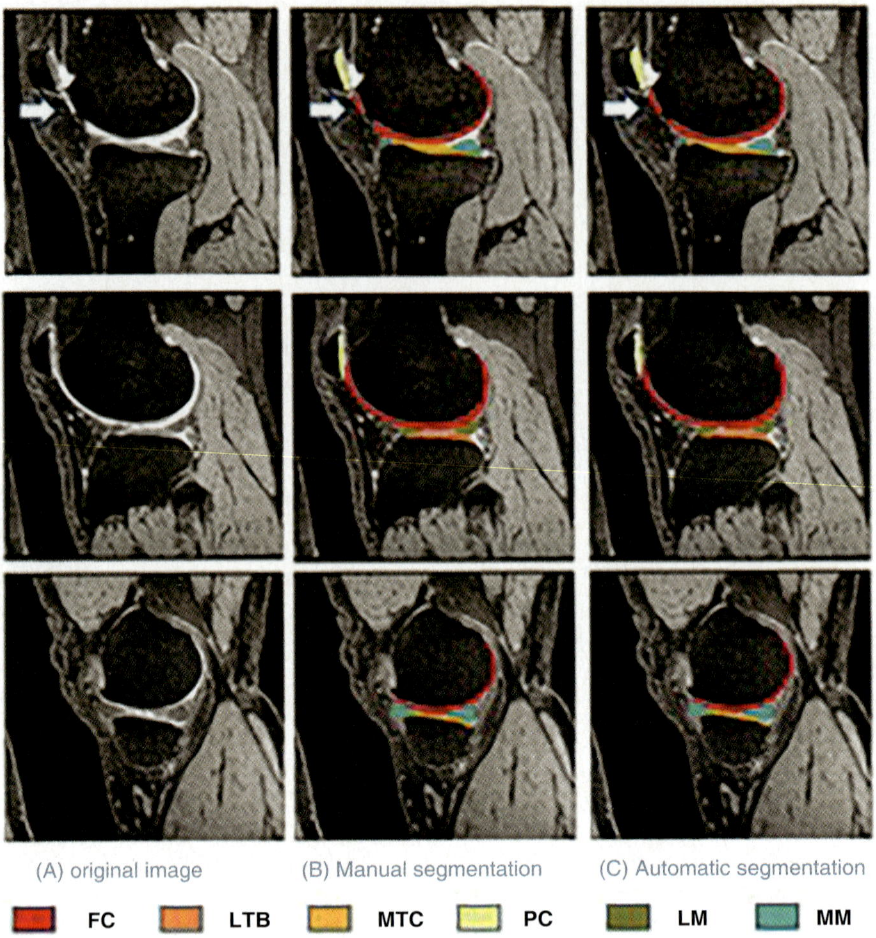

Fig. 11.10 Manual and automatic segmentation for femoral condyles (FC), lateral tibial (LTB), medial tibial cartilage (MTC), patellar cartilage (PC), lateral meniscus (LM), and medial meniscus (MM).[46] (From Gaj S, Yang M, Nakamura K, Li X. Automated cartilage and meniscus segmentation of knee MRI with conditional generative adversarial networks. *Magn Reson Med*. 2019;841:437–449. https://doi.org/10.1002/mrm.28111.)

A study published in 2019 was done on delayed gadolinium-enhanced MRI of cartilage utilizing a deep learning approach to develop hip cartilage segmentation technique that is fully automatic and enables an accurate, reliable, and reproducible analysis of cartilage thickness, surface area, and volume. This extremely efficient and objective evaluation of biochemical cartilage composition and morphology yields the potential to improve patient selection in femoroacetabular impingement surgery and help surgeons with planning.[47]

NONMUSCULOSKELETAL SEGMENTATION

AI can help radiologists to accurately measure the size of the different organs. Hu et al. performed multiorgan segmentation (liver, spleen, and both kidneys) on 140 abdominal CT images. They employed deep fully CNNs for organ detection. Average Dice overlap ratios for the liver, spleen, and both kidneys are 96.0%, 94.2%, and 95.4%, respectively. The computation time for a CT volume was 125 seconds in average. They achieved accuracies comparable to state-of-the-art methods with much higher efficiency.[48]

Classification

After a radiologist identifies the finding, the next step is to classify the disease and assess the severity of it. There are multiple deep learning models available to assess different benign and malignant diseases.

AUTOMATED OSTEOARTHRITIS EVALUATION

Antony et al. in 2016 demonstrate that classification accuracy can be significantly improved using deep CNN models pretrained on ImageNet and fine-tuned on knee osteoarthritis images. They used transfer learning techniques to existing CNN and extract features to create automated knee osteoarthritis quantification model, capable of classifying into mild, moderate, or severe grades.[49]

A study published in 2020 analyzed hip joints on weight-bearing AP pelvic radiographs from participants in the Osteoarthritis Initiative.[50] Femoral osteophytes, acetabular osteophytes, and joint space narrowing were graded as absent, mild, moderate, or severe. Subchondral sclerosis and subchondral cysts were graded as present or absent (Fig. 11.11). The accuracy of the model for assessing these five features was 86.7% for femoral osteophytes, 69.9% for acetabular osteophytes, 81.7% for joint space narrowing, 95.8% for subchondral sclerosis, and 97.6% for subchondral cysts in the internal test set of approximately 1500 hip joints, and 82.7% for femoral osteophytes, 65.4% for acetabular osteophytes, 80.8% for joint space narrowing, 88.5% for subchondral sclerosis, and 91.3% (95 of 104) for subchondral cysts in the external test set of approximately 100 hip joints.

AUTOMATED GRADING OF DEGENERATIVE SPINE DISEASE

Because MRI is the most used imaging modality to evaluate spine, a study published in 2017 evaluated MRIs of the lumbar spine using deep CNN twice, first for segmentation and then for characterization.[51,52] The 12,018 intervertebral discs, from 2009 patients, were graded by a radiologist and were then used to train (1) a system to detect and label vertebrae and discs in a given scan and (2) a CNN model that predicts several radiologic gradings. The detection system achieved 95.6% accuracy in terms of disc detection and labeling. The model can produce predictions of multiple pathological gradings that consistently matched those of the radiologist. On a test set of 203 patients, the model achieved accuracy of 95.6% in terms of disc detection and labeling. In addition to spinal canal stenosis grading, other capabilities of their model included grading of disc desiccation, degree of disc narrowing, spondylolisthesis, endplate defects, and marrow signal changes, with a processing time of only one to two min per lumbar MRI.[53]

SKELETAL BONE AGE ASSESSMENT

Bone age assessment is very common and important evaluation in pediatric musculoskeletal imaging but is extremely time-consuming. A study by Spampinato and colleagues compared several deep learning techniques to manual evaluation and found out that the discrepancy for deep learning techniques was only about 0.8 years, which is considered state of art.[54]

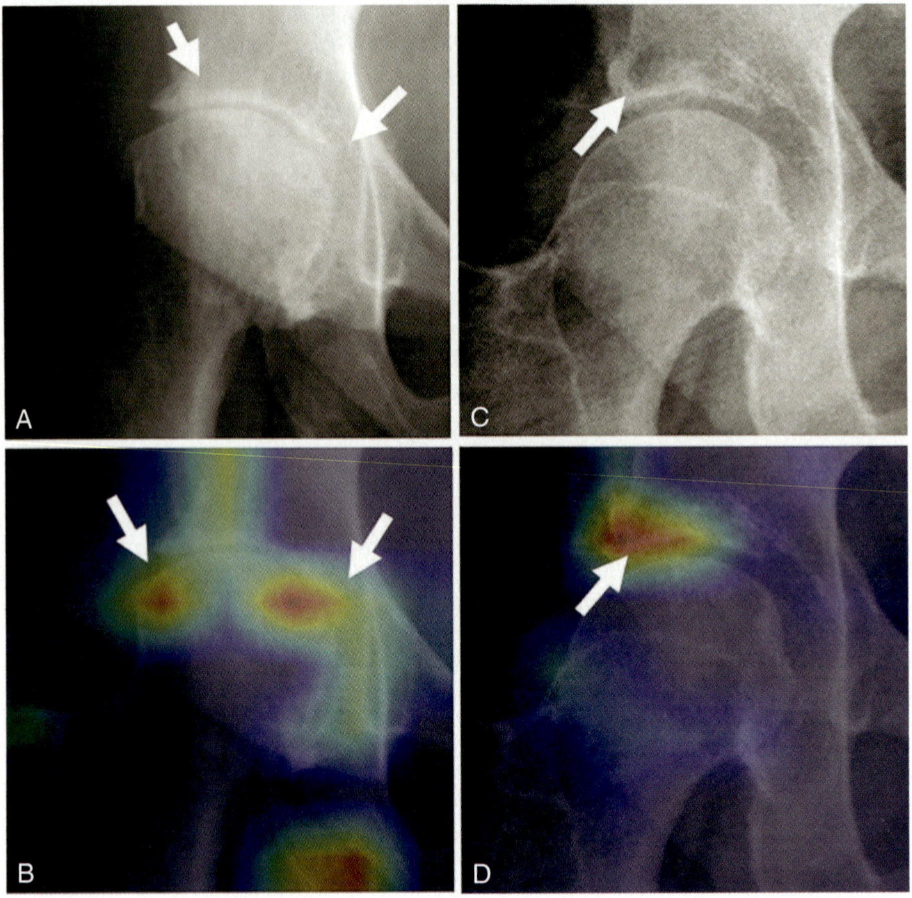

Fig. 11.11 Femoral and acetabular osteophytes, joint space narrowing, subchondral sclerosis, and cysts *(arrows)*, identified as hot spots.[50] (From von Schacky CE, Sohn JH, Liu F, et al. Development and validation of a multitask deep learning model for severity grading of hip osteoarthritis features on radiographs. *Radiology*. 2020;2951:136–145. doi:10.1148/radiol.2020190925.)

NONMUSCULOSKELETAL ASSESSMENT

A study performed by Yao et al. used texture analysis and machine classification on chest CT scans to distinguish between areas of acute infection and chronic fibrosis and quantify features to increase the CT precision for measuring severity and disease progression.[55]

Radiomics and AI from MRI may aid in the noninvasive differentiation of triple negative and luminal A breast cancers from other subtypes.[56]

CNN helping detect high-grade small bowel obstruction with sensitivity of 83% and specificity of 68%. Detection of high-grade small bowel obstruction on conventional radiography with CNNs.[57,58]

ORTHOPEDIC IMPLANT ASSESSMENT

Deep learning can assist musculoskeletal radiologists in the evaluation of orthopedic implants. Assistance can be in identification of implants/models, characterization based on anatomic type, and evaluation for positioning/complications. In addition, NLP can assist in getting relevant clinical information from the electronic medical record. Several proof-of-concept works have been published in the literature describing the application of deep learning toward these various tasks, with performance comparable to that of expert musculoskeletal radiologists.[59,60]

Noninterpretive

PROVIDERS ORDERING RELEVANT IMAGING EXAMINATION

AI algorithms can utilize various information from medical records, including history, laboratory values, physical examination findings, and prior imaging results, to recommend an appropriate patient-specific imaging examination tailored to the clinical question that needs to be answered.[60,61]

PROTOCOLLING EXAMINATIONS

Once the examination is ordered, a significant amount of a practicing radiologist's time is spent reviewing radiology orders and protocolling and planning examinations. Chosen protocols can be suboptimal depending on the expertise of the protocolling radiologist, fellow or resident. Appropriate protocol based on deep learning models could retrieve information on the appropriately ordered examination request but could also potentially mine the medical record, prior examination protocols, prior examination reports, scanner data, contrast agent and injection system data, the cumulative or annual radiation dose, and other quantitative data.[62]

So automated optimal protocol recommendation can help with the flow. A study published by Trivedi et al. utilized deep learning natural language classification system from IBM Watson to automatically determine the need for intravenous contrast for musculoskeletal MRI examinations. The model demonstrated 83% accuracy compared with original protocols.[63]

In another study published in 2018, a CNN-based MRI protocol determinations model was evaluated. Accuracies were evaluated by a radiologist-confirmed protocol as the reference protocols, with a sensitivity of 92.10%, a specificity of 95.76%, and an AUC of 0.977. All MRI protocols were correct in the pelvic bone, upper arm, wrist, and lower leg MRIs.[52]

SCHEDULING

No-shows, reschedules, or same day cancellations add up to lot of missed opportunities for all the radiology department and can lead to significant financial losses.[52] Using medical records data, some AI models can successfully predict imaging no-shows. Harvey et al. developed a model that used 16 data elements and had good ability to predict no-shows with AUC = 0.753.[64] In the future, this type of information can be appropriately utilized without any biases to engage these patients with more personal reminders or other patient-centric interventions.

SAFETY SCREENING

ML-based models are proposed for patient screening.[65,66] These applications have potential to be used for multiple radiology indications, for example, MRI safety screening or prior to contrast administration.

PRIORITIZATION OF STUDIES

Radiologists mostly read emergency department examinations first then they address inpatient and finally outpatient examinations. Some large hospital emergency room study volumes can be very large, and radiologists may not be able to read those examinations within 1 hour. In addition, at times outpatient studies may have emergent findings that cannot get interpretation for hours and at times days, especially on weekends or holidays. AI can help in the triage of all examinations for at least critical or lifesaving findings. There are Food and Drug Administration–approved software to detect pneumothorax.[67]

Critical Care Suite's overall AUC for detecting a pneumothorax is 0.96. Large pneumothoraxes are detected with extremely high accuracy (AUC = 0.99). Small pneumothoraxes are detected with high accuracy (AUC = 0.94) by program used by GE Healthcare 510k K183182, similarly there are commercially used AI tools for brain hemorrhage, which screen all the brain CTs and move suspicious CTs higher on the list to be read in the PACS system.

In 2015 at Ohio State University, a group developed an AI tool using deep learning algorithm to evaluate noncontrast head CT to detect for hemorrhage, mass effect, or hydrocephalus and to determine the performance for detecting suspected acute infarct. The results showed 90% sensitivity and 85% specificity with AUC of 0.91 with the brain window. For suspected acute infarct, the best performance was achieved with the stroke window showing 62% sensitivity and 96% specificity with AUC of 0.81. So, these type of AI features can be added to the workflow to identify cases to be read earlier (smart list) and can help and assist radiologist to pick subtle cases.[68]

AUTOMATED RADIATION DOSE ESTIMATION

AI can be employed to calculate radiation dose. A study by Cho et al. revealed accuracy of higher than 96% in organ mapping and organ-specific radiation dose estimation when employing a deep CNN classifier on CT data sets.[69]

RADIOLOGIST REVIEW OF CLINICAL INFORMATION

Most of the time, radiologists receive minimal clinical information (e.g., history such as fall or pain) with radiology examination request, probably because providers are very busy. It takes significant amount of time and effort for the radiologist to get relevant clinical information. These innovations can help radiologists to make relevant interpretations when they identify a finding and overall increase the sensitivity and specificity of the examinations. It can also assist junior residents to look for relevant finding based on history.[60,70]

IMAGE PRESENTATIONS AND HANGING PROTOCOLS

Radiologists work a lot more efficiently if the PACS systems (which radiologists use to view images) consistently, accurately, and automatically display images in the preferred position, orientation, magnification, window/level, syncing/cross-referencing, relevant modality, body part, laterality, and time (as radiologists hang images in certain way to compare with old images). One PACS vendor uses algorithms to learn how radiologists prefer to view examinations, collect contextual data, present layouts for future similar studies, and adapt after any corrections.[71]

In a study out of University of California–San Francisco, 1885 chest x-rays were identified as frontal or lateral x-rays with 100% accuracy using deep convoluted networks with a fast processing speed of 38 images per second. Interestingly the deep convoluted network used for this study was originally created for nonradiologic images.[55]

As discussed previously, radiology examinations often require comparing with previous studies to determine if the patient has gotten better or worse. AI can help radiologists in syncing, cross-referencing, and co-registering images that were performed in multiple points in time. Currently it is carried out manually by a radiologist, which is very time-consuming.[72,73]

INTEGRATED SMART REPORTS

AI can help integrate the data from images and genetic, laboratory, and clinical data to help make a clinical diagnosis, which is not easy for humans to perform since radiology reports contain a lot of information and most of this information is in free-text format. Due to variations in the reports, extraction of this information for clinical decision-making tools, quality improvement projects, and research is very limited.

Hassanpour et al. designed and developed an unsupervised ML approach to capture key concepts in the imaging reports and divide them based on focus areas. They applied this approach to close to 1.8 million reports, and their method identified 19 major radiology report topics (like chest x-ray, CT abdomen, CT brain, and so on).[74]

To convert free text into structured data, NLP in radiology has several applications like flagging/categorization of findings, imaging protocol generation, patient prioritization, and research. Recently deep learning-based NLP have outperformed traditional methods of NLP.[75]

ARTIFICIAL INTELLIGENCE–BASED RECOMMENDATION IN RADIOLOGY REPORT

Recommendations are integral component of radiology reports. Automatic extraction of recommendations would help with tasks such as recommendation tracking, quality improvement, and large-scale descriptive studies.

Steinkamp et al. presented a neural network architecture capable of extracting fully contextualized recommendations. They identified six major "questions" necessary to capture the majority of context associated with a recommendation: recommendation, time, reason, conditionality, strength, and negation. They annotated 2272 radiology reports and evaluated the performance of a long short-term memory architecture on the six-question task. The model achieves a performance of 89.2% at recommendation extraction and performances between 85% and 95% on extracting modifying features. The model extracts all types of recommendations, including follow-up imaging, tissue biopsies, and clinical correlation and can operate in real time.[76]

These advancements soon can summarize narrative report information, to generate the impression section automatically and suggest standard follow-up recommendation.[77]

Improving Image Quality and Faster Image Acquisitions

AI can assist with correcting imperfections in the images by removing artifacts. It can help with higher-resolution images in shorter acquisition times. AI can help in creating synthetic images within the same modality (like MRI) and can also help create images of one modality (MRI) by using images from other modalities (like x-ray or CT). Some published studies addressing these issues will be discussed in the following paragraphs.

ARTIFACTS

A study published in 2019 by Schilling et al. worked on improving diffusion MRI images, which typically suffer from spatial distortions due to susceptibility. Current state-of-the-art susceptibility correction algorithms typically require data acquired twice. Results show that distortion correction process results in better matching of the geometry of undistorted anatomical images and reduces variation in diffusion modeling in less time.[78]

Deep learning can help with artifact detection, patient motion, and removal of artifacts; alerts can be generated for technologist or radiologist, so they can acquire more images and help them to interpret false-positive clinical findings or correct images for motion after the examination is completed. Head motion during MRI is a significant challenge especially in patients with movement disorders. Duffy et al. presented a 3D CNN model that successfully diminished the severity of artifacts on real motion-affected data. After application of the correction algorithm, the number of quality control failures was reduced from 61 to 38 out of a total of 617 images. They also investigated whether motion correction resulted in statistically significant relationship between cortical thickness and Parkinson's disease. Before correction, significant cortical thinning was found to be restricted to limited regions within the frontal/temporal lobes. After correction, more widespread and significant cortical thinning was identified bilaterally across the frontal/temporal lobes.[79]

HIGHER RESOLUTION

MRI images with high resolutions and signal-to-noise ratios are desired in many clinical and research applications. However, acquiring such images takes a long time, which is both costly and susceptible to motion artifacts.[80]

In 2018 Chaudhari et al. develop a super-resolution technique using CNN (Deep Resolve) for generating thin-slice knee MRIs from thicker input slices and compared with alternative through-plane interpolation methods. Deep Resolve was trained using 124 double echoes in steady-state data sets with 0.7-mm slice thickness and tested on 17 patients. Two musculoskeletal radiologists ranked and reviewed the diagnostic quality of the three data sets (Deep Resolve, tricubic interpolation, and ground-truth images) for sharpness, contrast, artifacts, signal-to-noise ratio, and overall diagnostic quality. Deep Resolve significantly outperformed tricubic interpolation in all image quality categories and overall image ranking.[81]

Zhao et al. used a deep learning approach called Synthetic Multi Orientation Resolution Enhancement (SMORE) and demonstrated improved visualization of brain white matter lesions in fluid-attenuated inversion recovery images acquired from patients with multiple sclerosis. Then approach was shown to improve the visualization of scarring in cardiac left ventricular remodeling after myocardial infarction, obtain multiview images of the tongue, and improve performance in parcellation of the brain ventricular system. Both visual and quantitative metrics of resolution enhancement were demonstrated.[82]

SYNTHETIC IMAGES WITHIN THE SAME MODALITY

Synthesizing high-quality images (which are not acquired) from standard acquired sequences saves time and provides higher-quality evaluation.[83]

SYNTHETIC IMAGES FROM ANOTHER MODALITY

The relatively newer concept of synthesizing CT images from MRI will have a big impact in radiation oncology, although this technique still needs some improvement. Wang et al. in 2019 proposed that U-net algorithm was able to create synthetic CT images based on T2-weighted MRI in patients with nasopharyngeal carcinoma, which took on average 7 seconds per patient. Compared with true CT, mean absolute error of synthetic CT images in all tested patients was 97 ± 13 HU in soft tissue, 131 ± 24 HU in overall region, and 357 ± 44 HU in bone, respectively. The majority of soft tissue and bone region was reconstructed accurately, except the interface between soft tissue and bone and some delicate structures in nasal cavity, where the inaccuracy was induced by imperfect deformable registration.[84]

Deep learning with generative models is gaining interest. Galbusera et al. investigated if conditional generative adversarial networks can generate synthetic images of the lumbar spine (Fig. 11.12). Automated image-to-image translation was tested in the following tasks: (1) from T1-weighted to T2-weighted images and (2) vice versa; (3) from T2-weighted to short time

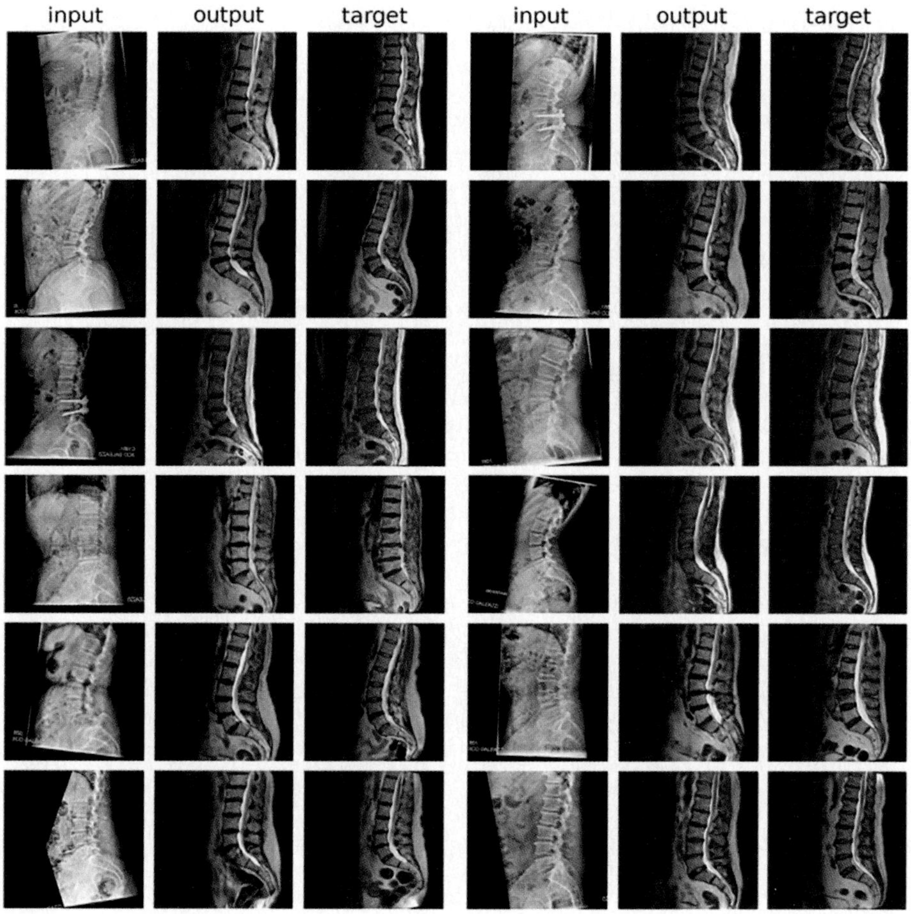

Fig. 11.12 Representative results (12 patients) of the translation from sagittal x-ray projections to T2-weighted (T2W) midsagittal magnetic resonance imaging (MRI) scans. Input: Original x-ray image, registered to match the alignment of the original MRI; output: synthetic T2W midsagittal MRI; target: original T2W midsagittal MRI. A few gross errors in the anatomy can be identified: the L1 in the first and fourth patients on the left; the sacrum in the first patient on the right; the thoracolumbar junction in the second patient on the right; L1 and the sacrum in the fourth patient on the right.[85] (From Galbusera F, Bassani T, Casaroli G, et al. Generative models: an upcoming innovation in musculoskeletal radiology? A preliminary test in spine imaging. *Eur Radiol Exp*. Published 2018. Accessed November 19, 2018. https://www.ncbi.nlm.nih.gov/pmc/articles/PMC6207611/.)

inversion-recovery images; (4) from T2-weighted to turbo inversion recovery magnitude images; (5) from sagittal standing x-ray projections to T2-weighted images. The training of the models was performed on MRI and x-ray images from 989 patients. The performance of the models was generally positive and promising, but with several limitations. Moderate to excellent concordance was found when translating T2-weighted to short time inversion-recovery and turbo inversion recovery magnitude images ($\kappa \geq 0.842$ regarding disc degeneration), although the agreement was poor when translating x-ray to T2-weighted images. Considering the limitations of the study, methods showed the potential to be an upcoming innovation.[85]

Technologist Workflow Improvements

There is a huge potential for AI assisting technologists who may be overworked or may not be well versed especially in performing complex examinations. AI can help technologists primarily in three ways: (1) during scanning, which can result into better image quality; (2) while postprocessing some of the acquired data, which can reduce variation (3); assisting technologists by some self-driving functions, which will improve efficiency and safety.

DURING SCANNING

A team of scientists from Mass General Hospital (MGH) developed an image reconstruction program automated transform by manifold approximation (AUTOMAP) based on data-driven supervised learning using 50,000 MRI brain scans. They found that the signal-to-noise ratio was better for AUTOMAP than conventional reconstruction (21.6 vs. 17.6). In addition, AUTOMAP takes few milliseconds versus conventional reconstruction, which can be very time-consuming. Since AUTOMAP provides instant feedback, it could prevent additional visits for repeat scans.[86,87]

POSTPROCESSING

In 2021, a group performed a study to develop and evaluate an algorithm that can automatically estimate the amount of coronary artery calcium from unenhanced (electrocardiogram)-gated CT cardiac volume acquisitions by using CNNs. The Agatston score (conventional coronary artery calcium scoring) was then computed and compared with the ground truth manually estimated by radiologists. The final model yielded a C-index of 0.951 on the testing set. Errors were mainly observed on small or low-density calcifications or calcifications located near the mitral valve or ring.[88]

SELF-DRIVEN OR PARTIALLY SELF-DRIVEN SCANNERS

AI can help with the lack of standardization in image acquisition between different scanners and sequences. In the world of self-driving cars, self-driving MRI is possible, which will select appropriate protocols based on patient size and clinical history. Similarly, telerobotic sonography is a new technology that can be used to increase access to sonography.[89]

Image Quality Analytics

One or more experienced radiologists in every group are responsible for image quality analysis, which can be very subjective and time-consuming. Using deep learning automated image quality evaluation has been attempted by researchers. For instance, work has been performed to evaluate liver MRI.[90]

Interventional Radiology

Recent development of AI applications also extended into the practice of interventional radiology, including the ability to offer prognostic information about interventional oncology procedures.[91,92]

If an interventional radiology team can use AI to classify patients prior to interventional procedures as a potential responder (complete or partial) or nonresponder with high accuracy, it could be used to decide whether a specific intervention should be performed. Abajian et al. published a study in 2018 in which they created AI framework using MRI and clinical patient data for the prediction of therapeutic outcomes of transarterial chemoembolization by applying ML model with overall predicted accuracy of 78%.[93]

Autonomous navigation during interventional procedures is possible. Fagogenis et al. created a robotic catheter and used it in the most difficult place, which is inside the beating heart. The catheter uses haptic vision, which is a hybrid sense using imaging for both touch-based surface identification and force sensing. Using in vivo animal experiments, they demonstrated that the performance rivaled that of an experienced clinician. It is a capability on which more sophisticated levels of autonomy can be built to perform procedures.[94]

Teaching and Education

Recent advances in virtual and augmented reality and its use in the entertainment and gaming industry led to its use in the field of medical imaging. Radiology services have started exploring the use of these technologies to help with radiology education and clinical care.[95]

Recent advancements in the use of NLP with AI led to a concept of a "virtual patient" for training students, residents, and junior technologists. A virtual patient develops several interactive computer-based clinical scenarios like MRI safety, contrast safety, or radiation exposure risk. This technology can promote a stress-free alternative learning environment.[96]

Conversational Applications

Radiologists spend a significant amount of time answering telephone scall from other physicians/providers, patients, and technologist related to patient safety, quality, or other inquiries. A smart device or web-based chatbots can help with some of these inquiries.

Chetlen et al. used chatbot technology to educate patients before breast biopsies. Survey results from 55 patients showed that a majority stated that the chatbot made it easier to understand their upcoming procedure (Fig. 11.13).[97]

The growing capability of AI and significant need for health care services led to the development of several conversational agents. Most of these agents use NLP so that users can speak or write to the agent as they would to a human. These conversational agents then analyze the input and respond appropriately in a conversational manner. Types of input that conversational agents can receive and interpret have also expanded, with some capable of analyzing movements, such as gestures, facial expressions, and eye movements.[98]

The concept of virtual radiologist is not far-fetched, and advanced conversational agents powered by AI may be able to answer patients', other clinicians', or technologists' questions and queries. Dimeff et al. developed an avatar system (Virtual Collaborative Assessment and Management of Suicidality System) for suicidal patients. Results show acceptance by patients and effectivity in reducing unnecessary hospitalization viewed by physicians.[99]

Virtual Multidisciplinary Conferences

Over the past few years, the approach to treat diseases has switched from a single specialist to treatment by a multidisciplinary team, with the intention of merging the opinions of various experts in an optimum way. Multidisciplinary teams or conferences are the backbone of the decision-making that forms the basis of modern medicine. AI methods can be used to help clinicians and surgeons with decision-making, to reduce errors in judgment and improve differential diagnosis, and thereby improve the choice of treatment and patient outcome. Continuous vigilance of AI models will still be of paramount importance to avoid physicians blindly following the AI-based pathway over the course of patient's treatment.[100]

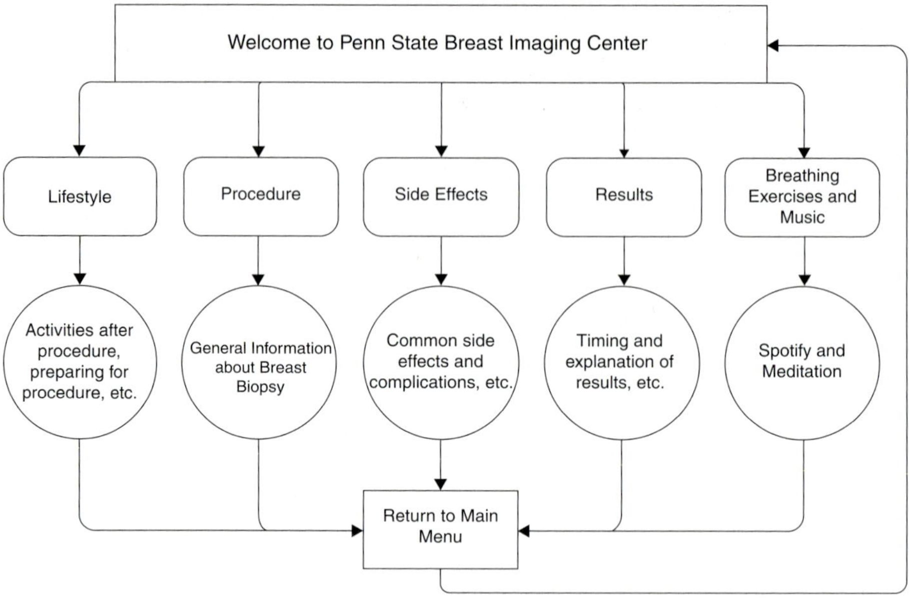

Fig. 11.13 Chatbot options available to patients before breast biopsy at Penn state.[97] (From Chetlen A, Artrip R, Drury B, Arbaiza A, Moore M. Novel use of chatbot technology to educate patients before breast biopsy. *J Am Coll Radiol*. 2019;16(9 Pt B):1305–1308. doi:10.1016/j.jacr.2019.05.050.)

Future Role of Artificial Intelligence and Radiology

It is also important to know the future role of the radiologist in the presence of AI, which could be beyond human perception. For example, a deep learning model by Yune et al.[101] outperformed human readers in determining the sex of a patient based only on hand x-rays, with an accuracy of 95.9% versus accuracies of 46% and 58% by two individual radiologists. The performance of this algorithm suggests that deep learning is capable of extracting or recognizing more imaging features than what is perceived by radiologists.

More use of quantitative data maybe be possible in the future, which is currently available on most of the imaging scans, but interpretation cannot be done due to technique, variability in data, and limited time available to radiologist.

In the future radiology information architecture can look like smartphone architecture, optimum for communication and integration, and could provide a large-channel backbone and many smaller feeding channels for basic functions, as well as those needing to innovate rapidly (Fig. 11.14).

Possible Issues of Artificial Intelligence

As radiologists adapt more and more AI models in their practices, there are some issues they need to be aware of as a consumer.

SENSIBLE ARTIFICIAL INTELLIGENCE

AI should make sense. Big data can be rich with variables, but it can be poor in providing the appropriate clinical context. Radiologists, therefore, must critically evaluate the predictions generated by AI and interpret the data in clinically meaningful ways.[103]

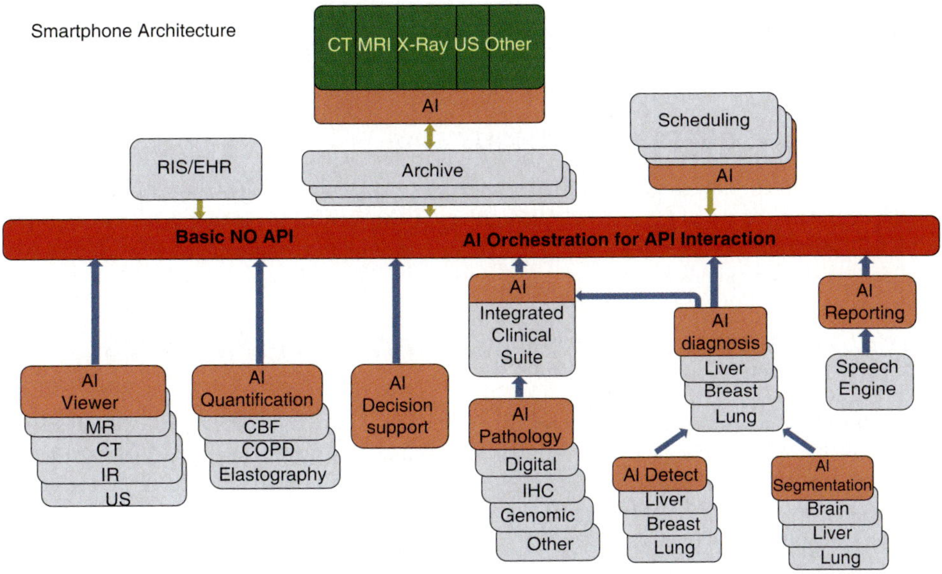

Fig. 11.14 Smartphone architecture. The basic backbone input/output operating system serves as an AI orchestration engine that connects one or more archives and AI-enhanced workflow engines to multiple best of breed applications. These applications with their own AI capabilities can perform tasks such as viewing, quantification, decision support, reporting. They could form integrated clinical suites that include AI-powered detection, diagnosis, segmentation, and genomic and pathology functionality. It is a large- and small-channel branched architecture. The main trunk (red bar) in this diagram provides API interfaces for all the major components of the picture archiving and communication systems (PACS) system, plus multiple other functions, each with its own integrated, embedded AI. It is equivalent to horizontal integration with standard API interfaces. The components with integrated AI can be swapped in and swapped out using best of breed, without the need for dealing with cumbersome specialized interfaces. These AI applications can be used in various ensembles to integrate their functionality and enhance their overall performances and efficacy. Arrow legend: orange = DICOM; aqua = HL7 or Fast Health Interoperability Resources; blue = API. AI, Artificial intelligence; API, application programming interface; CBF, cerebral blood flow; COPD, chronic obstructive pulmonary disease; CT, computed tomography; EHR, electronic health record; IHC, immune histochemistry; IR, interventional radiology; MRI, magnetic resonance imaging; RIS, Radiology Information System; US, ultrasound.[102] (From Enzmann DR, Arnold CW, Zaragoza E, Siegel E, Pfeffer MA. Radiology's information architecture could migrate to one emulating that of smartphones. *J Am Coll Radiol*. 2020;1710:1299–1306. doi:10.1016/j.jacr.2020.03.032.)

BROAD-RANGE UTILITY

The challenge currently for AI is that it is too specific for an organ or disease. For example, chest x-ray can have multiple abnormalities, which can affect bones, lungs, heart, soft tissues mediastinum, and each can have multiple pathologies. Most AI developers are working on one or two specific pathologies. For example, one of the major vendors is already using AI to detect pneumothorax as previously discussed, but that software will not detect any other pathology, for example, a lung nodule.[67]

Critical Care Suite's overall AUC for detecting a pneumothorax is 0.96. Large pneumothoraxes are detected with extremely high accuracy (AUC = 0.99). Small pneumothoraxes are detected with high accuracy (AUC = 0.94) by utilizing software by GE Healthcare 510k K183182. On the other hand, there are AI solutions that can detect nodules but cannot detect pneumothoraxes for example product named. ClearRead XRay by Riverain (riveraintech.com). Therefore, the future challenge will be to make sure that there is merger of all these solutions, otherwise it will not be cost- or time-efficient.

UNIVERSAL ACCEPTANCE WITHOUT BIAS

AI models should be able to work in different settings outside test settings. Clinical data collection biases can affect the type of patterns AI recognizes or the predictions it may make, and this can especially affect minorities and women due to long-standing underrepresentation in clinical trial and patient registry populations.[103]

INITIAL QUALITY AND MAINTENANCE OF QUALITY STANDARDS OF THE MODEL

Food and Drug Administration clearance for AI models is very difficult, because of the performance of their claimed accuracy outside test environment and the long-term maintenance of those models. It is even harder to obtain Food and Drug Administration clearance for an AI system that does not need a radiologist's supervision. For this reason, developers present AI systems as aid tools for radiologists rather than as tools that substitutes them.[104]

LEARNING AND EVER-CHANGING ARTIFICIAL INTELLIGENCE

AI systems are designed to be dynamic and learn from their experiences, and these are by their very nature unpredictable. It is impossible to predict all experiences a system will encounter, and it is not possible to foresee how the system will change. Given the evolving complexity of AI technology, it is almost inevitable that some of its inner workings will appear to be a "black box" to all but the very few who can comprehend how they work.[105]

How is a machine finding those signals? How can we be sure that it is right? How far should we trust deep learning? These are difficult questions, and one roboticist, Hod Lipson, described it very well; to paraphrase it here, imagine if there were aliens that had additional eye color receptors (other than red, blue, and green), then it would be difficult for humans to understand how aliens visualize the world and it would be difficult for aliens to describe it to the humans—it would be like explaining Shakespeare to the dog.

ETHICAL ISSUES

Since radiology will lead the development and implementation of AI algorithms, we should understand and learn how to manage the associated ethical and legal challenges. The white paper from the Canadian Association of Radiologists provides a framework for "the legal and ethical issues related to patient data (privacy, confidentiality, ownership, and sharing); algorithms (levels of autonomy, liability, and jurisprudence); practice (best practices and current legal framework); and finally, opportunities in AI from the perspective of a universal health care system."[106]

LIABILITY ISSUES

Who will be responsible if AI model miss something? Will it be the radiologist or the AI model? In the current malpractice setup, liability is evaluated based on common medical standards of care. The physician is liable if a patient is treated below the common medical standards. With respect to AI or algorithm models, the question is whether the patient would expect the physician to detect an algorithm error or not. If the physician cannot predict how the algorithms makes its decision, the physician will not be liable. If the physician could predict it, he or she will only be liable if the injury caused by the algorithm is more severe than what the patient is expected to tolerate, compared with the severity of the patients actual disease.[23,107]

Acknowledgment

Special thanks to Ms. Rania Khan.

References

1. Hounsfield GN. Computerized transverse axial scanning (tomography) part 1: description of system. *Br J Radiol.* 1973;46:1016–1022.
2. McCorduck P. Machines who think. *Homage to John McCarthy, the Father of Artificial Intelligence (AI)* (artificial-solutions.com). AK Peters: Natick, MA; 2004. 2nd ed. Originally published on June 2, 2017.
3. de Dombal FT, Leaper DJ, Staniland JR, McCann AP, Horrocks JC. Computer-aided diagnosis of acute abdominal pain. *Br Med J.* 1972;2(5804):9–13. https://doi.org/10.1136/bmj.2.5804.9
4. Deng J, Dong W, Socher R, Li L, Li K, Fei-Fei L. ImageNet: A large-scale hierarchical image database | *IEEE Conference Publication* | *IEEE Xplore.* 2009:248–255.
5. He K, Zhang X, Ren S, Sun J. Deep residual learning for image recognition. *2016 IEEE Conference on Computer Vision and Pattern Recognition (CVPR).* 2016:770–778. https://doi.org/10.1109/CVPR.2016.90
6. Syberfeldt A, Ekblom T. A comparative evaluation of the GPU vs. the CPU for parallelization of evolutionary algorithms through multiple independent runs. *Int J Comput Sci Inf Technol (IJCSIT).* 2017;9(3). https://doi.org/10.5121/ijcsit.2017.93011
7. Kim J. Deep learning vs. machine learning vs. AI: an in-depth guide. Readspeaker.ai. Published May 3, 2021. https://www.readspeaker.ai/blog/deep-learning-vs-machine-learning/
8. Borstelmann SM. Machine learning principles for radiology investigators. *Acad Radiol.* 2020;27(1):13–25.
9. Langs G, Röhrich S, Hofmanninger J, et al. Machine learning: from radiomics to discovery and routine. Radiologe. 2018;58(1):1–6. https://doi.org/10.1007/s00117-018-0407-3
10. Nemoto M, Masutani Y, Nomura Y, et al. Machine learning for computer-aided diagnosis. Igaku Butsuri. 2016;36(1):29–34. Japanese. https://doi.org/10.11323/jjmp.36.1_29
11. Lodwick GS, Keats TE, Dorst JP. The coding of Roentgen images for computer analysis as applied to lung cancer. *Radiology.* 1963;81:185–200.
12. Lodwick GS. Computer-aided diagnosis in radiology. A research plan. *Invest Radiol.* 1966;1(1):72–80.
13. van Ginneken B, Schaefer-Prokop CM, Prokop M. Computer-aided diagnosis: how to move from the laboratory to the clinic. Radiology. 2011;261(3):719–732. https://doi.org/10.1148/radiol.11091710
14. Sonka M, Hlavác V, Boyle R. *Image processing, analysis, and machine vision.* 3rd ed. Thomson Learning; 2007.
15. Do S, Song KD, Chung JW. Basics of deep learning: a radiologist's guide to understanding published radiology articles on deep learning. *Korean J Radiol.* 2020;21(1):33–41. https://doi.org/10.3348/kjr.2019.0312
16. Caudill M. Neural networks primer, part I. *AI Expert.* 1987;2(12):46–52.
17. Simonyan K, Zisserman A. Very deep convolutional networks for large-scale image recognition. Computer Vision and Pattern Recognition, Cornell University. Submitted on September 4, 2014 (v1), last revised on 10 Apr 2015 (this version, v6)]. https://ieeexplore.ieee.org/abstract/document/7486599
18. Szegedy C, Liu W, Jia Y, et al. Going deeper with convolutions. Computer Vision and Pattern Recognition. Cornell University. Submitted on September 17, 2014. https://ieeexplore.ieee.org/abstract/document/7486599
19. Lee C, Kim Y, Kim YS, Jang J. Automatic disease annotation from radiology reports using artificial intelligence implemented by a recurrent neural network. *AJR Am J Roentgenol.* 2019;212:734–740.
20. Girshick R, Donahue J, Darrell T, Malik J. Rich feature hierarchies for accurate object detection and semantic segmentation. Eprint arXiv, 2013. Accessed April 1, 2019. https://ui.adsabs.harvard.edu/abs/2013arXiv1311.2524G
21. Kazuhiro K, Werner RA, Toriumi F, Javadi MS, Pomper MG, Solnes LB, et al. Generative adversarial networks for the creation of realistic artificial brain magnetic resonance images. *Tomography.* 2018;4:159–163.

22. Goodfellow IJ, Pouget-Abadie J, Mirza M, et al. Generative adversarial networks. Eprint arXiv, 2014. Accessed April 1, 2019. https://ui.adsabs.harvard.edu/abs/2014arXiv1406.2661G
23. Chea P, Mandell JC. Current applications and future directions of deep learning in musculoskeletal radiology. *Skeletal Radiol.* 2020;49(2):183–197. https://doi.org/10.1007/s00256-019-03284-z
24. Aerts HJWL. The potential of radiomic-based phenotyping in precision medicine: a review. *JAMA Oncol.* 2016;2(12):1636–1642. https://doi.org/10.1001/jamaoncol.2016.2631.
25. Kumar V, Gu Y, Basu S, et al. Radiomics: the process and the challenges. *Magn Reson Imaging.* 2012;30(9):1234–1248. https://doi.org/10.1016/j.mri.2012.06.010
26. Lambin P, Rios-Velazquez E, Leijenaar R, et al. Radiomics: extracting more information from medical images using advanced feature analysis. *Eur J Cancer.* 2012;48(4):441–446. https://doi.org/10.1016/j.ejca.2011.11.036
27. Yin P, Mao N, Zhao C, et al. Comparison of radiomics machine-learning classifiers and feature selection for differentiation of sacral chordoma and sacral giant cell tumour based on 3D computed tomography features. *Eur Radiol.* 2019;29:1841–1847.
28. Gottumukkala RV, Le TQ, Duszak R Jr, Prabhakar AM. Radiologists are actually well positioned to innovate in patient experience. *Curr Probl Diagn Radiol.* 2018;47(4):206–208.
29. McDonald RJ, Schwartz KM, Eckel LJ, et al. The effects of changes in utilization and technological advancements of cross-sectional imaging on radiologist workload. *Acad Radiol.* 2015;22(9):1191–1198. https://doi.org/10.1016/j.acra.2015.05.007
30. Rosenkrantz AB, Hughes DR, Duszak R Jr. The U.S. radiologist workforce: an analysis of temporal and geographic variation by using large national datasets. Published October 28, 2015. https://doi.org/10.1148/radiol.2015150921
31. https://www.diagnosticimaging.com/articles/radiologys-future-rests-training-and-education
32. http://www.ajronline.org/doi/full/10.2214/ajr.12.10375
33. Brady AP. Error and discrepancy in radiology: inevitable or avoidable? *Insights Imaging.* 2017;8(1): 171–182. https://doi.org/10.1007/s13244-016-0534-1
34. Newman-Toker DE, Pronovost PJ. Diagnostic errors: the next frontier for patient safety. *JAMA.* 2009;301:1060–1062.
35. Johnson CD, Krecke KN, Miranda R, Roberts CC, Denham D. Developing a radiology quality and safety program: a primer. Published July, 1 2009. https://doi.org/10.1148/rg.294095006
36. Gore JC. Artificial intelligence in medical imaging. *Magn Reson Imaging.* 2020;68:A1–A4. https://doi.org/10.1016/j.mri.2019.12.006
37. Rajpurkar P, Irvin J, Bagul A, et al. MURA: large dataset for abnormality detection in musculoskeletal radiographs. Published 2017. Accessed April 8, 2019. https://arxiv.org/abs/1712.06957v4
38. Liang S, Gu Y Towards robust and accurate detection of abnormalities in musculoskeletal radiographs with a multi-network model. Sensors (Basel). 2020;20(11):3153. https://doi.org/10.3390/s20113153
39. Burns JE, Yao J, Summers RM Vertebral body compression fractures and bone density: automated detection and classification on CT images. Radiology. 2017;284(3):788–797. https://doi.org/10.1148/radiol.2017162100
40. Olczak J, Fahlberg N, Maki A, et al. Artificial intelligence for analyzing orthopedic trauma radiographs. *Acta Orthop.* 2017;88(6):581–586. https://doi.org/10.1080/17453674.2017.1344459
41. Urakawa T, Tanaka Y, Goto S, Matsuzawa H, Watanabe K, Endo N. Detecting intertrochanteric hip fractures with orthopedist-level accuracy using a deep convolutional neural network. *Skeletal Radiol.* 2019;48(2):239–244. https://doi.org/10.1007/s00256-018-3016-3
42. Liu F, Zhou Z, Samsonov A, et al. Deep learning approach for evaluating knee MR images: achieving high diagnostic performance for cartilage lesion detection. *Radiology.* 2018;289(1):160–169. https://doi.org/10.1148/radiol.2018172986
43. Bien N, Rajpurkar P, Ball RL, et al. Deep-learning-assisted diagnosis for knee magnetic resonance imaging: development and retrospective validation of MRNet. *PLoS Med.* 2018;15(11):e1002699. https://doi.org/10.1371/journal.pmed.1002699
44. Liu CF, Paddy S, Ramachandran S, et al. Using deep Siamese neural networks for detection of brain asymmetries associated with Alzheimer's disease and mild cognitive impairment. *Magn Reson Imaging.* 2019;64:190–199.
45. Lee H, Troschel FM, Tajmir S, et al. Pixel-level deep segmentation: artificial intelligence quantifies muscle on computed tomography for body morphometric analysis. *J Digit Imaging.* 2017;30(4):487–498. https://doi.org/10.1007/s10278-017-9988-z

46. Gaj S, Yang M, Nakamura K, Li X. Automated cartilage and meniscus segmentation of knee MRI with conditional generative adversarial networks. *Magn Reson Med.* 2019;84(1):437–449. https://doi.org/10.1002/mrm.28111
47. Schmaranzer F, Helfenstein R, Zeng G, et al. Automatic MRI-based three-dimensional models of hip cartilage provide improved morphologic and biochemical analysis. *Clin Orthop Relat Res.* 2019;477(5):1036–1052. https://doi.org/10.1097/CORR.0000000000000755
48. Hu P, Wu F, Peng J, Bao Y, Chen F, Kong D. Automatic abdominal multi-organ segmentation using deep convolutional neural network and time-implicit level sets. *Int J Comput Assist Radiol Surg.* 2017;12(3):399–411. https://doi.org/10.1007/s11548-016-1501-5
49. Antony J, McGuinness K, Connor NEO, Moran K. Quantifying radiographic knee osteoarthritis severity using deep convolutional neural networks. ArXiv160902469 Cs. Published 2016. Accessed January 21, 2019. http://arxiv.org/abs/1609.02469
50. von Schacky CE, Sohn JH, Liu F, et al. Development and validation of a multitask deep learning model for severity grading of hip osteoarthritis features on radiographs. *Radiology.* 2020;295(1):136–145. https://doi.org/10.1148/radiol.2020190925
51. Lee YH. Efficiency improvement in a busy radiology practice: determination of musculoskeletal magnetic resonance imaging protocol using deep-learning convolutional neural networks. *J Digit Imaging.* 2018;31(5):604–610. https://doi.org/10.1007/s10278-018-0066-y
52. Mieloszyk RJ, Rosenbaum JI, Hall CS, Raghavan UN, Bhargava P. The Financial burden of missed appointments: uncaptured revenue due to outpatient no-shows in radiology. *Curr Probl Diagn Radiol.* 2018;47(5):285–286. https://doi.org/10.1067/j.cpradiol.2018.06.001
53. Jamaludin A, Lootus M, Kadir T, et al. ISSLS Prize in Bioengineering Science 2017: automation of reading of radiological features from magnetic resonance images (MRIs) of the lumbar spine without human intervention is comparable with an expert radiologist. *Eur Spine J.* 2017;26(5):1374–1383. https://doi.org/10.1007/s00586-017-4956-3
54. Spampinato C, Palazzo S, Giordano D, Aldinucci M, Leonardi R. Deep learning for automated skeletal bone age assessment in X-ray images. *Med Image Anal.* 2017;36:41–51. https://doi.org/10.1016/j.media.2016.10.010
55. Yao J, Dwyer A, Summers RM, Mollura DJ. Computer-aided diagnosis of pulmonary infections using texture analysis and support vector machine classification. Acad Radiol. 2011;18(3):306–314. https://doi.org/10.1016/j.acra.2010.11.013
56. Leithner D, Mayerhoefer ME, Martinez DF, et al. Non-invasive assessment of breast cancer molecular subtypes with multiparametric magnetic resonance imaging radiomics. *J Clin Med.* 2020;9(6):1853. https://doi.org/10.3390/jcm9061853
57. Cheng PM, Tejura TK, Tran KN, Whang G. Detection of high-grade small bowel obstruction on conventional radiography with convolutional neural networks. *Abdom Radiol (NY).* 2018;43(5):1120–1127. https://doi.org/10.1007/s00261-017-1294-1
58. Cheng PM, Tran KN, Whang G, Tejura TK. Refining convolutional neural network detection of small-bowel obstruction in conventional radiography. *AJR Am J Roentgenol.* 2019;212(2):342–350. https://doi.org/10.2214/AJR.18.20362
59. Yi PH, Mutasa S, Fritz J. AI MSK clinical applications: orthopedic implants. *Skeletal Radiol.* 2022;51(2):305–313. https://doi.org/10.1007/s00256-021-03879-5
60. Gyftopoulos S, Lin D, Knoll F, Doshi AM, Rodrigues TC, Recht MP. Artificial intelligence in musculoskeletal imaging: current status and future directions. *AJR Am J Roentgenol.* 2019;213(3):506–513. https://doi.org/10.2214/AJR.19.21117
61. Lakhani P, Prater AB, Hutson RK, et al. Machine learning in radiology: applications beyond image interpretation. *J Am Coll Radiol.* 2018;15(2):350–359. https://doi.org/10.1016/j.jacr.2017.09.044
62. Kohli M, Dreyer KJ, Geis JR. Rethinking radiology informatics. *AJR Am J Roentgenol.* 2015;204(4):716–720. https://doi.org/10.2214/AJR.14.13840
63. Trivedi H, Mesterhazy J, Laguna B, Vu T, Sohn JH. Automatic determination of the need for intravenous contrast in musculoskeletal MRI examinations using IBM Watson's natural language processing algorithm. *J Digit Imaging.* 2018;31(2):245–251. https://doi.org/10.1007/s10278-017-0021-3
64. Harvey HB, Liu C, Ai J, et al. Predicting no-shows in radiology using regression modeling of data available in the electronic medical record. *J Am Coll Radiol.* 2017;14:1303–1309.

65. Marella WM, Sparnon E, Finley E. Screening electronic health record-related patient safety reports using machine learning. *J Patient Saf.* 2017;13(1):31–36.
66. Fong A, Howe JL, Adams KT, Ratwani RM. Using active learning to identify health information technology related patient safety events. *Appl Clin Inform.* 2017;8(1):35–46.
67. 08c67ebb6bc747ae953f39c061a93562.pdf (gehealthcare.com)
68. Prevedello LM, Erdal BS, Ryu JL, et al. Automated critical test findings identification and online notification system using artificial intelligence in imaging. *Radiology.* 2017;285(3):923–931. https://doi.org/10.1148/radiol.2017162664
69. Cho J, Lee E, Lee H, et al. Machine learning powered automatic organ classification for patient specific organ dose estimation. Paper presented at: SIIM 2017 Scientific Session. Thursday, June 1 - Saturday, June 3, 2017 at the David L. Lawrence Convention Center, Pittsburgh, PA.
70. Davatzikos C, Sotiras A, Fan Y, et al. Precision diagnostics based on machine learning-derived imaging signatures. *Magn Reson Imaging.* 2019;64:49–61.
71. Wang T, Iankoulski A Intelligent tools for a productive radiologist workflow: how machine learning enriches hanging protocols. GE Healthcare | Centricity Universal Viewer | White Paper.
72. Schemmel A, Lee M, Hanley T, et al. Radiology workflow disruptors: a detailed analysis. *J Am Coll Radiol.* 2016;13(10):1210–1214. https://doi.org/10.1016/j.jacr.2016.04.009
73. Doshi AM, Moore WH, Kim DC, et al. Informatics solutions for driving an effective and efficient radiology practice. *Radiographics.* 2018;38(6):1810–1822. https://doi.org/10.1148/rg.2018180037
74. Hassanpour S, Langlotz CP. Unsupervised topic modeling in a large free text radiology report repository. *J Digit Imaging.* 2016;29(1):59–62. https://doi.org/10.1007/s10278-015-9823-3
75. Sorin V, Barash Y, Konen E, Klang E. Deep learning for natural language processing in radiology-fundamentals and a systematic review. *J Am Coll Radiol.* 2020;17(5):639–648. https://doi.org/10.1016/j.jacr.2019.12.026
76. Steinkamp J, Chambers C, Lalevic D, Cook T. Automatic fully-contextualized recommendation extraction from radiology reports. *J Digit Imaging.* 2021;34(2):374–384. https://doi.org/10.1007/s10278-021-00423-8
77. Kahn CE Jr, Langlotz CP, Burnside ES, et al. Toward best practices in radiology reporting. *Radiology.* 2009;252(3):852–856. https://doi.org/10.1148/radiol.2523081992
78. Schilling KG, Blaber J, Huo Y, et al. Synthesized b0 for diffusion distortion correction (Synb0-DisCo). *Magn Reson Imaging.* 2019;64:62–70. https://doi.org/10.1016/j.mri.2019.05.008
79. Duffy BA, Zhao L, Sepehrband F, et al. Retrospective motion artifact correction of structural MRI images using deep learning improves the quality of cortical surface reconstructions. *Neuroimage.* 2021;230:117756. https://doi.org/10.1016/j.neuroimage.2021.117756
80. You X, Cao N, Lu H, Mao M, Wang W. Denoising of MR images with Rician noise using a wider neural network and noise range division. *Magn Reson Imaging.* 2019;64:154–159.
81. Chaudhari AS, Fang Z, Kogan F, et al. Super-resolution musculoskeletal MRI using deep learning. *Magn Reson Med.* 2018;80(5):2139–2154. https://doi.org/10.1002/mrm.27178
82. Zhao C, Shaoa M, Carassa A, et al. Applications of a deep learning method for anti-aliasing and super-resolution in MRI. *Magn Reson Imaging.* 2019;64:132–141.
83. Ryu K, Shin NY, Kim DH, Nam Y. Synthesizing T1 weighted MPRAGE image from multi echo GRE images via deep neural network. *Magn Reson Imaging.* 2019;64:13–20.
84. Wang Y, Liu C, Zhang X, Deng W. Synthetic CT generation based on T2 weighted MRI of nasopharyngeal carcinoma (NPC) Using a deep convolutional neural network (DCNN). *Front Oncol.* 2019;9:1333. https://doi.org/10.3389/fonc.2019.01333
85. Galbusera F, Bassani T, Casaroli G, et al. Generative models: an upcoming innovation in musculoskeletal radiology? A preliminary test in spine imaging. Eur Radiol Exp. Published 2018. Accessed November 19, 2018. https://www.ncbi.nlm.nih.gov/pmc/articles/PMC6207611/
86. Zhu B, Liu JZ, Cauley SF, Rosen BR, Rosen MS. Image reconstruction by domain-transform manifold learning. *Nature.* 2018;555(7697):487–492. https://doi.org/10.1038/nature25988
87. https://www.nmr.mgh.harvard.edu/lfi/pdf/AUTOMAP_NatureMethods.pdf
88. Gogin N, Viti M, Nicodème L, et al. Automatic coronary artery calcium scoring from unenhanced-ECG-gated CT using deep learning. *Diagn Interv Imaging.* 2021;102(11):683–690. https://doi.org/10.1016/j.diii.2021.05.004

89. Adams SJ, Burbridge B, Obaid H, Stoneham G, Babyn P, Mendez I. Telerobotic sonography for remote diagnostic imaging: narrative review of current developments and clinical applications. *J Ultrasound Med.* 2021;40(7):1287–1306. https://doi.org/10.1002/jum.15525
90. Esses SJ, Lu X, Zhao T, et al. Automated image quality evaluation of T2 -weighted liver MRI utilizing deep learning architecture. J Magn Reson Imaging. 2018;47(3):723–728. https://doi.org/10.1002/jmri.25779
91. Iezzi R, Goldberg SN, Merlino B, Posa A, Valentini V, Manfredi R. Artificial intelligence in interventional radiology: a literature review and future perspectives. *J Oncol.* 2019;2019:6153041. https://doi.org/10.1155/2019/6153041
92. Gurgitano M, Angileri SA, Rodà GM, et al. Interventional radiology ex-machina: impact of artificial intelligence on practice. *Radiol Med.* 2021;126(7):998–1006. https://doi.org/10.1007/s11547-021-01351-x
93. Abajian A, Murali N, Savic LJ, et al. Predicting treatment response to intra-arterial therapies for hepatocellular carcinoma with the use of supervised machine learning—an artificial intelligence concept. *J Vasc Interv Radiol.* 2018;29(6):850–857.e1. https://doi.org/10.1016/j.jvir.2018.01.769
94. Fagogenis G, Mencattelli M, Machaidze Z, et al. Autonomous robotic intracardiac catheter navigation using haptic vision. *Sci Robot.* 2019;4(29):eaaw1977. https://doi.org/10.1126/scirobotics.aaw1977
95. Uppot RN, Laguna B, McCarthy CJ, et al. Implementing virtual and augmented reality tools for radiology education and training, communication, and clinical care. *Radiology.* 2019;291:570–580. https://doi.org/10.1148/radiol.2019182210
96. Isaza-Restrepo A, Gómez MT, Cifuentes G, Argüello A. The virtual patient as a learning tool: a mixed quantitative qualitative study. *BMC Med Educ.* 2018;18(1):297. https://doi.org/10.1186/s12909-018-1395-8
97. Chetlen A, Artrip R, Drury B, Arbaiza A, Moore M. Novel use of chatbot technology to educate patients before breast biopsy. *J Am Coll Radiol.* 2019;16(9 Pt B):1305–1308. https://doi.org/10.1016/j.jacr.2019.05.050
98. Milne-Ives M, de Cock C, Lim E, et al. The effectiveness of artificial intelligence conversational agents in health care: systematic review. *J Med Internet Res.* 2020;22(10):e20346. https://doi.org/10.2196/20346
99. Dimeff LA, Jobes DA, Chalker SA, et al. A novel engagement of suicidality in the emergency department: virtual collaborative assessment and management of suicidality. *Gen Hosp Psychiatry.* 2020;63:119–126. https://doi.org/10.1016/j.genhosppsych.2018.05.005
100. Di Ieva A. AI-augmented multidisciplinary teams: hype or hope? *Lancet.* 2019;394(10211):1801. https://doi.org/10.1016/S0140-6736(19)32626-1
101. Yune S, Lee H, Kim M, Tajmir SH, Gee MS, Do S. Beyond human perception: sexual dimorphism in hand and wrist radiographs is discernible by a deep learning model. *J Digit Imaging.* 2019;32(4):665–671. https://doi.org/10.1007/s10278-018-0148-x
102. Enzmann DR, Arnold CW, Zaragoza E, Siegel E, Pfeffer MA. Radiology's information architecture could migrate to one emulating that of smartphones. *J Am Coll Radiol.* 2020;17(10):1299–1306. https://doi.org/10.1016/j.jacr.2020.03.032
103. Hashimoto DA, Rosman G, Rus D, Meireles OR. Artificial intelligence in surgery: promises and perils. *Ann Surg.* 2018;268(1):70–76. https://doi.org/10.1097/SLA.0000000000002693
104. Recht M, Bryan RN. Artificial intelligence: threat or boon to radiologists? *J Am Coll Radiol.* 2017;14(11):1476–1480. https://doi.org/10.1016/j.jacr.2017.07.007
105. Castelvecchi D. Can we open the black box of AI? *Nature.* 2016;538(7623):20–23. https://doi.org/10.1038/538020a
106. Jaremko JL, Azar M, Bromwich R, et al. Canadian Association of Radiologists white paper on ethical and legal issues related to artificial intelligence in radiology. *Can Assoc Radiol J.* 2019;70(2):107–118. https://doi.org/10.1016/j.carj.2019.03.001
107. Aagaard L. Artificial intelligence decision support systems and liability for medical injuries. *J Res Pharm Pract.* 2020;9(3):125–127. https://doi.org/10.4103/jrpp.JRPP_20_65

12

The Future of Robots in Medicine

Douglas P. Murphy

KEY POINTS

- Robotics and artificial intelligence (AI) are radically changing rehabilitative medicine and medicine in general.
- The near future of robotics in medicine exists now in various start-up companies across the world.
- Robotics and AI may displace some workers but in general they are meant to enhance, extend, and complement the operations of health-care workers.

On a city side street at night a body lies motionless on the sidewalk. A passerby notes the fallen individual, a man in a coat with the top open revealing a dark suit and white shirt, and after shaking the man without any response, calls 911. The passerby waits for several minutes and then an ambulance shows up with its lights flashing, easing to a stop in front of the unconscious individual. The doors in the back of the ambulance split open and from inside a stretcher is lowered to the sidewalk with two robotic arms that place it parallel to the motionless form.[1] The stretcher is merely inches from the surface of the cement. The robotic arms lower a cloth over the man, and this cloth, with billions of nanosensors, immediately starts reading a multitude of physiologic parameters that are connected via Bluetooth to the artificial intelligence (AI) systems on the ambulance and simultaneously to a central cloud that registers in the emergency room of a nearby hospital. Pulse is rapid, blood pressure is low, but oxygen saturation levels are good. The electrocardiogram registers a potential myocardial infarction. The robotic arms lift the man swiftly onto the stretcher and then pull the stretcher into the ambulance as the back doors close automatically. Electric and driverless, the ambulance moves off without a sound. Inside the ambulance robotic arms grab the man's arm and slip it into a machine that quicky locates a vein through its ultrasound system and then inserts an intracatheter, which is connected to intravenous saline. Another robotic arm ensures oxygen is being delivered to the man through a mask.

When the ambulance arrives at the emergency room, a robotic transport vehicle is waiting, and the transfer from ambulance to the robotic vehicle goes smoothly and quickly, and soon the vehicle has taken the man into one of the treatment bays. Monitors light up with the patient's vital statistics, which are as comprehensive as any intensive care unit. Electrocardiogram, heart rate, oxygen levels, respiratory rate, and so on are all displayed.

Within minutes the doctor arrives. The doctor has already downloaded the transport and arrival information from the cloud system and has begun to process clinical information from its databank of millions of chart records and journal articles and textbooks. The doctor is a robot with its own AI system that is also connected to a hospital AI system. Orders are nearly instantaneously transmitted to the cloud system to notify pharmacy so that treatment can begin almost immediately. Hours later the man opens his eyes to find himself in a hospital bed with a friendly and caring nurse bending over him and smiling.

"How are you feeling, Mr. Smith?" The man's identity through a flawless facial recognition system had already been determined and his wife notified. His wife stood on the other side of the bed.

From the previous chapters, one can see that robots are rapidly making inroads into the health-care industry. From the previous chapters, one can also see that several categories of robots are impacting the health-care sector. These types include surgical, modular, service, social, mobile, and autonomous robots. However, these inroads are barely if at all perceptible to most people accessing medical care. In the future, most likely, this status will change and almost everyone will encounter robots either directly or indirectly when going through the medical system either on an inpatient or an outpatient basis. Robots with autonomous or semiautonomous operating systems using AI will provide advantages for service and health delivery that will be too hard to pass up. These robotic systems could come in virtually any form or potentially without form. These systems will offer benefits of speed and technical efficiency and will bring greater depths and ranges of scientific expertise into clinics and outpatient offices.

But exactly what do experts in these areas anticipate these advantages to be? Certainly, now the germs of the future 5, 10, and 20 years from now have been created. In the following pages the future of robotics can be seen through companies that have started to create that future. An article in *Fortune* on March 3, 2019, by Jeremy Khan indicated that funding for AI-assisted drug discovery had increased by 4.5 times to $13.8 billion compared with the previous year.[2] In an article in *Towards Data Science* on December 2, 2019, by Henri Heinomen, the amount of revenue growth from the use of AI software will increase from $9.5 billion in 2018 to $118.6 billion in 2025.[3] In an article in *Cision* on November 2, 2020, the future growth of the US robotics market would extend from $76.6 billion in 2020 to $176.8 billion in 2025 with a compound annual growth rate (CAGR) of 18.2%.

A sure indicator for the global interest, commitment, and level of development for robotics and AI would include the amount of funding being poured into academic programs as well as businesses rushing to compete in this market. An article in *National Defense* on February 10, 2021 by Jon Harper indicated a figure of around $6 billion of federal money being applied to these areas.[4] Undoubtedly this amount will grow.

Of course, one could not talk about the future of robots in medicine without talking about AI, as the two areas are inextricably linked together and, in many cases, AI provides the operating system for robots. AI itself is experiencing tremendous growth through an outpouring of funding and research activity. AI is based in computer chips and mechanistic constructions, but in process are also biomechanistic models with intelligent operating systems based both in biological constructs such as DNA as well as computer chips. AI benefits from the attributes of both worlds. AI has traditionally run under two models: the rules-based one or the neural networks type. The latter has resulted in the deep learning systems that have taken the field forward in quantum leaps. Rules-based systems operate on a series of rules such as if x is true then y. However, this type lacked the complexity to handle many real-world problems. The neural networks approach attempts to duplicate the actual functioning of the brain and mind. The computer structure consists of layers of neural networks. Large quantities of data are fed to the computer to allow the computer to establish the patterns within the data. Three factors comprise the key to successful deep learning: (1) computing power; (2) technical expertise; (3) the amount of data available for programming. China at this point has a reservoir of data greater than the United States and Europe combined.[5] Also, there are four factors that underpin the commercial development of AI: (1) governmental supports; (2) engineers with technical expertise; (3) entrepreneurial grittiness; (4) abundant data. Through its deep-rooted system of managing social and commercial intercourse through apps such as WeChat, China has surpassed all other nations in its collection of data that can be employed in the development of AI.[6] In addition to elite scientists leading discoveries and innovation, there must also be a large cadre of competent but not necessarily brilliant engineers and scientists to provide real-world practical applications. The seven giants of the AI age include Google, Facebook, Microsoft, Baidu, Alibaba, and Tencent.[7]

So, let us delve into the future and see what current projections tell us about the relationship of mankind to robots and AI in the area of health care. Undoubtedly there could be many versions of this future, but we will try to look at the most promising ones. Currently speculation or perhaps concerns arise that robots or AI systems will replace doctors, nurses, and pharmacists. Developers have already stated that radiologists are no longer necessary because AI systems have achieved a capacity for accuracy in reading images that surpasses human physicians. This statement was made years ago and yet it has not happened. Most envision a world where AI and robot systems enhance the capabilities of humans in the delivery of health care rather than the future where humans are replaced. Part of the capacity for achieving the current feats in narrow AI come from the ability of new computers to handle vast quantities of data. Interestingly the gaming world has contributed the graphics processing unit, or GPU, to make such feats possible particularly in the processing of images. The current GPU has a greater capacity than a supercomputer of several years ago and is small enough to be carried in your hands. Other concerns center around the machines developing social biases that would not and should not be tolerated in the workforce. Timnit Gebru, a computer scientist with undergraduate and graduate degrees from Stanford and who has interests and expertise in algorithmic biases and data mining, felt that large AI systems could develop racial biases and that having AI teams of diverse racial backgrounds would help curtail that possibility.

Surgical robots have captured a lot of media attention, and for the most part, these are controlled through surgeons to ensure good technique and outcomes. However, the additional input of robots adds advantages of fatigue and tremor resistance, scalability, and greater axial movement. These enhancements have decreased morbidity for certain procedures.[8] However, the emergence of autonomous, surgical robots driven by AI systems has opened an interesting new development. For example, in an experimental setting, Shademan et al.[9] performed experiments where an autonomous robot anastomosed porcine intestine using the Smart Tissue Autonomous Robot (STAR) with a capacity that exceeded the reach of human surgeons. Currently systems that include some level of autonomy include the da Vinci (Intuitive Surgical, Sunnyvale, California), which has a master-slave control, the TSolution-One orthopedic robot (THINK Surgical, Fremont, California), and the Mazor X spinal robot (Mazor Robotics, Caesarea, Israel). Undoubtedly in the future certain surgical procedures will be performed autonomously by robots controlled through advanced AI systems.

Any discussion of the future of robotics in medicine would not be complete without a thorough discussion of the role of AI. As it stands now, many robotic machines are enhanced through the integration of AI and machine learning (ML). ML involves the integration of algorithms whereby the AI learns through data and experiences and enhances its own functionality through the newly learned information. Therefore, the evolutionary destination of any AI system fitted with ML has a certain level of unpredictability. A neuron in the human brain can fire at a rate of 200 Hz, whereas a computer can have its transistors fire in the gigahertz range. These aspects raise the long-standing question of whether robots and AI will outstrip humans in autonomous intellectual skills and in the ability to manipulate and control the environment and instigate the fear that these machines may ultimately gain control of humanity and its cultures. Certainly, it would make sense to incorporate safeguards and controls at these early stages before such a reality ever presented itself.

AI generally falls into two different categories: narrow AI and artificial general intelligence. One burgeoning area is for AI to take a hand in its own development to accelerate the advancement of AI capacities. It is natural that self-aware machines with intelligence would have goals that would not be human goals. AI is constructed to adopt our goals. However, even with performances that outshine radiologists, the algorithm in AI will eventually make a mistake, which will fall back on the doctor.

Constance Lehman, MD, PhD, professor of radiology at Harvard Medical School, is working toward the integration of AI technology into breast imaging and sees these opportunities for the future: (1) an increase in patient access to imaging; (2) an increase in safety through the reduction of errors; (3) an increase in the opportunities for radiologists to directly engage with patients; (4) the provision of cost reductions for these services.[10] A recent Stanford study found that AI could read fractures in wrist and finger x-rays better than radiologists, although the latter performed better with elbows, forearms, and other areas.[11,12] At the present time AI is good at solving single problems (narrow AI). However, artificial general intelligence, in which more complex problems are solved, is still a long way away. One issue with using this technology is automation bias. Doctors take advice from computers and fail to pay attention to potential errors due to an over-reliance on the technology.

So currently most AI systems are specific in their functions and directed toward accomplishing very specific tasks. However, researchers are directing efforts toward creating artificial general intelligence. To this end, individuals such as Ben Goertzel, PhD, are developing open-source AI code and an AI mind cloud that all robots can use. Thus, the robots can access their own individual memory systems but also the vastly larger one of the cloud. One robot can learn something and then transfer that knowledge to another robot. Many factors are contributing to an exponentially accelerating growth in robot/AI systems that affect all aspects of our culture including the delivery of health care. In addition to learning from one another through being linked into a type of hive mind through a cloud system, robots can train one another and can develop their own systems such as AlphaGo 2 (the successor to AlphaGo, which defeated the world's best player) did. AlphaGo was trained through copious quantities of data; AlphaGo 2 did not go through this process but instead became much more proficient through developing its own systems.

Computer engineers are also undergoing a phenomenal acceleration in learning through a global cross-pollination in ideas and technical know-how. Many AI algorithms are open source. In a joke familiar to Chinese scientists, when they are asked how far behind Silicon Valley the Chinese are, they say 16 hours, the time difference between China and California. There are many public forums where new papers are published such as www.ariv.org where the latest developments can be examined by anyone in the world. There are many global organizations that foster the exchange of ideas and technology such as the World Artificial Intelligence Organization, Global AI, Global Partnership on AI, AI Global, AI-Organization for Economic Cooperation and Development, Global AI Action Alliance of the World Economic Forum, and Artificial Intelligence in Society-European Commission.

Integrating AI and robotics with all the complexities of the health-care system represents quite a challenge. Nevertheless, this challenge is being addressed. The new systems will affect pharmacies in an out of the hospital, the delivery of medications, communications within a hospital, the robotic transport of laboratory materials, the nature of radiologic imaging and assessment, and even the provider-patient interaction. The following represents an example of the latter potential. Imagine a war veteran with posttraumatic stress disorder walking into an office in a mental health clinic. There is a large screen before him, which lights up, and on the screen is the picture of a woman dressed conservatively and professionally. She is smiling encouragingly and empathically. She is not any specific human being, but an AI construct designed to listen to your issues, to sympathize with them, and to offer insights and guidance. Such systems exist and are currently being refined to provide the psychological help and support for those who need it.

Another area of burgeoning promise is the field that crosses over between biological systems and electrical/mechanical/computer ones. In Sweden a new type of supercomputer is being developed at the University of Lund that combines components of muscle and more traditional electrical systems to develop a computer whose power could rival the potential of quantum computers. The muscle component used is the myofibril. This biological component is used to propel a nanobot down a logic system that results in analytic capabilities that are fast and vast in scope. Refer to the article "Parallel Computation With Molecular-Motor-Propelled Agents in Nanofabricated Networks," by Dan V. Nicolau Jr. from the University of California at Berkeley, California, and several of his colleagues.[13]

Tying into the area of robotics and AI, smart devices are upgrading the immediacy of early detection and intervention for health issues as well as creating a means for prediction of future health trends in any given individual. An example of such capabilities is the smart fabric of Nanowear, a company[14] founded by the father-son team of Vijay Varadan and Venk Varadan. Nanosensors are integrated into wearable fabrics, and these nanosensors can communicate wirelessly to a mobile telephone or laptop to convey real-time physiological information to a physician or nurse for monitoring, prevention, and early intervention in various disease processes such as heart or lung disease. The noninvasive sensors are augmented with AI technology to give the most precise and advanced recordings of physiological information within a fabric that is comfortable to wear. The technology is completely inapparent due to its small size.

AI can have numerous applications in health care and affect all specialties, but the top three broad categories are: (1) quality control, (2) customer care, and support (3) monitoring and diagnostics. In MIT Technology Review, A New Rx: AI for operations in health care by MIT Technology Review Insights.[15] July 15, 2020, the author states the top benefits for the use of AI include (other than the ones already mentioned): inventory management, personalization of products or services, cybersecurity, asset management, fraud detection, finance processes and analysis, and pricing.

Of course, the development of AI is not only dependent on the quality of algorithms designed for its software, but also dependent on the capability of the chips for expressing algorithms. To this end numerous companies are racing to create the optimal chips for such a purpose. Leaders in this field operate both in the United States and in China and range from the large well-known companies to the smaller boutique ones. Large and familiar Silicon Valley denizens such as Facebook, Intel, Qualcomm, Nvidia, Google, and Microsoft are pushing ahead alongside lesser-known start-ups. In China the Ministry of Science and Technology is incentivizing start-ups to compete in the AI chip market and the boutique companies include Horizon Robotics, Bitmain, and Cambricon Technologies. With large amounts of investment capital these companies can make competitive strides to fill this market. For example, Bitmain Technologies advertises "advanced tensor acceleration for deep learning, Bitmain's AI chips can be used for a wide range of applications such as facial recognition, automatic driving, smart cities, smart governance, smarter security, medical services."[16] Horizon Robotics has focused on AI chips for autonomous vehicles. Cambricon[17] advertises chips that combine with cloud systems for more effective and broad-based AI computing systems.

Some of the most fascinating questions that arise as humanity watches the growth of AI concern the possibility of machines developing self-awareness and the ability to think in a manner like humans. The Turing test arose many decades ago to assess machine intelligence in this fashion. While working at the University of Manchester in 1950, Alan Turing published "Computing Machinery and Intelligence,"[18] in which he initially proposed a test to determine if machines can think. In the test an interrogator must submit written questions and then receives responses from a human and a machine, and the interrogator must determine solely from the responses which response came from the machine and which came from the human. If the human interviewer determines that the response from the machine is from a human, then the machine has passed the threshold for entering the realm of human intelligence. The machine, however, must pass the test repeatedly. Turing, himself, bet that a machine would pass the test by the year 2000. The test has supporters and detractors but is frequently cited.

Have machines advanced sufficiently to fool a human observer with its responses? Look at following history of some famous examples.[19]

From 1964 to 1966 Joseph Weizenbaum (a computer scientist and MIT professor) created ELIZA, a natural language processing program, at the MIT Artificial Intelligence Laboratory. This program looked for keywords in typed comments and developed them into sentences. ELIZA used different scripts to process and provide responses. One of these was the DOCTOR script, which was patterned after Carl Rogers, a psychotherapist who often would simply parrot back what a patient had said to him. ELIZA in this context could fool some observers, one of whom was Weizenbaum's secretary.

In 1972, the chatbot PARRY emerged from the lab of the Stanford scientist Kenneth Colby, who described his creation as "Eliza with attitude." Colby designed his program so that it mimicked the behavior of a paranoid schizophrenic. Parry performed so well during the Turing test that two groups of psychiatrists mistook Parry's responses for those of patients 48% of the time.[20]

Eugene Goostman is a chatbox that presents itself as a 13-year-old boy from Odessa, Ukraine. His answers followed the pattern of a boy who did not speak English that well and whose thought patterns resembled those of a young boy. In 2014 Goostman managed to fool a panel of three judges 33% of the time into believing his cover story. In other words, the bot was able to make at least some claim to having passed the Turing test. Three programmers (two from Russia and one from Ukraine) developed Goostman in St. Petersburg in 2001.

In a rather stunning display of AI capabilities the Google Duplex voice AI first called a hairdresser in 2018 and then secured an appointment with that hairdresser without that individual ever recognizing that she was talking to a machine. Although this program performed well in this circumstance, it does not necessarily have the capability to perform well within some other, significantly different context.

For the future in health care, AI systems will need to be more flexible and adjust to context and will need to handle novel situations and adjust to novel input to function well in this environment. Currently systems are headed in that direction, and when those goals are achieved, robotic nurses and doctors will certainly make a more successful debut and be of a greater aid in the deliverance of health-care services.

Another area that has been initiated but has yet to achieve even a small part of its potential is the 3D printing of robots.[21] At this point many different types of 3D printed robots exist for a multitude of purposes. A lot of these have been and potentially could be adapted to different health-care environments such as in rehabilitation medicine.

Let us explore some categories of these robots and see what their current potentials are, and thus it will be an easy leap to understand the future directions of this type of technology. Many of these creations are open source. These types of robots include humanoid ones, robotic arms, zoomorphic robots, robotic hands (Fig. 12.1).[22] There are 3D printed arms that can themselves serve the functions of a 3D printer, which can print robotic arms and serve functions that other robotics arms can perform. Some of these creations have generic functions that one could see easily translating into a rehabilitation environment. To some extent these robots are customizable, and that flexibility allows the adjustment of the machines to address individual patient needs. Robotic arms could easily serve purposes in the area of assistive technology. The whole idea of comfort robots has achieved some level of acceptance, and the 3D printed robots offer possibilities here as well. An example of this type is ASPIR, an acronym which stands for Autonomous Support and Positive Inspiration Robot. The creation of John Choi, this device is around 30 pounds in weight and 4 feet tall with 22 motors. It is completely open source with an estimated build time of several months and a cost of around $2500. Jimmy the 21st Century Robot could serve the functions of emotional support and education. Applications to special needs children has been suggested. It is bipedal with a customizable shell over an endoskeleton and employs an Intel Edison chip. An open-source Linux C++ system drives the robot.

In a different tact, 3D robot makers have pursued a difficult but frequently approached goal of duplicating the abilities of the human hand. The Biomimetic Mechatronic Hand (Fig. 12.2) with

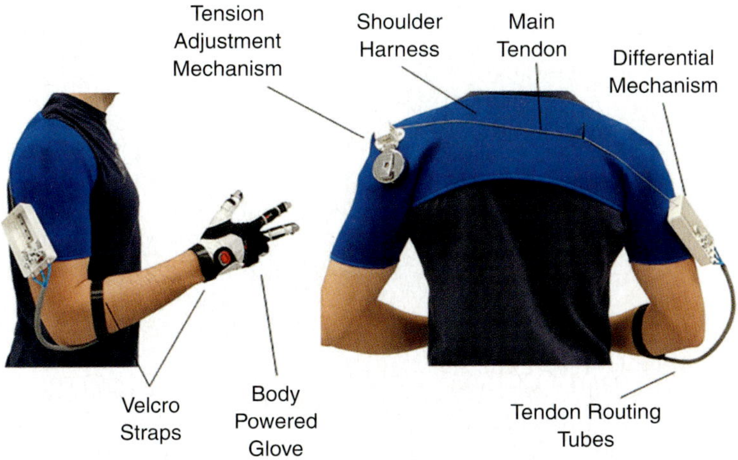

Fig. 12.1 3D printed soft robotic glove.[22] (OpenBionics by www.openbionics.org is licensed under a Creative Commons Attribution-ShareAlike 4.0 International License.)

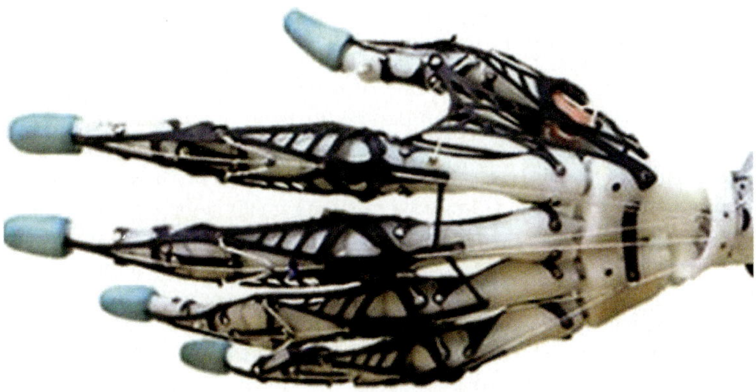

Fig. 12.2 Mechatronic hand. (From Ultra-high-performance robot hand that completely imitates the movements of human fingers, the world of the Ghost Inner shells reality. Gigazine.)

23 degrees of freedom has made great strides in this direction under the guidance of Will Cogley. There is also a robotic hand controlled by hand gestures created by Eben Kouao. The robotic arm that is controlled is 3D printed as well as the controller that fits over the hand of the human controlling the robotic arm. All of these are steps toward assistive technologies that can be assembled easily, locally, and inexpensively with the hopes of significantly enhancing the options of someone hindered by paralysis or some other disability to interact and manipulate the environment in a beneficial and reinforcing way.

At Stanford University Giada Gerboni[23–26] has pushed the vanguard in soft robotics in ways that will benefit and change many different specialties in medicine.[27] One of her primary and current areas of research concerns the use of ultrasound and soft robotics for needle guidance for procedures of various types. She is cultivating a robotic needle that allows for a single puncture for multiple tumor radio frequency ablation (RFA) ablations through a robotic needle that can be steered through a tight curvature. Soft robots create movement and action through a controlled

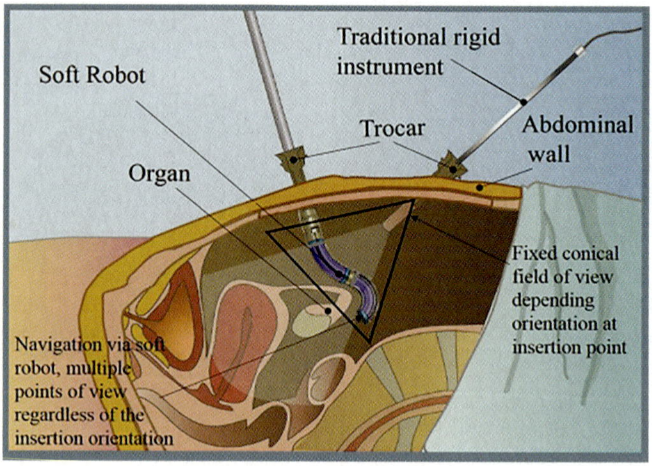

Fig. 12.3 Soft robotics from highly dexterous two-module soft robot for intraorgan navigation in minimally invasive surgery. (From Abidi H, Gerboni G, Brancadoro M, et al. *Int J Med Robot* 2018.[28])

series of deformations directed to a given goal. Combining this technology with thin, sometimes deformable needles under ultrasound guidance can allow safer and more effective procedures that can advance to a target without disturbing the tissues in the surrounding areas. These tools enhance accuracy and maneuverability. Minimally invasive surgery with soft robots (Fig. 12.3)[28] improves the dexterity of the surgeon and can decrease the chances of harm during the procedure. Soft robots allow surgery to progress toward a more minimally invasive model. Current systems with rigid or semirigid tools have difficulty maneuvering around organs in intraabdominal procedures or require multiple ports leaving multiple scars. The soft robot surgical devices have the potential for improving tissue compliance and thus increasing safety. One cadaver study involved the use of a two-module soft robot unit with flexible fluid actuators to access difficult to reach organs. The potential of reducing risk is evident. The EU funded the STIFF-FLOP manipulator, which is a soft robotic mechanism with a bendable tip about 14.7 mm in diameter, a bendable base, and a camera in the tip. The tip portion can elongate. It can be inserted through a standard 15-mm trocar port. The goal is ultimately to combine this with haptic technology in the future to allow surgeons to operate with a minimally invasive device that can negotiate around organs and yet still provide the advantages of an open technique. Further capabilities include the capacity to increase and decrease the stiffness of the device. Professor Kaspar Althoefer is project coordinator, and Helge Wurdemann is project manager in the London-based research.

After years of training and exposure to hundreds if not thousands of patients, physicians often base their diagnoses on correlations between clear-cut indicators of specific diseases and ignore data that appear irrelevant to the diagnosis of disease. AI on the other hand does not make any judgments on the relevance of data and can form associations and correlations between historical, examination, and laboratory findings that normally would not impress a clinician or be considered relevant. This capacity of AI can result in an earlier and potentially more precise diagnosis. There are many examples of this phenomenon. For example, a Stanford AI system was able to diagnose melanoma accurately 95% of the time compared with an accuracy rate of 87% for physicians. IBM's Watson can perform at a similar level of accuracy.

Currently deep learning systems have been primarily applied to image assessment in both radiology and dermatology. The AI systems can drill down to tiny differences in images to find correlations with disease and hence improve accuracy and reliability. Several studies have demonstrated this capability. Liu et al.[29] applied a deep learning (DL) system capable of distinguishing 26 common skin conditions and subsequently compared the accuracy of the machine to the assessments of panels of dermatologists, primary care physicians, and nurse practitioners. In all, 963 cases were assessed. The machine scored in a comparable fashion to the dermatologists and better than the primary care physicians and the nurse practitioners. The authors cite the importance of this development as enhancing the quality and timeliness of the diagnosis of skin conditions to improve outcomes in patient care. With around 1.9 billion people suffering from skin conditions, the number of dermatologists falls short and primary care physicians must then handle the overload. Thus, potentially the AI systems could favorably reduce the burden on dermatologists and primary care physicians for providing a high level of care to these individuals.

The capabilities of DL/AI in interpreting radiologic images have advanced so far that Geoffrey Hinton,[30] PhD, a well-known developer of such technology, made several years ago the now well-known quote, "We should stop training radiologists now. It's just completely obvious that within five years, deep learning is going to do better than radiologists." This situation has not occurred, and many researchers feel that it will never occur. Instead, the computer systems will enhance the activity of radiologists both in scope and quality of activity.

As mentioned, this system of DL occurs through the provision of thousands of examples and providing corrections when the AI system gets a wrong result. DL consists of layers of neural connections and the AI can improve these connection points in a way analogous to the human brain. It is a trial-and-error method that requires millions of trials. In this case 16,114 cases were used.

Even though a lot of DL diagnostic systems have focused on the fields of dermatology and radiology, such applications are also showing up in other fields as well in areas related to physiatry, rheumatology, and orthopedics,[31,32] DL systems are being developed to assess the probability of requiring a total knee replacement based on radiographs. In a retrospective study by Leung et al., a large group of patients who underwent total knee replacement for osteoarthritis were compared with a matched control population who did not. DL systems were developed to assess the radiographs of these two groups and to look for differences that could serve as predictors. The conclusion of the study was that the DL system provided a more accurate prediction of total knee replacement than standard predictive systems.

Countries across the globe have different levels of robotic development and penetration into the functioning of their culture and economy. Although China, the United States, and Japan are well known for their advances in this field, other countries also have advanced this technology quite extensively. So, what are the top 10 countries in this field?[33] The number one country for automation is South Korea followed by Japan, Germany, Sweden, Denmark, Hong Kong, Chinese Taipei, United States, Belgium, and Luxemburg. This ranking comes from statistics from the International Federation of Robotics. Another method of assessing a country's use of robotics comes through robot density (i.e., the number of robots per employees). In this category Singapore tops the list with a robot density of 918 robots per 10,000 employees in 2019. South Korea closely trails Singapore with 868 robots per 10,000 employees. Japan and Germany take the next spots. Japan is the foremost manufacturer of robots, and 47% of the world's robots come from Nippon. Robots are even used to manufacture robots.

Another Chinese company that is trying to reshape the way medicine is practiced is RXThinking. With a background in AI research and a work history in Silicon Valley, Kan Deng, PhD, founded the company and is its chief executive officer. The company has developed a medical management platform that can transform natural language unstructured records into structured records.[34] With the concentration of the most sophisticated medical care in urban centers, China has a need for extending the level of health care in the urban centers to the more rural ones to thus equalize medical care among its citizens. Through a diagnostic app the company intends on enhancing the capabilities of the more rural health-care practitioners through an AI system based on somewhere around 400 million medical records. The AI system can rapidly and thoroughly scan journals and other sources for medical care for the latest and best treatments. As information is fed into the app about a given patient, the app in turn asks for more information, more tests, and then ultimately provides recommendations for diagnosis and treatment. The latter are suggestions, and doctors always retain their autonomy and ability to override the app. The management of medical records systems allows the company to establish a large data base as support for the above purposes.

Ali Parsa is the founder and chief executive officer of Babylon Health. His aim was to build an AI that does a better diagnostic examination than human physicians. Babylon Health offers a service that could represent a growing future trend of health-care services. It attempts to address problems that resemble those RXThinking tries to address in China such as being able to access health care of high quality in situations or locations where the old model does not work as well. Its solutions are dependent on AI. Consequently, to create an AI system that works efficiently and accurately, immense amounts of data are fed into AI programs from sources such as deidentified medical records, laboratory tests, traditional medical reference sources, and so on. The function of the AI system is patterned after how a physician is trained to assess and analyze clinical situations. The options of the company offer an alternative to traditional face-to-face ones. One should not confuse these offerings with telemedicine per se as the technology has stepped further into the future than telemedicine, which itself has grown considerably and still to some extent could be considered a vanguard type of technology. At the time of this writing three products comprise their services to their customers: Babylon 360, see a healthcare provider 24-7, and digital health tools. These products are directed not just to solving a current health issue but also to maintaining health and preventing illness. Care can be accessed from a mobile device or laptop at any time. The services provide a timely care interaction as well as cost savings.[35]

With a growing population of citizens aged 65 and older, South Korea struggles to meet the needs of these individuals.[36] The South Korean president implemented funds for robotics research and development in 2020 that included 250 million for service-oriented robotics in health care, rehabilitation, and disaster relief. There are hopes of establishing a $13 billion robotic industry.

South Korea is taking a lead in the cultivation of robots for the delivery of health care. The president of this country has devoted funds to promote this area in the hopes of getting a $13 billion industry. Part of the impetus in this direction came from the needs of citizens over 65 years of age and the shortfall of human resources to meet those needs. Yonsei University Medical Center opened a robotic surgical training center. CUVIS-spine from CUREXO, a company in Seoul, Korea, is one the robotic surgical devices that will be used for training as well as Revo-i from the Korean Meerecompany.[37]

So how else is South Korea paving the way for a future in robotics? The government intends for the country to become the fourth largest center for robotics in the world by the year 2023 and the country's president plans to foster the top 20 robotics companies.[38] The road to such an achievement will be built through the infusion of funds and a game plan that includes the infusion of funds and less dependence on the United States and Japan for parts and software. These plans do not just target industry and manufacturing but also the service sector as well. Some consider South Korea the most robot-friendly country in the world with a higher robot density than Japan.

To assess the global drive toward the use of robotics and AI[39] across the full spectrum of cultural, business, and health-care activities, the results of the AI readiness Index[40] conducted by Oxford and the International Development Research Centre in 2019 provide some interesting perspectives. Topping the list, Singapore comes in with a score of 0.9186 and is followed by the United Kingdom, Germany, the United States, Finland, Sweden, Canada, France, Denmark, and Japan. China was 21st in these rankings. India held third place in the Asia Pacific region after Singapore and Hong Kong. Lack of creativity, innovation, and technicians with strong AI skills hinder to some extent the country's advancement. On the other hand, countries leading the field of AI research include, China, the United States, Japan, the United Kingdom, and Germany. The United States heads this list but unless certain systemic issues are corrected China stands to overtake the United States for multiple reasons. Contributing factors toward China's race to the top include having the latest electronics such a smartphones, computers, and other electronic devices as well as having a systemwide approach with autonomous cars, robotics, and advanced medical equipment. Data-driven science that fuels AI also is accelerating their push forward and companies like UBTECH Robotics (humanoid robots) and SenseTime (facial recognition) represent some of these efforts. UBTECH promotes its ADIBOT for its potential contributions to the control of the COVID-19 pandemic through the machine's ability to disinfect rooms and locations with its ultraviolet-C light and its ability to navigate multiple floor plans. With the growth in these areas, skill sets that will take priority include those for AI, ML, and data science.

The future of robotics in health care would not be complete without a discussion on the opportunities that nanotechnology offers. Nanotech and nanobots excite the imagination with their immense potential for influencing our health for the better. Here are some of the ways this technology can benefit the delivery of health care both to cure individuals of various diseases but also in the areas of prevention. Nanotechnology has an important role in the areas of diagnostics, treatment, and monitoring, and these areas will be explored.

So just how big or how small is nanotech? One nanometer is one-billionth of a meter and health-care devices range from 1 to 100 nm. The small size puts them on the same scale as molecules and atoms. The field of nanotechnology has affected nearly all if not all areas of science and technology, and the medical world also has begun to feel the profound repercussions of this kind of tech. At this point, however, the types of opportunities it provides is only beginning to appear and the future looms with exciting new possibilities.

Let's take an easy example. Suppose you love salting your food and have high blood pressure and thus have been told to restrict your salt intake. The salt particles can be fractured into nanograins and that process greatly increases the surface area of the salt particles. With far less salt the perception of saltiness is increased. Reduction of salt intake can occur without a reduction in salt flavoring. Nanotechnology can also increase the absorption of nutrition. With its antibacterial properties, nanosilver has been incorporated into food cutting boards but also has been applied to medical bandages and dressings for the clear-cut advantages there.

One of the most frequently cited areas for the application of nanotechnology is in the treatment of cancer. Quantum dots are being deployed to precisely localize tumor cells through the incorporation of inorganic fluorophores. The characteristics that make them useful are a broad spectrum of excitation, brighter imaging signals, the ability to operate without lasers, and stable fluorescence with simple excitation. Quantum dots can be used in cancer diagnosis and in multiplexed diagnostics and in therapeutics (Fig. 12.4).[41] Molecular diagnosis and genotyping are other applications. Nanoparticles may allow the destruction of cancer cells with complete specificity and thus not interfere with other cells and tissues.

Currently nanotech is being used in vaccine development to make vaccines more effective and efficient. China, the United States, Russia, India, and Brazil have taken a lead in this direction. In a similar vein these particles can help in the optimal delivery of drugs and medications. Nanotech can be attached to drugs or liposomes to confer various advantages. These formulations offer a host of refinements in the treatment of patients through the enhancement of the transport of medications across endothelial layers, specific targeting of pathology and avoidance of healthy tissue, retention of the medication at the target site for more prolonged benefit, bypassing the issue of poor water solubility of some medications and providing the ability to provide therapeutics and diagnostics in one system. The nanoparticles cluster in the tumor selectively due to the rapid growth of blood vessels with pores the nanoparticles can slip through. Additionally, since the tumor generally lacks a lymphatic system, the nanoparticle is not washed away but retained for longer periods.[42] A similar mechanism can enhance the effect of antibiotics on infections.

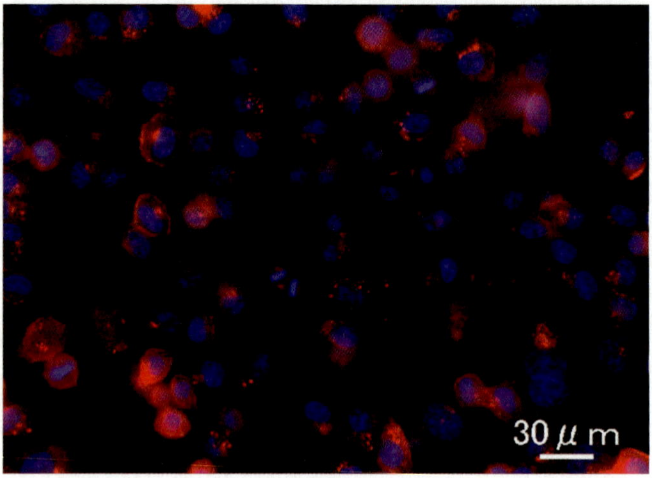

Fig. 12.4 Quantum dots lighting up breast tumor cells.[41]

In the case of coronary heart disease, nanotechnology delivery systems could target the effects of statins to the cellular level and potentially avoid some of the side effects of this type of medication when it is distributed in a more systemic fashion. Controlled release of the medication represents another opportunity for this area and either internal or external mechanisms can trigger the release of the medications. Potential internal triggers might include changes in the environment of the tumor compared with normal tissue. External triggers might involve temperature changes, light, or ultrasound as stimuli.[43]

Technological advances have greatly increased the reach and sophistication of health monitoring, and nanotech has shown promise in this area as well using graphene wearables that transmit basic information such as heart rate. These graphene wearables can consist of radio frequency identification (RFID) tags that have already been deployed in some health systems for inpatients.

In the preceding paragraphs, AI and nanotech have been discussed separately as two technologies that exist independently. But can they be combined for novel technological developments that can provide unique advantages in health care or related disciplines? The answer of course is yes, and this fusion of two technologies is a nascent but growing area. One obvious area is the combination of nanotech and AI computational capacities, and this area has already been discussed before. Researchers at the University of Texas Rio Grande have utilized microchannels, surfaces with nanotech that bind breast cancer cells, and AI to categorize such cells using data banks of information on these cells. Cells are extracted, imaged, and categorized.[44]

Not all developments in robotics have to do with technological advances. Sociological advances also hold great promise as well. Michelle Johnson, PhD, at the GRASP Laboratory in the University of Pennsylvania pioneers advancements in rehabilitation robots but also has initiated programs to serve third-world countries and populations where resources and trained personnel are scare.[45,46] Her efforts are contained within the Rehabilitation Robotics Lab and coordinated with the Department of Physical Medicine and Rehabilitation at this university. Her laboratory has a partnership with a university in Latin America and is reaching out to African countries as well. Her area of interest and expertise concerns neurorehabilitation robots, particularly for stroke patients undergoing rehabilitation. Dr. Johnson continues to explore the use of her rehabilitation robots to serve stroke patients in countries such as Mexico to improve and extend the rehabilitation services that are available. Using such robots, she has helped to upgrade the availability of rehabilitation for underserved areas across the world. This application is perhaps a less obvious but nonetheless extraordinary application with immense future potentials.[47]

In the deep of night an elderly man is sleeping when abruptly a device lights up on his night table. Almost immediately a robot attendant enters the room. The robot has already analyzed innumerable data points from the nanosensors in the man's pajamas that have alerted the robot to a rapid and irregular pulse and a large clot that had has formed in the man's middle cerebral artery. Without pausing, the robot signals a hospital ambulance, starts an intravenous line, loads the man onto a stretcher and lift, covers him with blankets, and wheels him to the side door and from there to the driveway. His brain is rapidly swelling, and the man has remained unconscious. At the hospital, the robotic drone ambulance, after collecting the data from a cloud system from the attendant, has loaded up appropriate supplies and medicine and then has started the flight to the man's house. There it lands in the driveway where the attendant robot quickly loads the man into the ambulance, which promptly takes off for the return trip to the hospital. During the flight oxygen is delivered, physiological signs continue to be measured, and the initial round of medications are slipped into the intravenous line. Upon arrival to the hospital the man is rushed to the magnetic resonance imaging machine and then to the intensive care unit. The magnetic resonance imaging scan shows that the clot has already started to dissolve, allowing blood flow into the ischemic brain tissue. Monitors show that the heart rate has come down. Ultimately the man recovers with minimal sequela from the stroke and can return to his home where his robotic attendant will continue to keep a watchful eye on him. Before he leaves the hospital, a rehabilitation program tailored to the man's physical deficits is downloaded into his home robot so that the program for upper-extremity restoration, self-care skills, and gait can start immediately. The robot automatically registers the patient's progress and performance and relays that information to a central computer where the information can be reviewed. If necessary, from that central source the rehabilitation program can be adjusted or ended as necessary. In the central computer, data are accumulated from robots across the country performing similar tasks and eventually analyzed by an AI program that looks for opportunities to improve the entire process.

References

1. Pentagon Seeks Robo-EMS to Rescue Wounded Warriors. Wired.
2. Khan J. Money is pouring in to A.I.-assisted drug discovery, while fewer A.I. startups are getting VC backing. Fortune. March 3, 2019. https://fortune.com/2021/03/03/artificial-intelligence-ai-index-venture-capital-startup-funding/
3. Heinonen H. Artificial Intelligence AI-Over 100 Billion in Revenues By 2025. Towards Data Science, December 2, 2019. https://towardsdatascience.com/artificial-intelligence-ai-over-100-billion-in-revenues-by-2025-e737459a345e
4. Harper J Federal AI. Spending To Top $6 Billion. National Defense/ February 10, 2021. https://www.nationaldefensemagazine.org/articles/2021/2/10/federal-ai-spending-to-top-$6-billion
5. Lee K-F. AI Superpowers: China, Silicon Valley, and the new world order. Mariner Books. 2018
6. Allison G, Schmidt E. Is China Beating the US to AI Supremacy? Harvard aKennedySchool. Belfer Center for Science and International Affairs. August 2020. https://www.belfercenter.org/publication/china-beating-us-ai-supremacy#:~:text=The%20%E2%80%9CSeven%20Giants%20of%20the,either%20side%20of%20the%20Pacific
7. Association for the Advancement of Artificial Intelligence. https://www.aaai.org/
8. Panesar S, Cagle Y, Chander D, Morey J, Fernandez-Miranda J, Kliot M. Artificial intelligence and the future of surgical robotics. *Ann Surg*. 2019;270(2):223–226.
9. Shademan A, Decker RS, Opfermann JD, Leonard S, Krieger A, Kim PC. Supervised autonomous robotic soft tissue surgery. Sci Transl Med. 2016;8(337):337ra64. https://doi.org/10.1126/scitranslmed.aad9398.
10. Lehman C. AI and the future of breast cancer detection and risk prediction. Executive Education at HMS. https://executiveeducation.hms.harvard.edu/thought-leadership/webinar-series/recorded-presentations/ai-future-breast-cancer-detection-risk-prediction

11. Jackie Snow, AI is continuing its assault on radiologists. *MIT Technology Review*. January 18, 2018. https://www.technologyreview.com/2018/01/18/146133/ai-is-continuing-its-assault-on-radiologists/
12. Rajpurkar P, Irvin J, Bagul A, et al. Large dataset for abnormality detection in musculoskeletal radiographs. Arxiv.org. https://arxiv.org/pdf/1712.06957.pdf
13. Nicolau DV Jr, Lard M, Korten T, et al. Parallel computation with molecular-motor-propelled agents in nanofabricated networks. Proc Natl Acad Sci USA. 2016;113(10):2591–2596. https://doi.org/10.1073/pnas.1510825113.
14. Nanowear. Smarter care. Anywhere. https://www.nanowearinc.com/
15. MIT Technology. Review Insigths A New Rx: AI for operations in health care. MIT Technology Review. July;15:2020. https://www.technologyreview.com/2020/07/15/1004743/a-new-rx-ai-for-operations-in-health-care/.
16. About us. Bitmain. https://www.bitmain.com/about
17. About us. Cambricon. https://www.cambricon.com/index.php?m=content&c=index&a=lists&catid=7
18. Turing AM I.—COMPUTING MACHINERY AND INTELLIGENCE, Mind. 1950;LIX(236):433–460. https://doi.org/10.1093/mind/LIX.236.433
19. Panova E. Which AI has come closest to passing the Turing test. Dataconomy. Published March 9, 2021. https://dataconomy.com/2021/03/which-ai-closest-passing-turing-test/
20. Garber M. When PARRY Met ELIZA: a ridiculous chatbot conversation from 1972. The Atlantic. Published June 9, 2014. https://www.theatlantic.com/technology/archive/2014/06/when-parry-met-eliza-a-ridiculous-chatbot-conversation-from-1972/372428/
21. 3D printed robot: most advanced projects in 2021 | All3DP 3D Printed Robot: Most Advanced Projects in 2021 | All3DP. https://all3dp.com/2/3d-printed-robot-print-robots/
22. Defusco E. Researchers Studying Wearable Technology for Stroke Patients. Katz School of Science and Health. Yeshiva University. September 8, 2022. https://blogs.yu.edu/katz-school/2022/09/08/researchers-study-wearable-technology-for-stroke-patients/
23. Gerboni G, Greer JD, Laeseke PF, Hwang GL, Okamura AM. Highly articulated robotic needle achieves distributed ablation of liver tissue. *IEEE Robot Autom Lett*. 2017;2(3):1367–1374. https://doi.org/10.1109/LRA.2017.2668467
24. Abidi H, Gerboni G, Brancadoro M, et al. Highly dexterous 2-module soft robot for intra-organ navigation in minimally invasive surgery. *Int J Med Robot*. 2018;14(1):10.1002/rcs.1875. https://doi.org/10.1002/rcs.1875
25. De Falco I, Gerboni G, Cianchetti M, Menciassi A. Design and fabrication of an elastomeric unit for soft modular robots in minimally invasive surgery. *J Vis Exp*. 2015;105:53118. https://doi.org/10.3791/53118
26. Ranzani T, Gerboni G, Cianchetti M, Menciassi A. A bioinspired soft manipulator for minimally invasive surgery. *Bioinspir Biomim*. 2015;10(3):035008. https://doi.org/10.1088/1748-3190/10/3/035008
27. Gundersen OE Standing on the feet of giants — reproducibility in AI. AI Magazine. 2019;40(4):9–23. https://doi.org/10.1609/aimag.v40i4.5185.
28. 111040892.pdf. core.ac.uk
29. Liu Y, Jain A, Eng C, et al. A deep learning system for differential diagnosis of skin diseases. *Nat Med*. 2020;26(6):900–908. https://doi.org/10.1038/s41591-020-0842-3
30. Harvard Business. AI will change radiology—NOT replace radiologists. https://human-centered.ai/2018/04/18/ai-will-change-radiology-not-replace-radiologists/
31. Leung K, Zhang B, Tan J, et al. Prediction of total knee replacement and diagnosis of osteoarthritis by using deep learning on knee radiographs: data from the osteoarthritis initiative. *Radiology*. 2020;296(3):584–593. https://doi.org/10.1148/radiol.2020192091
32. Sharifi Renani M, Myers CA, Zandie R, Mahoor MH, Davidson BS, Clary CW. Deep learning in gait parameter prediction for OA and TKA patients wearing IMU sensors. *Sensors (Basel)*. 2020;20(19):5553. https://doi.org/10.3390/s20195553
33. Robot race. the world's top 10 automated countries. International Federation of Robotics. https://ifr.org/ifr-press-releases/news/robot-race-the-worlds-top-10-automated-countries.
34. Pitchbook. https://pitchbook.com/profiles/company/437580-73#overview.
35. Our services. Babylon Health. https://www.babylonhealth.com/en-us/services
36. A boom of healthcare robotics in South Korea. Hospital Insights Asia. Published March 2, 2020. Hospital Management Asia. https://hospitalmanagementasia.com/tech-innovation/healthcare-robotics-in-south-korea-sun-medical-center-ceo-dr-sun-seung-hoon/

37. Behn C. South Korean health system opens surgical robot training center. Becker's Spinereview. Accessed December 22, 2020. https://www.beckersspine.com/robotics/50754-south-korean-health-system-opens-surgical-robot-training-center.html
38. Shin Ji-hye. S. Korea aims to become No. 4 robotics player by 2023. The Korea Herald. Accessed March 22, 2019. http://www.koreaherald.com/view.php?ud=20190322000576
39. Countries leading the way in AI. Xaltius. https://xaltius.tech/countries-leading-the-way-in-ai/
40. https://www.idrc.ca/en/news/2020-government-ai-readiness-index-governments-must-prioritise-responsible-ai-use
41. Riken Research Highlights. Quantum dots light up cancer with a little help. It ain't magic. Published November 27, 2017. https://itaintmagic.riken.jp/research-highlight/quantum-dot/
42. Nanotechnology for drug delivery applications. AZO Nano. Published November 1, 2017. https://www.azonano.com/article.aspx?ArticleID=4668#:~:text=The%20application%20of%20nanotechnology%20for%20drug%20delivery%20provides,delivery%20systems%20from%20nanoscale%20molecules%20such%20as%20liposomes
43. *Nanotechnology in medicine—thematic research*. Report produced by GlobalData Thematic Research. https://www.globaldata.com/store/report/nanotechnology-in-medicine-theme-analysis/.
44. https://www.azonano.com/article.aspx?ArticleID=5116
45. Mohan M, Mendonca R, Johnson M Towards quantifying dynamic human-human physical interactions for robot assisted stroke therapy. International Conference Rehabilitation Robotics (ICORR). 2017;913–918.
46. Johnson M, Mendonca R, Venditti N, Jordan A, Barathi S. Do therapists use object affordances to develop functional activities for task-oriented therapy: Implications for robot-assisted task-oriented therapy. Arch Phys Med Rehabil. 2016;97(10):e59.
47. Deng Y, Zhang X, Shen H, et al. Application of the nano-drug delivery system in treatment of cardiovascular diseases. Front Bioeng Biotechnol. 2020;7:489. Published January 31, 2020. https://doi.org/10.3389/fbioe.2019.00489.

INDEX

Page numbers followed by "*f*" indicate figures and "*t*" indicate tables